...e Book for 2007

The Johns Hopkins University Press gratefully acknowledges members of the 2007 Director's Circle for supporting the publication of works such as *Public Health and Human Rights: Evidence-Based Approaches.*

Anonymous
Alfred & Muriel Berkeley
John & Bonnie Boland
Darlene Bookoff
Sylvia Bookoff
William & Charlotte Cronin
Jack Goellner & Barbara Lamb
Willard Hackerman
Charles & Elizabeth Hughes
James D. Jordan & Angela von der Lippe
John & Kathleen Keane
Ralph S. O'Connor
Peter Onuf
Eric R. Papenfuse & Catherine A. Lawrence
Douglas R. Price
Anders Richter
David Ryer
Dorothy McIlvain Scott
R. Champlin & Debbie Sheridan
Winston & Marilyn Tabb
Daun & Patricia Van Ee
Robert L. Warren & Family

Public Health & Human Rights

Evidence-Based Approaches

Edited by

Chris Beyrer, M.D., M.P.H.

and H. F. Pizer

THE JOHNS HOPKINS UNIVERSITY PRESS

Baltimore

The Johns Hopkins University Press
2715 North Charles Street
Baltimore, Maryland 21218-4363
www.press.jhu.edu

Library of Congress Cataloging-in-Publication Data

Public health and human rights : evidence-based approaches / edited by Chris Beyrer
and H. F. Pizer.
p. ; cm.
Includes bibliographical references and index.
ISBN 13: 978-0-8018-8646-1 (hardcover : alk. paper)
ISBN 10: 0-8018-8646-5 (hardcover : alk. paper)
ISBN 13: 978-0-8018-8647-8 (pbk. : alk. paper)
ISBN 10: 0-8018-8647-3 (pbk. : alk. paper)
1. Social medicine—Cross-cultural studies. 2. Human rights—Health aspects—
Cross-cultural studies. 3. Public health—Cross-cultural studies. 4. Health—Cross-
cultural studies. I. Beyrer, Chris. II. Pizer, Hank. [DNLM: 1. Health Policy. 2. Health Care
Reform. 3. Human Rights. 4. Public Health.   WA 525 P9747 2007]
RA418.P8343 2007
362.1—dc22   2006039837

A catalog record for this book is available from the British Library.

*This book is offered with deep thanks to my parents,
Dr. Charles R. Beyrer and Nancy Beyrer,
and to my partner, Michael Smit.*
C.B.

For Chris, Katie, and Bruce.
H.F.P.

Contents

III. Policy

Foreword

Just over a decade ago, Jonathan Mann opened his new journal, *Health and Human Rights*, with the sentence "Health and human rights have rarely been linked in an explicit manner" (1994, p. 1). To the extent that public health policies had a relationship to human rights, moreover, Mann and his colleagues saw it as so problematic that they declared, "For the present, it may be useful to adopt the maxim that health policies and programs should be considered discriminatory and burdensome on human rights until proved otherwise" (p. 16). So he proposed means by which health policies such as mandatory testing and quarantine could be subjected to special human rights scrutiny.

How far have we come? Thanks to the thinking, insights, and analysis of many who have built on the foundation laid by Mann, the human rights lens—and the idea of human dignity at its center—has become essential to understanding major public health challenges. No serious discussion of the transmission of HIV can take place without examining the human rights violations that fuel it: the discrimination and lack of economic and social power among women in Africa that result in their accounting for two-thirds of new infections; the moral stigma attaching to intravenous drug users and sex workers that limits harm-reduction programs in Asia and the former Soviet Union; and patterns of poverty, marginalization, and discrimination that have led HIV/AIDS in the United States to be a predominantly African American disease. Even responses to public health problems with less ideological freight than HIV/AIDS, such as severe acute respiratory syndrome (SARS), cannot be fully understood without taking into account the lack of freedom of expression in China.

Human rights has also proven to be a powerful tool for broadening and deepening the assessment of the effectiveness and legitimacy of policies and programs designed to advance public health. For example, the field of public health often focuses on the most effective use of available but often scarce resources in effective ways to promote population health; a human rights analysis, which includes the right to the highest attainable standard of health, goes further, demanding not only that current resources be well deployed but also that investments be increased if needed to fulfill rights. Public health policies often focus on the health of the population as a whole, an approach acceptable from a human rights viewpoint only if it also zeroes in on those who are so often left out: the vulnerable, the poor, the marginalized. Public health pays close attention to health infrastructure such as clean water, sanitation, and primary health care; human rights, too, pays heed to these, but also to social policy on access to education, protection of civil rights, rights of political participation, and availability of economic opportunities, all of which affect the access to that infrastructure.

At the same time, public health methodologies have had a profound influence on human rights documentation and analysis. In the past, the central means of human rights fact-finding was taking testimony of victims and witnesses and placing the evidence in a framework of human rights law. Public health provides a new set of methodologies for documenting human rights and can shed light on the scope and extent of human rights violations within a population, assess the strength of factors that may contribute to them, and point to policy solutions. These methods have been employed, for example, in epidemiological and other population-based studies on rape during conflicts, the extent of war crimes committed, the extent of and mechanisms of discrimination against marginalized groups, and in many other circumstances of severe and widespread violations of human rights.

That is why this volume is so important and timely. However strong the connections between public health and human rights, understanding them in their full complexity is enormously challenging. It takes rigor, sophisticated research design, grounding in human rights law, and understanding of the dynamics of policy. This volume is a pioneering effort at showing where we are in meeting those challenges, and it is full of ideas, insights, and learning. It deepens our understanding of the "doing" of public health and human rights and demonstrates in concrete ways how that work can help us move toward a more just world.

Leonard S. Rubenstein, J.D.
Executive Director, Physicians for Human Rights

Preface

How do human rights violations affect the health of populations? How can such complex interactions best be studied, analyzed, and remedied? How can the efforts of human rights advocates further affect health outcomes? And, finally, can the tools of modern public health better assist in documenting, understanding, and preventing human rights violations? These are the linked and difficult questions that the authors you are about to read have asked of themselves and their disciplines.

The good news is that there do appear to be powerful synergies between human rights work and public health practice. It helps to understand health outcomes in eastern Burma if we first assess the effect of human rights violations perpetrated by the Burmese junta against ethnic minority families and communities. And we cannot understand the enormous iatrogenic (human-made) epidemic of HIV among rural blood donors in China without examining the role of state suppression of medical inquiry in this human tragedy. The first section of this book, Case Studies, explores these realities in Thailand, Burma, China, and Russia and in U.S. prisons, to help elucidate the many interactions of public health and human rights.

We begin with a case study from Thailand and, most appropriately, with the extraordinary work done by the Thai Drug Users' Network, TDN, a grass-roots organization formed by a group of Thai drug users facing the harsh "War on Drugs" policy of the Thai government. What makes TDN so important for this emerging field, and the chapter they've written with Canadian colleagues so important for this book, is that they show us that defending the human rights of marginalized communities can be done effectively when those affected by rights violations partner with public health. TDN shows us the power of people facing rights violations and health threats to organize, work for their rights, and protect themselves and their communities. That they are now a grantee of the Global Fund to Fight AIDS, Tuberculosis, and Malaria, to provide HIV/AIDS services to Thai drug users demonstrates that rights-based approaches to funding decisions are critical too.

Doing health work in conflict settings is always challenging. The long-standing Burmese civil conflict is no exception. In their case study, Thomas Lee and colleagues describe the work of the Backpack Health Workers Program in providing health care and measuring vital statistics for the large population of internally displaced Karen, Karenni, Mon, and Shan ethnic minority families in eastern Burma's civil conflict zones. The Backpack Program, like TDN's, is particularly relevant here because it was built by the ethnic groups themselves and is one of a handful of examples of refugees crossing back into their homeland (at great personal risk) to provide services for internally displaced communities.

The China case study raises some fundamental issues for those concerned about public health and rights. In this case, provincial government involvement in unsafe (but profitable) blood-collection schemes generated what may be the most severe iatrogenic epidemic of HIV/AIDS yet recorded. The suppression of scientific information around this disaster, including the jailing of the lead author of this chapter, Wan Yanhai, for posting HIV information on a website, reminds us that scientific freedom is fundamental to the public's right to know. And as SARS would later demonstrate, limitations on this freedom in one state can quickly become a health threat to others, and violations of political rights can make epidemics harder to control.

Julie Stachowiak and Alena Peryshkina show us in clear terms how the rights of women are human rights and how damaging to health their abrogation can be. They share with us the special threats to health faced by women in Russia's burgeoning sex industry, and the critical role these women play at the center of this rights and health nexus.

That human rights violations and their health effects might apply to conflict settings or repressive states is much less controversial than asserting that these same complex synergies might be relevant in the wealthy democracies of the First World. Julie Samia Mair, a lawyer and public health researcher, takes us for the last case study into men's prisons in the United States, where rape is an ever-present threat to dignity and health. She demonstrates that prison rape is all too often tolerated by prison authorities and that the protection provided by condoms from at least some harms is routinely denied those subject to this brutality.

From case studies we move to Part II, Methods and Approaches, where we explore new tools and new uses of existing tools for rights-based public health research. This section may be of most interest to students and practitioners of public health for doing work in difficult security and political contexts. We have struggled to keep the scientific language as nontechnical as possible, such that those with human rights or civil society backgrounds will also find this section useful in their work. My own work in using the molecular epidemiology of HIV as an investigative tool provides the first methods chapter. This is not the place to learn how to do molecular analyses, but it may help those seeking to understand how a genetic analysis might greatly add to a human rights investigation. We need only think of the way DNA testing has transformed criminal law to grasp how this powerful tool might be used in a variety of health and rights settings. These methods confirmed, for example, that the epidemic of HIV among ethnic minorities in southwest China was directly linked to the heroin export routes out of Burma. Whatever denials either state wished to put forward regarding this reality, the double helix does not lie—and it made a convincing case in documenting this cross-border outbreak.

Investigating human trafficking is one of the toughest tasks in this field. Cathy Zimmerman and Charlotte Watts lay out the challenges for us and provide enormously helpful guidance for research and programmatic work in this arena. They share experience on interviewing victims of trafficking, security concerns for both participants and staff members, and approaches to the provision of services and meeting the needs of trafficked women at each stage in the life-threatening trafficking continuum.

Physicians for Human Rights (PHR) has done groundbreaking work in the development and refinement of tools to measure the health effects of rights violations. Chen Reis describes the methods PHR developed and used to investigate the prevalence and incidence of rape and sexual violence in the civil conflict in Sierra Leone. Rape in this context had been used as a tool of war against civilian populations, and it required population-based methods to document it.

Genocide is the most extreme threat to the life of communities and peoples. That it is a mortality and morbidity problem as much as a legal one is starkly evident, yet genocide has been little investigated using the population tools of health research. Jennifer Leaning, whose work is an exception to this omission, uses the unfolding tragedy of the Darfur region of the Sudan to explore a medical approach to the diagnosis of genocide. This critical work could lead to a preventive approach rather than a prosecutorial one, move the global effort toward identifying the early warning signs of this "problem from hell," and prevent its recurrence.

Human rights contexts are not static and can change abruptly. In a methods chapter linked to the Thai case study, the research group led by David Celentano describes their responses to the dramatic change in rights status brought about by Thai crackdown on drug use. They demonstrate how researchers can adapt their efforts to work in deteriorating rights contexts, maintain crucial channels to their study participants, and document the health effects of rights violations.

Skillful adaptation of field methods is called for in rights-challenged environments. This theme runs throughout the book but is made explicit in Lynn Lawry's chapter. She uses vivid examples from her work on women's access to health care under the Taliban regime in Afghanistan, from work in Iraq, and in Sudan, to demonstrate practical methods and approaches to collecting good-quality data in some of the most challenging settings there are.

There is considerable debate in public health circles about the impact of conflict on the spread of disease. Some have argued that wars can limit the spread of disease by restricting population movement and mixing. Whatever the case in any given conflict, it is true that much more is known about the health status of populations living in stability and peace than about those in conflict. In the last methods section here, we describe a novel approach to measuring not the impact of conflict on public health, but the impact of conflict on *health research,* and do so using a 25-year review of research efforts from the Democratic Republic of Congo. This work demonstrates that the vigorous malaria and AIDS research efforts in the Democratic Republic of Congo were destroyed by the late years of the Mobutu regime and had almost entirely ceased several years before the 1998–2002 war in the Congo, the bloodiest since World War II.

Finally, we have to ask, if human rights and public health do have many profound connections, how can they be used to improve human lives? Part III, Putting Policy into Practice, attempts to do just this. Here we confront a range of current policy approaches, from Brazil's integration of rights into HIV/AIDS programming to the contradictory and confounding global policies on illicit drugs, and look to future directions with programmatic recommendations and strategies. The health challenges outlined here are devilishly difficult. Those who advocate for human rights know all too well that these are battles for which new fronts open with terrible regularity. Nevertheless, our objective here is to explore the ways in which successful campaigns and programs have been built which have improved health and rights for people facing threats to both.

Brazil provides a clear case of the benefits for individuals and society of building human rights considerations into HIV prevention and care programs. As Varun Gauri, Denise Vaillancourt, and I argue, Brazil is particularly heartening because the demand for rights in the context of HIV/AIDS led to a wider demand for universal access to health care for all Brazilian citizens, arguably the most equitable way to ensure access to HIV care.

It is hard to find a more contentious policy arena than the swirl of conflict surrounding the use of illicit drugs. Whereas narcotics policies have been influenced less by health concerns than by political, criminal, and security ones, these policies have profound and far-reaching public health effects. As Daniel Wolfe and Kasia Malinowska-Sempruch demonstrate, conflicting drug policies have had as wide a range of human rights implications as they have effects on disease. Skillfully unpacking the policy conundrums around this issue, they make a compelling case that rights-based policies in this arena are essential to disease control from Eastern Europe to Southeast Asia.

Modern medical ethics and the human rights movement share a common origin: both developed in response to the Nazi atrocities of World War II, and both fields continue to be driven by shared ideals of justice, fairness, and beneficence. Yet the fields do differ, and their professional practice regarding public health can differ widely. In "Responding to the Global HIV/AIDS Pandemic: Perspectives from Human Rights and Public Health Ethics," a human rights lawyer and investigator (Jonathan Cohen), a public health ethicist (Nancy Kass), and an epidemiologist (your coeditor) discuss how human rights and ethics frameworks do and do not overlap and where the synergies might lie for further cross-fertilization of these disciplines.

We know that women often bear disproportionate burdens when either rights or public health are threatened. In a policy piece linked to the Burma case study, a Thai, Burmese, and U.S. group discuss the gender and sexual and reproductive health rights of women and girls and describe how building gender rights into programs might help mitigate these synergistic threats. It is only fitting that the senior author here, Cynthia Maung, a refugee herself, should also have been the recipient of the first Jonathan Mann Prize for Health and Human Rights.

Finally, while the public health efforts described here may be well done, the science valid, and the rights concerns well documented, it takes advocacy to change policy and to begin to have "real world" impacts. Few advocates have more experience, and have had more success, in this arena than Holly Burkhalter. She tells here about how moving policy forward gets done, the uses of different kinds of health data to affect decision makers, and how best to advocate for needed change.

THIS BOOK BEGAN IN DISCUSSIONS WITH THE PARTICIPANTS in an international seminar held at Johns Hopkins University in 2004 entitled "Public Health and Human Rights in the Era of AIDS." It was jointly sponsored by the Johns Hopkins Fogarty AIDS International Training and Research Program (Grant 2D43 TW000010-18-AITRP), the Open Society Institute, and the Institute for Asian Democracy. The editors would like to thank all three organizations for their support and encouragement of this work.

A portion of the proceeds of this book, should there be any, will be donated to the Institute for Asian Democracy for their work on behalf of health and human rights in Burma.

We would like to thank the staff of the Fogarty program at Johns Hopkins, Denise Carolan and Molly McHugh, for their efforts on behalf of the conference and this book.

Contributors

Editors

Chris Beyrer, M.D., M.P.H., is a professor in the Departments of Epidemiology and International Health at the Johns Hopkins Bloomberg School of Public Health. He serves as director of Johns Hopkins Fogarty AIDS International Training and Research Program, which provides advanced training in HIV/AIDS research for scientists and health care providers from Africa, Asia, Latin America, and the Russian Federation. He is the founder and director of the Center for Public Health and Human Rights at Johns Hopkins. The center is engaged in research, teaching, and advocacy on a range of public health and human rights issues. Dr. Beyrer is active in HIV vaccine research and serves as chair of the Injecting Drug Use Working Group of the HIV Vaccine Trials Network, supported by the Division of AIDS of the National Institutes of Health.

Dr. Beyrer has worked on Tibetan refugee health at the Tibetan Delek Hospital, in Dharamsala, India, and in Sarnath, India. He has served as epidemiologist for the Pan American Health Organization working on measles and polio surveillance systems in the Caribbean and Guyana. He has done considerable work with Native American health and has lived and worked on the White Mountain Apache, Zuni, and Gila River Reservations. From 1992 to 1997, Dr. Beyrer was the field director for the collaborative HIV/AIDS research programs between the Johns Hopkins University, Chiang Mai University, the Royal Thai Ministry of Public Health, and the Royal Thai Army and was based in Chiang Mai, northern Thailand. He became active in health and human rights issues related to Burma and the region during those years, and he published some of the first reports on the emerging HIV epidemic in Burma in the 1990s. He subsequently served as advisor on health issues to the elected leadership in Burma, and he currently works on improving public health services with the Karen, Shan, Mon, Karenni, and other ethnic nationalities in the Burmese civil conflict, supported by the Bill and Melinda Gates Population Institute at Johns Hopkins. He also has HIV/AIDS and public health training programs under way in Laos, supported by the Fogarty International Center. He is actively engaged in health and human rights advocacy in China, in collaboration with the Beijing Aixhing Educational Foundation and supported by the Levi Strauss Foundation.

As a medical epidemiologist working on infectious diseases, Dr. Beyrer currently has research or training activities in Thailand, China, Burma, India, Laos, Malawi, Uganda, Ethiopia, South Africa, Russia, Tajikistan, and the United States. He is the author of the 1998 book *War in the Blood: Sex, Politics and AIDS in Southeast Asia* (Zed Books), which has been translated into Thai, Chinese, and Vietnamese. Dr. Beyrer has published extensively on HIV/AIDS epidemiology and prevention research, HIV vaccine research, and public health and human rights. He has served as a consultant on health in developing countries to the World Bank Institute, the World Bank Thailand Office, the Office for AIDS Research of the NIH,the U.S. Military HIV Research Program, the Henry M. Jackson Foundation for the Advancement of Military Medicine, the Open Society Institute, the Royal Thai Army, the Thai Red Cross Program on AIDS, and numerous other organizations. He serves on the Advisory Board to the Sexual Health and Rights Program of the Open Society Institute; on the Scientific Advisory Committee of the International Partnership for Microbicides; on the Advisory Committee of the Asian Social Issues Program of the Asia Society; on the Advisory Board of the Fisher Center for the Study of Women and Men at Hobart and William Smith Colleges. He is a trustee of the Institute for Asian Democracy and serves on the Committee for Human Research of the Johns Hopkins Bloomberg School of Public Health.

H. F. Pizer is a medical writer, health care consultant, and physician assistant. He has written and edited fourteen books and numerous articles about health and medicine. With Kenneth Mayer, he coauthored the first book about AIDS for the general public, *The AIDS Fact Book* (Bantam Books, 1983) and most recently *The AIDS Pandemic: Impact on Science and Society.* His other works cover a variety of subjects in health and medicine, including the first books for the general public on organ transplants (*Organ Transplants: A Patient's Guide with the Massachusetts General Organ Transplant Teams,* Harvard University Press, 1991) and stroke (*The Stroke Fact Book,* with Conn Foley, Bantam Books, 1985, and the American Heart Association), and in women's health and family planning (*The New Birth Control Program,* with Christine Garfink, R.N., Bolder Books, 1977), parenting (*The Post Partum Book,* with Christine Garfink, R.N., Grove Press, 1979), miscarriage (*Coping with a Miscarriage,* with Christine O'Brien Palinski, Dial Press, 1980), and artificial insemination (*Having a Baby Without a Man,* with Susan Robinson, M.D., Simon & Schuster, 1985). He also coauthored *Confronting Breast Cancer* (with Sigmund Weitzman, M.D., and Irene Kuter, M.D., Random House, 1987). From 1984 to 1994, he was founder and president of New England Medical Claims Analysts, a health care cost-containment consultancy in Cambridge, Massachusetts. During that time, he wrote and lectured on health care cost containment. He is cofounder and principal of Health Care Strategies, Inc., a consulting firm in Cambridge, Massachusetts, that provides program monitoring and evaluation services and management consulting services to community health care providers, health care systems, educational programs, and social service providers. He is a former president of the Massachusetts Association of Physician Assistants.

Contributors

Apinun Aramrattana, M.D., Ph.D., is a medical epidemiologist and a leading researcher on drug use in Thailand. He is a deputy director of the Research Institute of Health Sciences at Chiang Mai University. Dr. Apinun is the Thai principal investigator on several NIH-supported HIV-prevention trials for injection drug users and methamphetamine-using youth, and he is directing a study for the HIV Prevention Trials Network on buprenorphine/naloxone substitution maintenance therapy versus buprenorphine/naloxone detoxification as a strategy for preventing HIV.

Holly Burkhalter is vice president for governmental affairs at the International Justice Mission, a human rights service organization that provides assistance to victims of abuse and accountability for the perpetrators in ten countries of Latin America, Asia, and Africa. Before joining the International Justice Mission, Ms. Burkhalter was the U.S. policy director of Physicians for Human Rights and she served as advocacy director for Human Rights Watch. Ms. Burkhalter is a frequent witness before Congress and publishes regularly on issues of HIV/AIDS, women's rights, genocide, and U.S. foreign policy. She was appointed by President Clinton to serve on the board of the U.S. Institute of Peace in 1999 and continues to serve in that capacity.

David D. Celentano, Sc.D., M.H.S., is professor and director of the Infectious Diseases Epidemiology Program and deputy chair of the Department of Epidemiology at the Johns Hopkins Bloomberg School of Public Health. He is principal investigator of the HIV Prevention Trials Unit for Thailand, for the National Institute of Mental Health Collaborative HIV/STD Prevention Trial in India, and for a series of investigator-initiated National Institutes of Health grants in Thailand. He has been working on social and behavioral factors in HIV/AIDS since 1983 and has conducted a series of epidemiological and behavioral intervention trials in the United States, Thailand, India, and Vietnam. He serves as chair of the Behavioral Sciences Work Group for the HPTN and has been a consultant to the Office of AIDS Research (NIH) and to various institutes and centers of the NIH.

Jonathan Cohen, J.D., is the director of the Law and Health Initiative at the Open Society Institute. He oversees a range of legal assistance, litigation, and law-reform efforts to advance public health goals worldwide. Mr. Cohen was previously a researcher with the HIV/AIDS and Human Rights Program at Human Rights Watch, where he conducted numerous investigations of human rights violations linked to AIDS epidemics in sub-Saharan Africa, Southeast Asia, and North America. A Canadian lawyer, Mr. Cohen served as a law clerk at the Supreme Court of Canada in 2001 and was coeditor-in-chief of the *University of Toronto, Faculty of Law Review.*

Noya Galai, Ph.D., is an associate professor in the Department of Epidemiology at the Johns Hopkins Bloomberg School of Public Health. Dr. Galai has worked since 1991 as a biostatistician on the large cohort studies of the natural history of HIV in the United States, Italy, and Thailand. She has also worked on national studies evaluating the quality of care in Israel and currently also has a position at Haifa University, Israel. Dr. Galai has a strong interest in the translation of epidemiological research to health policy, in particular, concerning disadvantaged populations.

Varun Gauri, Ph.D., is a senior economist in the Development Research Group of the World Bank. Dr. Gauri's research interests include the enforcement and impact of legally codified social and economic rights, the political economy of government responses to HIV/AIDS, the governance of nongovernmental organizations in developing countries, the effect of AIDS treatment, the use of vouchers for basic education, and immunization in developing countries. He has also worked on and led a variety of operational tasks in the World Bank, including operational evaluations, investments in privately owned hospitals in Latin America, a social sector adjustment loan to Brazil, several health care projects in Brazil, a study of the decentralization of health care in Nigeria, and the 2007 World Development Report. Mr. Gauri has taught courses on health policy, bioethics, and education policy in the United States and in Chile.

Karyn Kaplan is the international advocacy coordinator of the Bangkok-based Thai AIDS Treatment Action Group and advocacy advisor to the Thai Drug Users' Network. Karyn has worked in Thailand since 1988 on HIV and human rights issues, primarily with drug users and sex workers, and coconducted the first human rights documentation project among Thai injectors with Paisan Suwannawong. Before moving back to Thailand in 2002, Karyn was the HIV/AIDS program officer with the International Gay and Lesbian Human Rights Commission.

Nancy Kass, Sc.D., is Phoebe R. Berman Professor of Bioethics and Public Health at the Johns Hopkins Bloomberg School of Public Health and the Johns Hopkins Berman Bioethics Institute. She also is a faculty affiliate of the Kennedy Institute of Ethics, Georgetown University, and a fellow of the Hastings Center. Dr. Kass conducts empirical work in bioethics, public health, and health policy. Her publications are primarily in the fields of U.S. and international research ethics, public health ethics, HIV/AIDS policy, and genetics policy. She is coeditor (with Ruth Faden) of *HIV, AIDS and Childbearing: Public Policy, Private Lives* (Oxford University Press, 1996). Dr. Kass has fifteen years' experience designing and conducting quantitative and qualitative empirical research studies in bioethics and health policy. She directs the Johns Hopkins Fogarty Bioethics Training Program for African professionals.

Thomas Kerr, Ph.D., is a research scientist with the British Columbia Centre for Excellence in HIV/AIDS and a clinical assistant professor with the Department of Medicine at the University of British Columbia. He is also currently the coprincipal investigator of the Vancouver Injection Drug Users Study and the Scientific Evaluation of Supervised Injecting Project. Dr. Kerr has had a working partnership with the Thai Drug Users' Network (TDN) since 2003 and was the principal author of TDN's successful submission to the Global Fund to Fight AIDS, Tuberculosis and Malaria.

Alice Khin, M.B.B.S., M.Med. (Int. Med.), is a faculty lecturer at University of Alberta, Edmonton, Canada. She is a health and human rights activist, and returns to Mae Sot, on the Thai-Burma border, every year to work with the Mae Tao Clinic and Burma Medical Association. She has organized health and human rights training and workshops for health workers of various ethnic groups along the border. She is a former personal physician to the 1991 Nobel Peace Laureate Aung San Suu Kyi and executive member of the Burma Medical Association, chaired by Dr. Cynthia Maung.

Heather Kuiper, M.P.H., works in national and international reproductive health research, policy, and evaluation. Since 1997, she has worked with the Global Health Access Program to develop health information and reproductive health initiatives for displaced Burmese populations served by the Mae Tao Clinic and Backpack Health-worker Team Program of Mae Sot, Thailand.

Lynn Lawry, M.D., M.S.P.H., M.Sc., is director of Evidence-based Research for the International Medical Corps and director of the Initiative in Global Women's Health at the Brigham and Women's Hospital, of Harvard Medical School. She is a special-ist in internal medicine, women's health, and epidemiology. Located in Washing-ton, D.C., the International Medical Corps is a global humanitarian nonprofit or-ganization dedicated to relieving suffering through health care training, relief, and development programs that build local capacity. As senior medical researcher with Physicians for Human Rights, she conducted population-based health and human rights investigations in Afghanistan, Pakistan, Sierra Leone, Nigeria, and Iraq. With the International Medical Corps, she has completed population-based studies in Dar-fur and Afghanistan. Dr. Lawry also has served as a volunteer medical director and consultant providing emergency medical care and public health programming for humanitarian aid organizations in Kenya, the former Zaire, Rwanda, Albania, and Kosovo.

Jennifer Leaning, M.D., S.M.H., is professor of the practice of international health at the Harvard School of Public Health and directs the Program on Humanitarian Crises and Human Rights, based at the François-Xavier Bagnoud Center for Health and Human Rights. She is an assistant professor of medicine at Harvard Medical School and an attending physician in the Emergency Department of Brigham and Women's Hospital. She also is senior advisor in international and policy studies at the Radcliffe Institute for Advanced Study and is codirector of the Harvard Humani-tarian Initiative. Dr. Leaning teaches disaster management, human rights, and re-sponse to humanitarian crises. She has field experience in problems of disaster re-sponse and human rights (particularly in the Middle East, former U.S.S.R., Somalia, the African Great Lakes area, Albania, Kosovo, Afghanistan, and Sudan) and has written widely on these issues. She is lead editor of *Humanitarian Crises: The Medical and Public Health Response* (Harvard University Press, 1999). She currently serves on several nonprofit boards, including Physicians for Human Rights and Oxfam America.

Thomas J. Lee, M.D., M.H.S., is cofounder of Global Health Access Program and an adjunct assistant professor of medicine at the University of California at Los An-geles. He has been working on the Thai-Burma border with the Backpack Health Workers since 1998 providing support for their health programs. His prior experi-ence includes working with similarly displaced populations in El Salvador at the end of their civil war. Dr. Lee received his medical degree from the University of California at San Francisco.

Sara Lowther, M.P.H., is a doctoral candidate in the Department of Epidemiology at the Johns Hopkins Bloomberg School of Public Health. She received her M.P.H. at Emory University and has been a consultant to the Centers for Disease Control and Prevention, the World Health Organization, and the United Nations Children's Fund working in the areas of viral diseases, child health, and immunization. At Johns Hopkins she has continued her training in epidemiology while assisting on projects for the Johns Hopkins Center for Public Health and Human Rights.

Mahn Mahn is a senior medic with the Backpack Health Worker Team based along the Thai-Burma border. He has been active in providing health services and in training health workers since he was forced to flee his homeland in 1988. He has played a leadership role in developing the Backpack Health Worker Program with special emphasis on malaria prevention, treatment, and care for internally displaced persons in Burma.

Julie Samia Mair, J.D., M.P.H., is an assistant scientist in the Department of Health Policy and Management at the Johns Hopkins Bloomberg School of Public Health and a core faculty member of the Center for Law and the Public's Health at Johns Hopkins and Georgetown Universities, the Johns Hopkins Center for Public Health and Human Rights, and the Johns Hopkins Center for Gun Policy and Research. Ms. Mair is involved in several research areas related to violence prevention, including: the use of law as a public health tool; prevention and control of violence through environmental modifications; incarceration policies; firearm injury prevention; and strategies to prevent the proliferation and use of biological weapons. Before joining the faculty at Johns Hopkins, Ms. Mair practiced law for more than eight years; she is currently a member of the Washington, D.C., Maryland, and Pennsylvania Bars. She has a Certificate in Health and Human Rights, a Certificate in Humanitarian Assistance, and a Certificate in Injury Control from the Bloomberg School of Public Health.

Kasia Malinowska-Sempruch is the director of the International Harm Reduction Development (IHRD) program at the Open Society Institute. Under her direction, IHRD has expanded its support to underserved communities such as prisoners, street children, Roma communities, and sex workers. She has also developed donor consortia and a policy initiative, and collaborates actively with UNAIDS and UNDP. She is a member of the Technical Review Panel of the Global Fund to Fight AIDS, Tuberculosis and Malaria and vice chair of the board of the International Council of AIDS Service Organizations. Ms. Malinowska-Sempruch has been a member of the Task Force Millennium Project on HIV/AIDS, TB, Malaria, and Access to Essential Medicines, as well as the U.N. Reference Group on HIV/AIDS Prevention and Care among Injecting Drug Users. Before joining the Open Society Institute, she worked with the UNDP's HIV and Development Program in both New York City and her native Poland. In Poland she managed a $2.5 million program that supported HIV initiatives by the government and civil sectors; she also coauthored that country's first National AIDS Program and designed training courses for nurses, physicians, social workers, teachers, local policy makers, prison personnel, and psychologists.

Cynthia Maung, M.B.B.S., is the founder of the Mae Tao Clinic in Mae Sot, along the Thai-Burma border, serving the health needs of Burmese migrants. An ethnic

Karen, she was born in Rangoon and graduated in medicine from Rangoon University and practiced in Karen State. Following the 1988 uprising, she was forced to flee to the border and subsequently to Thailand, where she founded the clinic in 1989. For her work, she is the recipient of numerous honors, including the Jonathan Mann Health and Human Rights Award in 1999, the Foundation for Human Rights in Asia's Special Award from Japan in 2001, the Van Heuven Doedhart Award from the Netherlands in 2001, and the Magsaysay Award for Community Leadership in 2002; she was a nominee for the Nobel Peace Prize in 2005.

Mwandagalirwa Kashamuka Melchior, M.H.S., is a Congolese HIV/AIDS researcher in Kinshasa, Democratic Republic of Congo, and was for many years the laboratory manager for Projet SIDA, the long-standing HIV/AIDS research center in Kinshasa. A former Fogarty Fellow at the Johns Hopkins University Bloomberg School of Public Health, he now serves as Fogarty in-country project coordinator for the Democratic Republic of Congo at Johns Hopkins and the University of North Carolina. In 2000, he was awarded a certificate in tropical medicine and public health and in 2001 a master's in health science degree in molecular microbiology and immunology from the Johns Hopkins University. He has studied the transmission of HIV in the Democratic Republic of Congo between mother and child, and hospital employees and their spouses.

Htee Moo is one of the cofounders and current leaders of the Backpack Health Worker Team. He is also the secretary of the Karen Health and Welfare Department and currently manages more than twenty clinics providing services for more than 80,000 ethnic Karens. He has been a health worker for more than thirty years and has played a critical role in serving the health needs of internally displaced persons in eastern Burma.

Luke C. Mullany, Ph.D., M.H.S., is an assistant professor at the Johns Hopkins Bloomberg School of Public Health and a technical consultant for Global Health Access Program. He has been providing technical support on the Thai-Burma border for the Backpack Health Worker Team since 2000. Prior experience with internally displaced populations includes work in northern Angola during 1998–99.

Alena Peryshkina is a cofounder of AIDS Infoshare and a long-time HIV/AIDS and human rights advocate in Russia. Ms. Peryshkina currently represents the European region on UNAIDS Programme Coordinating Board and is on the steering committee of the Russian Round Three Global Fund NGO consortium. She has overseen all aspects of research at AIDS Infoshare, including qualitative and quantitative data collection, ethics, and recruitment. Ms. Peryshkina serves as the Russian principal investigator for several international collaborative research projects, in both Russia and Central Asia. Her organization publishes the leading AIDS journal in Russia as well as Russia's largest journal for people living with AIDS.

Chen Reis, J.D., M.P.H., was senior research associate with Physicians for Human Rights. In that role, she was primarily responsible for developing research projects on HIV/AIDS and human rights in Africa and for working on research relating to women's health and human rights. Ms. Reis has extensive experience in the field of international human rights law and policy, with a focus on health and human rights issues relating to women and children.

Adam K. Richards, M.D., M.P.H., is a resident in the Social Internal Medicine Residency Program of the Department of Family and Social Medicine of the Montefiore Medical Center, in the Bronx, New York. He has provided technical support for the Global Health Access Program and has served as associate director of the Malaria Program since 2001. His experience in parasitic and infectious disease includes research in the Peruvian Amazon, and he has promoted human rights in Burma since 1992.

Susan G. Sherman, Ph.D., M.P.H., is an associate professor in infectious diseases epidemiology at the Johns Hopkins Bloomberg School of Public Health. Dr. Sherman is a behavioral scientist and social epidemiologist whose work focuses on epidemiological studies of and socioeconomic interventions with drug users. She has worked on several randomized behavioral interventions with drug users in the United States, Thailand, and Pakistan. She has studied IDU dyads, social networks, gender differences in illicit drug use patterns and disease acquisition, and factors related to transition to injection drug use. She has also evaluated several overdose-prevention interventions in many U.S. cities. She uses both quantitative and qualitative methods in conducting research.

Terrence Smith, M.D., M.P.H., has previously worked in the Maternal and Child Health Program of the California State Health Department and as a physician and technical advisor with Doctors of the World projects in Vietnam and Chiapas, Mexico. In recent years, he has worked with the Reproductive Health Department at the Mae Tao Clinic.

Julie Stachowiak, Ph.D., is a cofounder and president of AIDS Infoshare Russia, a Moscow-based nongovernmental organization. Her research focuses on the risk factors and prevalence of sexually transmitted diseases, HIV, and hepatitis C in female sex workers in Moscow and on the risk factors and prevalence of HIV among injection drug users in Tajikistan.

Voravit Suwanvanichkij, M.D., M.P.H., is an internist and research associate with the Center for Public Health and Human Rights, Johns Hopkins Bloomberg School of Public Health. He received both his master's and medical degrees from Johns Hopkins and has served as a volunteer physician at the Mae Tao Clinic, helping to train medics and caring for migrants from Burma. He is currently based in Chiang Mai, northern Thailand, where he works in HIV/AIDS clinical care and research. He also continues to investigate and write about issues involving Burma, human rights, migration, and public health, in addition to continuing to provide and coordinate medical care for migrants from Burma.

Paisan Suwannawong is the director of the Thai AIDS Treatment Action Group and cofounder of the Thai Drug Users' Network. He was the founding chair of the Thai Network of People Living with HIV/AIDS and a founding partner of Alden House, a shelter and community-based organization that serves people living with HIV/AIDS, primarily drug users, where he managed programs for ten years.

Arpi Terzian, M.P.H., is a doctoral candidate in the Department of Epidemiology at the Johns Hopkins Bloomberg School of Public Health. Ms. Terzian is a recipient of the 2005 National Institute of Drug Abuse's Drug Abuse Dissertation Research Fellowship. Collaborating with the STATEPI Research Group in the Department of Epidemiology, she is examining how HIV, hepatitis C virus infection, and history of drug use influence physical functioning among participants of the Women's Intragency HIV Study. As principal investigator, Ms. Terzian is responsible for study design and analysis as well as overseeing the implementation of physical functioning protocols, data collection, and management.

Denise Vaillancourt, B.A., M.I.P.P., is a senior health evaluation officer in the Operations Evaluation Department of the World Bank. Her research interests include health sector policy and management capacity; results-based management for tracking and improving health sector performance and outcomes; and the development effectiveness of health and HIV/AIDS programs. She has also led the World Bank's health sector policy dialogue, lending, and project supervision work in a number of African countries, including, Benin, Burkina Faso, Côte d'Ivoire, and Niger and provided technical inputs and peer review support to numerous other teams and countries on health and HIV/AIDS. While in the World Bank Institute, Ms. Vaillancourt collaborated on a multiple-agency initiative to strengthen and use African management capacity through the establishment and support of African professional networks for management training, consulting, research, and marketing.

Wan Yanhai is a prominent leader in the global campaign against HIV/AIDS. He is the director of Beijing AIZHIXING Institute of Health Education, which advocates for HIV/AIDS education and treatment, reducing drug harm, and protecting the human rights of people living with AIDS and others affected by the disease. In 1992, while working for China's National Health Education Institute, he launched China's first HIV/AIDS counseling hotline. In 1994, he founded AIZHI Action Project, a nongovernmental organization that uses health education, research, publishing, and conferences to confront the growing HIV/AIDS crisis in China. Central to his message is the belief that widespread social prejudice against gays, lesbians, bisexuals, and intravenous drug users exacerbates the suffering of HIV-positive individuals in China and undermines efforts to combat the spread of the disease. His role in bringing public attention to the public health crisis in China's Henan Province, where hundreds of thousands of rural villagers became infected with HIV through faulty blood collection practices, won him widespread international acclaim.

Charlotte Watts, Ph.D., is head of the Health Policy Unit and a senior lecturer in epidemiology and health policy. She heads a multidisciplinary research group working on Gender and Women's Health and has published widely on HIV, domestic and sexual violence, trafficking, methodological and ethical issues associated with conducting research on violence, and the importance of female-controlled methods of HIV prevention. Her publications include scientific and policy papers in the *Lancet*, *Science*, and *BMJ*. She headed the Rockefeller Foundation Public Health Working Group on microbicides, is senior technical advisor to the WHO Ten Country Study on Women's Health and Domestic Violence, and was on the organizing committee for the 2002 and 2004 International Microbicides Conference.

Daniel Wolfe is a community scholar at the Center for History and Ethics of Public Health at Columbia University and an AIDS advocate whose work has focused on HIV policy and community response. He is the author of a 2002 survey of HIV and primary care in Eastern Europe and the former Soviet Union, a consultant to Open

Society Institute on issues related to illicit drug policy and media representations of people with HIV, and the author of the acclaimed *Men Like Us: The GMHC Complete Guide to Gay Men's Sexual, Physical, and Emotional Well-Being* (Ballantine Books, 2000). He was the longtime director of communications for Gay Men's Health Crisis, the world's oldest and largest AIDS organization. His writing has appeared in publications including the *Nation*, the *Guardian*, *POZ*, the *Advocate*, the *New York Times Book Review*, and the *Village Voice*.

Evan Wood, Ph.D., is research scientist with the British Columbia Centre for Excellence in HIV/AIDS and is an assistant professor with the Department of Medicine at the University of British Columbia. Dr. Wood is the principal investigator of several cohort studies involving injection drug users and street youth, including the Vancouver Injection Drug Users Study. He has extensive research experience in the area of clinical epidemiology, especially in evaluating the treatment of HIV/AIDS, addiction, and epidemiological study design, particularly among injection drug-using populations. Dr. Wood is also the associate editor of the *International Journal of Drug Policy*.

Xiaorang Li, Ph.D., joined the Institute for Philosophy and Public Policy at the University of Maryland in 1993. Her specialty is in human rights and democracy with a focus on developing countries, particularly China. She has written on subjects including the integrity of civil-political and social-economic-cultural rights, "Asian values," women's rights, distributive justice, world hunger, development ethics, Confucianism, civil society, cultural pluralism, and tolerance. Dr. Xiaorang is the author of a forthcoming book, *Ethics, Human Rights and Culture* (Palgrave Macmillan). She helped found the New York-based group Human Rights in China and served on its board until 2005. She created and edited the organization's journal, *Humanity and Human Rights (ren yu renquan)*.

John A. Zambrano, M.H.S., is a research associate at the RAND Corporation working with the Center for Domestic and International Health Security. His research focuses on national preparedness and response to emerging health threats. During Mr. Zambrano's time at Johns Hopkins, he was the recipient of the Paul and Marianne Gertman Fellowship in Public Health and Human Rights and directed an evaluation of access to incarcerated women's health care in the Washington, D.C., Correctional Facilities. In 2004, Mr. Zambrano received the Protecting Health and Human Rights Community Service Award from the D.C. Prisoners' Legal Services Project on behalf of the Johns Hopkins Center for Public Health and Human Rights.

Cathy Zimmerman, M.Sc., is a research fellow in the Health Policy Unit at the London School of Hygiene and Tropical Medicine, where she is part of an interdisciplinary research team working on violence against women. She has carried out qualitative and quantitative multiple-country studies examining the physical and mental health of women trafficked in Europe. She is the coauthor of the WHO Ethical and Safety Recommendations for Interviewing Trafficked Women. In Cambodia, she founded and managed a local nongovernmental organization, Project against Domestic Violence, where she conducted primary research, including a national household survey, qualitative studies, and a legal analysis on domestic violence.

Acronyms

ACT-UP	AIDS Coalition to Unleash Power
AIDS	acquired immune-deficiency syndrome
ALRC	Asian Legal Resource Center
ALTSEAN	Alternative Association of Southeast Asian Nations Network on Burma
AOR	adjusted odds ratios
AZT	azidothymidine (zidovudine), an anti-HIV drug that reduces the amount of virus in the body
BPHWT	Backpack Health Worker Team
CCM	The Global Fund "Country Coordinating Mechanism"
CCR	Centers for Capacity Building and Referral Care
CDC	Centers for Disease Control and Prevention
CEDAW	Convention on the Elimination of All Forms of Discrimination against Women
CEEHRN	Central and Eastern European Harm Reduction Network
CHALN	Canadian HIV/AIDS Legal Network
CHANGE	Center for Health and Gender Equity
CI	confidence interval
CIA	Central Intelligence Agency
CIOMS	Council for International Organizations of Medical Sciences
CND	Commission on Narcotic Drugs

CRF	circulating recombinant form
CRT	State Reference and Treatment Center for AIDS
CSIS	Center for Strategic and International Studies
CTA	Center for Testing and Counseling
DFID	Department for International Development
DLHPRN	Drug Law and Health Policy Research Network
ECOMOG	Peacekeeping mission of ECOWAS
ECOWAS	Economic Community of West African States
ECRE	European Council on Refugees and Exiles
EMBASE	biomedical and pharmacological database with information about medical and drug-related subjects
ERI	Earth Rights International
EU	European Union
FEWSNET	Famine Early Warning Systems Network
FNC	Federal Narcotics Council
GAPA	Brazilian NGO, support group for AIDS prevention
GHAP	Global Health Access Program
GDP	gross domestic product
GFATM	Global Fund to Fight AIDS, Tuberculosis, and Malaria
GPS	global positioning system
HAART	highly active antiretroviral therapy
HAV	hepatitis A virus
HBV	hepatitis B virus
HCV	hepatitis C virus
HIV	human immunodeficiency virus
HRW	Human Rights Watch
HURFOM	Human Rights Foundation of Monland
IAS	International AIDS Society
ICCPR	International Covenant on Civil and Political Rights
ICESCR	International Covenant on Economic, Social and Cultural Rights
ICF	International Classification of Functioning, Disability and Health
ICG	International Crisis Group
ICBL	International Campaign to Ban Landmines
ICPD	International Conference on Population and Development

ICTR	International Criminal Tribunal for Rwanda
ICTY	International Criminal Tribunal for Yugoslavia
IDP	internally displaced person
IDU	injection drug user
ILO	International Labor Organization
IMC	International Medical Corps
IMR	infant mortality rate
INAMPS	Instituto Nacional de Assistência Médica da Previdência Social, Brazil's social security institute during military rule
INCB	International Narcotic Control Board
IOM	International Organization for Migration
IRB	institutional review board
ISI	scientific journal database
JLI	Joint Learning Initiative
KHRG	Karen Human Rights Group
KWAT	Kachin Women's Association Thailand
MDG	millennium development goals
MEDLINE	scientific journal database
MSF	Médicins sans Frontière
MMR	maternal mortality ratio
MSM	men who have sex with men
MTC	Mae Tao Clinic, a health clinic operating on the Thai-Burma border
NAP	Brazil's National AIDS Program
NASCP	National AIDS and STDs Control Program
NCGUB	National Coalition Government of the Union of Burma
NGO	nongovernmental organization
OHCHR	Office of the High Commissioner for Human Rights
PAB	Piso ambulatorial básico, primary care municipal system
PAHO	Pan American Health Organization
PAVE	Preparation for AIDS Vaccine Evaluations
PCR	polymerase chain reaction
PEPFAR	U.S. President's Emergency Program for AIDS Relief
PHR	Physicians for Human Rights
PIH	Partners in Health
PLWHA	People Living with HIV/AIDS

PMTCT	prevention of mother-to-child transmission
Projet SIDA	AIDS project
PUBMED	U.S. National Library of Medicine's search service
RUF	Revolutionary United Front
SANAM	(Russian name) Moscow-based NGO with a clinical and services focus
SARS	severe acute respiratory syndrome
SAS	Statistical Analysis Software
SF	Short Form Health Survey
SHRF	Shan Human Rights Foundation
SIECUS	Sexuality Information and Education Council of the United States
SPDC	State Peace and Development Council of Burmese military junta
STARHS	serologic testing algorithm for recent HIV seroconversion
STATA	statistical analysis software
STI	sexually transmitted infection
SUS	Sistema Único da Saúde, Brazil's government health system
SWAN	Shan Women's Action Network
TB	Tuberculosis
TBA	traditional birth attendant
TBBC	Thailand Burma Border Consortium
TDN	Thai Drug Users' Network
TNP+	Thai Network of People Living with HIV/AIDS
TRC	Truth and Reconciliation Commission
TTAG	Thai AIDS Treatment Action Group
U5MR	under age 5 mortality rate
UAE	United Arab Emirates
UDHR	Universal Declaration of Human Rights (1948)
UNAIDS	Joint United Nations Programme on HIV/AIDS
UNAMSIL	United Nations Mission for Sierra Leone
UNCESCR	United Nations Committee on Economic, Social and Cultural Rights
UNDAW	United Nations Division for the Advancement of Women
UNDP	United Nations Development Program
UNECOSOC	United Nations Economic and Social Council

UNESCO	United Nations Educational, Scientific, and Cultural Organization
UNFPA	United Nations Population Fund
UNGASS	United Nations General Assembly Special Session
UNHCR	United Nations High Commissioner for Refugees
UNHCHR	United Nations High Commissioner for Human Rights
UNICEF	United Nations Children's Fund
UNOCHA	United Nations Office for the Coordinator of Humanitarian Affairs
UNODC	United Nations Office on Drugs and Crime (formerly UNODCCP)
UNOMSIL	United Nations Observer Mission in Sierra Leone
URF	unique recombinant form
USAID	United States Agency for International Development
USCR	United States Committee for Refugees
US DHHS	United States Department of Health and Human Services
VCHR	Vietnam Committee on Human Rights
WCRP	Woman and Child Rights Project
WEO	Western European and Other Governments
WHO	World Health Organization
WLB	Women's League of Burma
WMA	World Medical Association

Introduction

Human Rights and the Health of Populations

Chris Beyrer, M.D., M.P.H.

Social justice and the protection of human rights do not ensure good health—free people can make poor choices, and affluence carries its own burdens of morbidity and mortality. But social injustice and limits on basic rights and freedoms, on human dignity itself, can have direct and indirect effects on the health of individuals, communities, and populations (Mann, 1995). A recent dictionary definition for human rights reads: "universal rights held to belong to individuals by virtue of their being human, encompassing civil, political, economic, social, and cultural rights and freedoms, and based on the notion of personal human dignity and worth" (Columbia Electronic Encyclopedia). This captures the essence of human rights, as distinct from civil liberties, which are freedoms derived from the laws of given states. Human rights are universal, relevant for all persons, and derived from the inherent dignity of being human.

That violations of an individual's human rights, such as torture or forced labor, can have health consequences is well described in both the medical and the rights literatures. That abrogation of social, economic, and cultural rights, such as those that pertain to gender equity, education, access to health information, and food and water have wide-ranging effects on health is also well accepted in the medical literature, in development work, and in international human rights law (United Nations, 1976). The population-level health effects of rights violations, the methods needed to assess them, and the interventions required to mitigate them are less well studied and understood.

Public health, the discipline that deals with the health of populations, is arguably the health field most affected by human rights realities and by governmental successes or failures to respect, protect, and fulfill those rights. This has become increasingly clear in the context of epidemic diseases, especially in the case of the greatest infectious disease threat of our time, HIV/AIDS, which has emerged as a remarkably sensitive and specific marker of injustice, discrimination, gender inequality, government negligence, and the social disruptions of civil strife, conflict, and war (Tomasevski et al., 1992). Yet the tools of modern public health, from risk assessment to demography to molecular epidemiology, have rarely been applied to human rights violations affecting populations. Much of the "tool kit" of human rights investigations derives from legal approaches, not epidemiological ones. In an era of ethnic cleansing and of military tactics such as rape as a tool of ethnic terror, population-level crimes require population-level methods and approaches. And it can be argued that public health has underused the frameworks, tools, and instruments of human rights to shape investigative questions, design programs, and address the health outcomes of rights violations. In a swiftly globalizing world, where both threats to public health and violations of human rights are increasing, and increasingly interconnected, methods and approaches that integrate the strength of these disciplines are clearly called for.

Our thesis is that a fundamental component of moving forward on the realization of global health and human rights goals is the need to focus the powerful population-based tools of public health science on the intersections of rights and disease. The health needs of vulnerable populations demand this, and public health efforts are clearly needed when and where rights violations occur for scientific approaches to remain relevant to decision makers. While concern has mounted in the political and human rights arenas over rights violations such as trafficking in women and children, gender-based and sexual violence in conflict zones, human slavery, and the impact of lack of scientific freedom on public health (so painfully demonstrated by China's initial response to severe acute respiratory syndrome), hard data on the population-level health effects of these violations have been strikingly limited (Beyrer, 2004a, b). And while epidemiology has played pivotal roles in elucidating mechanisms of disease spread in populations, the field has been largely silent on political and rights-associated risk factors for disease. A key scientific problem we now face is how best to investigate, mitigate, and ultimately reduce the health consequences of human rights violations. Work on the intersection of rights and public health can be challenging, as the authors included in this volume certainly attest, but the effects on human well-being can be enormous.

Public Health and Human Rights

Because public health is concerned with the health and well-being of populations, its scope and scale are directed beyond the clinic and the consulting room to encompass communities, workplaces, environments, and the wider world. A public health approach wants to see not only that each individual child in a community is fully immunized for her or his own protection, but also that the coverage of immunizations across all children in a population is sufficient to prevent a measles outbreak or a polio epidemic. Because public health interventions seek to improve health outcomes by operating at population levels, this has generally meant engagement with the body politic, and has made public health among the most inherently political of medical fields. Indeed, most public health professionals work in national, state, or municipal public health departments and programs. It should not be surprising that public health threats from emerging diseases to land mines to childhood malnutrition should be so consistently connected to political and social realities, or that human rights and civil liberties should be so intertwined with public health interventions. So we should acknowledge that public health mandates and governments' responsibilities for the health of the public have sometimes placed public health squarely in opposition to individual rights. Public health has tools such as mandatory isolation and quarantine backed by state power that can limit individual and community rights from free association to freedom of movement and beyond. Less onerous, but equally limiting to the freedoms of some, are public health measures like smoking bans, seat belt and child car seat laws, and immunization requirements for schools, day care settings, or workplaces. All have in common that they may limit individual rights for perceived public goods. These measures also share the recognition that states have a responsibility to enforce measures with evidence for efficacy for the well-being of the public. This active agency has proven critical to investigating state failures to respond to health threats and protect citizens.

The founding document of the modern human rights movement, The Universal Declaration of Human Rights of 1948, articulates in Article 25 that "everyone has the right to a standard of living adequate for the health and well-being of himself and of his family, including food, clothing, housing and medical care and necessary social services, and the right to security in the event of unemployment, sickness, disability, widowhood, old age or other lack of livelihood in circumstances beyond his control." It has been argued that both the medical care standard and the social services standard here ensure a right to minimum standards of public health as well as access to health services.

The International Covenant on Social Economic and Cultural Rights of 1966 articulates in greater detail those rights that relate to health. Article 12 of the covenant reads:

1. The States Parties to the present Covenant recognize the right of everyone to the enjoyment of the highest attainable standard of physical and mental health.
2. The steps to be taken by the States Parties to the present Covenant to achieve the full realization of this right shall include those necessary for:
    (a) The provision for the reduction of the stillbirth-rate and of infant mortality and for the healthy development of the child;
    (b) The improvement of all aspects of environmental and industrial hygiene;
    (c) The prevention, treatment and control of epidemic, endemic, occupational and other diseases;
    (d) The creation of conditions which would assure to all medical service and medical attention in the event of sickness.

Parts a (infant and child survival), b (environmental and industrial hygiene), and c (prevention, treatment, and control of epidemic diseases) are all broadly public health rights, whereas only part d (medical attention) is entirely medical in nature. The covenant clearly articulates a signatory state's responsibility to take steps toward the full realization of these health goals, and hence of its public health duties.

The International Covenant on Civil and Political Rights (1967) begins with "Recognizing that these rights derive from the inherent dignity of the human person." This inherent dignity has come to be seen by many as the core value from which minimal standards of health and public health derive, a position that the late Jonathan Mann was actively working on at the end of his life. So it is a violation of the dignity of persons to starve while food is plentiful, or for the children of the poor to die of preventable diseases for which affordable vaccines exist. The ICCPR addresses civil liberties that might appear outside the health arena, yet many of these rights, including the right to free expression, freedom from censorship of information, violence and discrimination against women, and freedom from incarceration without due process, can have marked public health implications, which this book will explore.

Building on these covenants, and on widely ratified conventions such as the Declaration on the Rights of the Child and the Convention on the Elimination of All Forms of Discrimination against Women (CEDAW), which further explicitly link health and rights, using a "rights-based approach" to health has become standard language in global health. Great strides have been made in this area, and a growing body of work continues to build the movement for health and human rights. But we would argue that rights-based approaches specific to *public health* challenges, and rights-oriented analyses of public health problems, are in urgent need of further development, articulation, and use. We remain in the early stages of operationalizing rights-based approaches to public health. This book is an attempt to bring together a range of groups and individuals working on rights-based approaches to public health, and to move the field further in thinking about methods, analytic approaches, and practical solutions to working with individual and communities in some of the most challenging settings known.

The limited use of rights-based approaches and analyses in public health remains common. And stalled and failed responses to population-level health threats are all too common as well, as the many millions of deaths each year from preventable causes such as diarrheal diseases and childhood illnesses attests. In some settings, the simple lack of resources—human, scientific, and financial, is sufficient to explain the failure of a state to respond to malaria or toxic waste or AIDS. We live in a world fraught with economic injustice, and the distribution of wealth grows more skewed each year. But plain poverty has rarely been the sole or primary cause of failure in public health. Using a rights-based framework it becomes clear, if we look at those states with the worst health status among citizens, that dictatorship, civil conflict, corruption, malfeasance, and human rights violations are all too common partners in public health failures. This was true in the Stalinist destruction of the environment in Central Asia, the health status of the black majority in Apartheid South Africa, and the man-made famines of Mao's China and British India. The great economist of famine, Amartya Sen, has gone further, in showing that all modern famines have occurred in the absence of democracy—that civil society, and not food aid, is the best prevention for mass hunger (Sen, 1999).

Public Health, Human Rights, and AIDS

Where civil society is abrogated and democracy denied, human rights violations from sexual violence to famine are more likely to occur. And it is in just such settings, unfortunately, that many infectious diseases are most likely to flourish. AIDS is the obvious example. We have drawn heavily on examples and discussions from the HIV/AIDS pandemic in this book because the pandemic continues to provide, unfortunately, so many examples of how rights violations can drive disease spread, and of limitations on human freedom and dignity that assist the virus, not its control.

When we take a critical look at the global responses to two decades of HIV/AIDS we see arguably the most glaring string of failures of public health policy and implementation of our time. HIV is almost entirely preventable, and numerous examples from Australia to Brazil, the United Kingdom, Senegal, and Scandinavia have shown us how prevention can be achieved and care provided. AIDS epidemics do not need to happen. Yet the pandemic surges ahead, with new hot zones in Russia, in Eastern Europe and Central Asia, and across the great populations of China, Indonesia, and India, threatening to make the third decade of AIDS the worst we have seen. How can this be? Again, the question is not simply of resources, or of limited use of tools like condoms and sex education. The next round of HIV/AIDS failures have to do with issues as fundamental and contentious as the lasting gender bias of Asian societies, the limits on scientific inquiry and freedom imposed by dictatorship, the denial of basic rights to care for drug users across Eurasia, and the refusal of first and third world political elites to let evidence, not prejudice, drive public health policy. In short, human beings, particularly those with political power, have too often aided and abetted the HIV virus. Those of us who remember the early days of the stalled U.S. responses to HIV/AIDS in the early 1980s will find chilling reminders of the same denial and obfuscation in too many countries now facing the spread of AIDS. These issues are compounded where citizens have limited rights, where information is restricted, the press censored, and dissidents, political or medical, are silenced.

Limitations

One of the compelling arguments against bringing human rights concerns into health programs is that health workers, like humanitarian relief workers, ought to remain nonpartisan. Bringing a political or human rights framework into public health has been seen as taking sides—and incurring the risks that partisanship can entail. Proponents of this view argue that public health practice could be weakened, not strengthened, by bringing human rights considerations into the field. There are certainly examples of where this might be true, or cases where engagement with human rights concerns could put practitioners in the field at risk. There is also the potential risk of undermining the objectivity of scientific research. The counterargument is not that we should be partisan in our work. Rather, it is to say that if human rights violations are under way and the populations we are attempting to work with around a given health threat are subject to those violations, it is simply bad science and poor public health practice not to investigate the potential interactions at work. Put simply, we ignore the political realties and human rights dimensions of threats to health at our peril. Further, well-intentioned public health efforts that seek to depoliticize threats to health in coercive and repressive settings risk the possibility that our very presence can lend political support to repressive regimes that are at the root of problems we seek to address. This has been the programmatic dilemma for more than a decade in Mugabe's Zimbabwe, in Burma, and in past contexts like the Mobutu dictatorship in Democratic Republic of Congo, then Zaire.

All sides of this debate would likely agree that, when rights violations are occurring, we are all on the side of the suffering, not the violators. When those guilty of rights violations are in power and their assent is necessary for our work, the dilemmas begin. Perpetrators will always resist documenting human rights violations on the part of state actors. Increasing the kinds of evidence available and measuring the population-level effects of flawed policies can be potent tools for advocacy and can meet resistance, hostility, and denial precisely because these kinds of data can be so compelling to policy makers. We hope the examples from Afghanistan, Iraq, China, Burma, and other states with limited rights for citizens will be helpful for those working toward improving public health in the toughest of contexts.

Taken together, these realities argue that rights-based analyses of public health challenges are demanded by the complexity of our time—where resources alone may do little to improve the health of people facing ongoing rights violations. This may lead to new territory for public health, but the benefits could be substantial, and, sadly, human rights violations and the health effects they can induce are unlikely to decline in scale or scope.

References

Beyrer, C. 2004a. Is trafficking a health issue? *Lancet* 363:564–65.

Beyrer, C. 2004b. Public health, human rights, and the beneficence of states. *Human Rights Reviews* 5(1):28–33.

The Columbia electronic encyclopedia, www.cc.columbia.edu/cu/cup/ (accessed November 16, 2005).

Mann, J. 1995. Human rights and the new public health. *Health and Human Rights* (1)3:229–33.

Sen, A. 1999. *Development as freedom.* New York: Knopf, 160–69.

Tomasevski, K., Gruskin, S., Lazzarini, Z., and Hendriks, A. 1992. AIDS and human rights. In *AIDS in the world,* ed. J. Mann, D. Tarantola, and T. Netter. Cambridge: Harvard University Press.

United Nations. 1976. International Covenant of Economic, Social, and Cultural Rights, G.A. res. 2200A.

PART I

Cases & Contexts

1

Health and Human Rights in the Midst of a Drug War

The Thai Drug Users' Network

Thomas Kerr, Ph.D., Karyn Kaplan,
Paisan Suwannawong, and Evan Wood, Ph.D.

On January 14, 2003, the then prime minister of Thailand, Thaksin Shinawatra, officially launched Thailand's "war on drugs" (BBC News, 2003). "There is nothing under the sun which the Thai police cannot do" in the effort to make Thailand "drug free," Thaksin declared (Amnesty International, 2003; Cohen, 2004). These orders resulted in a cascade of human rights violations and public health effects throughout Thailand. Within a few years, approximately 50,000 people, mostly young and poor, were sent to military-style boot camps, several thousand were tortured, and many executed without due process. Many more were driven underground and out of reach of essential health services (Kerr et al., 2004). Despite criticism and pressure from various international observers and organizations from both the human rights and health communities, this initiative has persisted since 2003 and received considerable support from high-ranking officials within the Thai government and from Thai society in general. The full extent to which these events contributed to widened epidemics of HIV/AIDS and other infectious diseases is still not known, but we can expect that the health effects of this brutal campaign will be far reaching. Our colleagues working in northern Thailand, Drs. Celentano, Sherman, and Aramrattana, have studied these health effects (see Chapter 10).

Thailand's drug war was described by officials as targeting the country's drug dealers, and the official prime minister's order called for total suppression of drug trafficking through various means, ranging from "soft to harsh," and went on to say, "If a person is charged with a drug offence, that person will be regarded as a dangerous person who is threatening social and national security" (Government of Thailand, 2003). This initial order was followed by orders from the Thai interior minister, who gave each province targets for the number of arrests of drug dealers and the amount of drugs to be seized. Politicians and police were offered incentives to comply with these orders, and more senior officials were threatened with dismissal if they failed to meet their assigned targets (Cohen, 2004).

Throughout the Thai drug war thousands of individuals suspected of using drugs were ordered to or coerced into attending addiction treatment facilities (Kerr et al., 2004). However, the quality of treatment was highly questionable because it typically consisted of attending a military-style boot camp and participating in military drills (Cohen, 2004). A more complete description of these camps is provided in Chapter 10. It was estimated that as many as 50,000 suspected drug users were sent to such military treatment camps (Cohen, 2004). In some cases, family members were allowed to attend as proxy for their child, who had run away from his province out of fear for his life. Reports from various observers later indicated that there were more than 2,200 extrajudicial killings of alleged drug dealers during the first three months of the drug war (Adams, 2003; Asia Times, 2003; BBC News, 2003), although evidence from various sources suggested that many of those arrested and killed were either current or former drug users, and in some instances, individuals with no drug use or trafficking history (Cohen, 2004). As the death toll continued to rise, the Thai government came under considerable international pressure as human rights organizations and various national governments such as Amnesty International, Human Rights Watch, and the U.S. government criticized the brutal campaign (Adams, 2003; Amnesty International, 2003; BBC News, 2003).

In response to criticisms of the drug war, the prime minister of Thailand repeatedly assured the Thai public that such criticisms were not to be taken seriously, and several other high ranking officials made comments that were supportive of the extreme measures taken by Thai police (Cohen, 2004). For example, the Thai interior minister responsible for providing arrest and seizure targets for individual provinces stated, "They will be put behind bars or even vanish without a trace. Who cares? They are destroying our country." The prime minister himself was quoted as saying, "Drug dealers are ruthless to our children, so being ruthless back to them is not a bad thing. . . . If there are deaths among traders, it's normal" (Ehrlich, 2003). A pro-business governor renowned for his "CEO" approach to ruling the country, he is also the only prime minister never to attend a National AIDS Committee meeting, of which he is the chair.

In sum, the Thai drug war resulted in an array of human rights violations among drug users and non-drug-using individuals who were suspected of illicit drug use or dealing by police. The consistency of reporting from various sources within and outside of Thailand confirms that this drug war was not only unsuccessful in making Thailand drug free, but it also resulted in various health-related harms, including death for thousands of individuals.

Setting the Stage for a National Drug War

Thailand, which shares borders with Burma, Cambodia, Laos, and Malaysia, has a long history of producing opium in its northern mountainous regions. The famous designation "Golden Triangle" refers to the area of opium cultivation in Burma, Thailand, and Laos. However, following U.S.-sponsored efforts to eradicate the crops in the 1960s, there was an increase in the trade of heroin between Thailand and other Golden Triangle countries. This, in turn, prompted a rise in the number of Thai opium users who began injecting heroin and sharp increases in HIV infection throughout the country (Celentano, 2003). A further significant change in illicit drug use trends in Thailand occurred in the late 1990s with the widespread emergence of methamphetamine, or "ya baa" (translated as "crazy pills") (Beyrer et al., 2004).

Consistent with experiences in other settings, illicit drug users in Thailand, in particular injection drug users (IDUs), are known to be at heightened risk for various adverse health outcomes (Beyrer et al., 2003; Srisurapanont et al., 2003; Srirak et al., 2005). For example, as indicated in Figure 1.1, there has been a long-standing HIV epidemic among IDUs in Thailand that has been characterized by persistently elevated HIV incidence rates and current HIV prevalence levels in the range of 30–50 percent (Mastro et al., 1994; Celentano et al., 1999; Vanichseni et al., 2001; Razak et al., 2003). Although there has been considerable investment and political commitment devoted to addressing HIV/AIDS in Thailand among sex workers, their clients, women and children, the Thai government has not initiated an evidence-based strategy to address the specific HIV prevention and care needs of IDUs (Celentano, 2003). In particular, despite the evidence supporting the efficacy of interventions such as provision of sterile syringes and methadone maintenance in reducing HIV risk behaviors, these programs have not been well supported by the Thai government (Beyrer et al., 2003; Celentano, 2003). In response to the persistently high rates of HIV infection among IDUs, several grassroots organizations mobilized their memberships to make a collective call for an evidence-based response to the HIV epidemic among Thai IDUs. Among the more vocal and active groups that rose up to protest a lack of HIV prevention services for Thai IDUs was the Thai Drug Users' Network.

The Thai Drug Users' Network

The Thai Drug Users' Network (TDN) formed in Bangkok on December 10, 2002, on International Human Rights Day, to address the health and human rights situation facing drug users in their country. The organization arose out of a meeting set up to discuss the findings of a human rights documentation project based on 33 first-hand testimonials of Thai injection drug users (Kaplan and Suwannawong, 2002). The project was undertaken in May 2002 by Karyn Kaplan of the International Gay and Lesbian Human Rights Commission (New York) and Paisan Suwannawong, the acting chair of the Thai Network of People Living with HIV/AIDS (TNP+), and focused on barriers to health care among IDUs, as well experiences with Thai police and the judicial system before the drug war (Kaplan and Suwannawong, 2002). The testimonials obtained before the 2003 drug war revealed an array of rights violations including instances of arbitrary arrest and torture, discrimination in judicial and health care settings, and a lack of access to essential health information and materials (Kaplan and Suwannawong, 2002). The results of the project were presented to indigenous leaders within the Thai IDU community, and later presented to the National Human Rights Commission and the

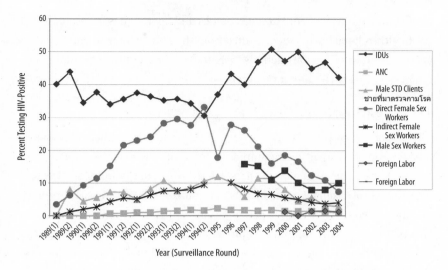

Figure 1.1. The median prevalence of HIV in Thailand: National Sentinel Surveil-lance, 1989–2004. *Source*: Ministry of Public Health, Thailand. Modernizing Health Care Systems in Thailand: Diseases Prevention in the Areas Devastated by Tsunami (accessed at eng.moph.go.th)

Thai Parliament. In response to the findings and persistently high rates of HIV infection, leaders from the Thai IDU community, who had for years informally discussed the need to band together to respond to government neglect and the abysmal legal and social status of IDUs, decided to establish the Thai Drug Users' Network, an organization that is now national in scope and includes more than 100 current and former drug users from various regions in Thailand. The mission of the organization is to "promote the dignity and human rights of people who use drugs."

The birth of TDN was timely, given that only a few months later the Thai government initiated its drug war. From their first meeting, which included training in human rights methods and harm-reduction approaches, much of the early work of TDN involved exposing the human rights violations and health-related harms caused by the state-sponsored drug war. This work included collaborations with various national and international institution partners, generating media coverage of the drug war, organizing direct actions and advocacy campaigns, and developing capacity to deliver peer-driven interventions for IDUs. Through their efforts, TDN repeatedly employed human rights and harm-reduction discourses and approaches in responding to the health-related harms that resulted from the Thai drug war. The following is a description of various actions TDN took to address the harmful consequences of this particular government-led campaign.

TDN's Response to the Drug War

TDN's work in response to the drug war began almost immediately following the announcement of the initiative. In April 2003, at the International Conference on the Reduction of Drug-related Harm in Chiang Mai, TDN took a first and brave step when its members organized a peaceful "silent protest" during a plenary welcoming presentation by the Thai Minister of Public Health, Sudarat Keyurophan (Valdimarsson, 2003). This early event proved to be pivotal for TDN, as the membership was forced to consider the potential implications of their first public appearance as a drug user organization.

During the protest TDN members and international allies from the United Kingdom, Australia, and Russia quietly filtered into the room holding bright yellow signs protesting the killing of drug users, the lack of harm-reduction policies in Thailand, and statements made by Thai politicians to cover up the crises facing drug users in Thailand. Despite their fear of potential backlash from Thai officials and local conference organizers who invited the Minister of Health to speak, TDN members held up large signs that said "clean needles save lives" and "drug users have rights too." TDN also wore shirts made by drug users living in a residential therapeutic community which included in Thai and English the words "Protect the Rights of Drug Users, Thai Government Drug Policy = Drop Dead." The T-shirts proved to be hugely popular and quickly sold out, leading TDN to make and distribute hundreds of the T-shirts at other events in the coming year.

In recognition of the harms caused by the drug war, the continuing high rates of HIV infection among IDUs, the lack of harm-reduction programming in Thailand, and the fact that many drug users had gone into hiding and thereby had become difficult to reach with prevention and treatment initiatives, TDN decided to build their capacity to deliver peer-driven care and support programs. In undertaking this effort TDN worked with the Canadian HIV/AIDS Legal Network (CHALN) and others in developing a comprehensive proposal for a peer-driven HIV/AIDS prevention, care, and support project that was submitted to the Global Fund to Fight AIDS, Tuberculosis, and Malaria (GFATM). The project included an array of activities, including: capacity building within TDN; provision of education concerning injection drug use and HIV/AIDS for health care providers, police, prison staff members, and policy makers; the establishment of four harm-reduction centers from which TDN members would provide peer-based outreach, education, counseling, and referrals, and support with voluntary HIV testing; and community-based, research-focused program evaluation, policy research, and ongoing documentation of the harms experienced by Thai IDUs.

TDN knew the GFATM proposal would be highly sensitive because of the ongoing drug war and the public support for this approach, the peer-driven nature of the proposed activities, and the fact that the Thai Global Fund "Country Coordinating Mechanism" (CCM) that oversaw previously funded GFATM projects included members who did not support an IDU-focused proposal.

Of particular relevance, therefore, was the fact that the Global Fund normally requires that all proposals be supported by a national CCM. Exceptions are granted only if (1) countries are without a legitimate government; (2) countries are in conflict or facing a natural disaster; and (3) countries suppress or have not established partnerships with civil society and nongovernmental organizations (NGOs) (Kerr et al., 2004). In light of these facts, TDN decided early on to present the proposal structure to various local stakeholders to persuade them of the need for the project, obtain feedback, and garner support through coalition building.

TDN did eventually submit the non-CCM proposal requesting 1.3 million U.S. dollars in funding, along with the numerous letters of support, to the GFATM Secretariat as a round 3 application in late April 2003. In the proposal, TDN gave the following reasons for applying without the normally required CCM approval:

(1) The government of Thailand, and Thai society in general does not currently recognize the value of harm reduction; (2) While there are public health officials in government positions who support harm reduction, they are currently unable to express this support publicly given the current policy environment; (3) the applicants made contact with the Thai CCM, and it was indicated clearly that the proposal would not receive the required support from all CCM members; (4) in light of current Thai drug policies, harm-reduction programming is ur-

gently needed, and it is drug users themselves who are in the best position to deliver harm-reduction programming as their peers may be reluctant to participate in similar government-initiated programs, as participation could be perceived to carry the risk of arrest, mandatory treatment and HIV testing-fears that could be further exacerbated given many existing practices, such as the sharing of information concerning drug users between hospitals and police; and (5) the applicants firmly believe that the Thai government will permit the proposed pilot project to proceed. (Kerr et al., 2003)

As reports of the deadly consequences of the drug war continued to emerge, TDN decided to follow up on the success of the April 2003 silent protest on June 12, 2003, by organizing and leading a mock-funeral demonstration in front of Thailand's Government House. The demonstrators carried body bags and funeral wreaths, and signs decrying the violence and injustice of the drug war. Due to growing reports of the significant number of casualties in children resulting from the drug war, TDN members also carried child-size body bags. Protestors also carried signs displaying statements such as "The next corpse could be . . . your relative" and "Does forced rehabilitation really work, Mr. Prime Minister?" TDN made several specific demands that were outlined in a letter submitted to the prime minister's office. The specific demands, which were echoed by TDN and their allies many times in the following months, were:

1. Eliminate the policies that promote violence in addressing the drug problem. Investigate each case of murder or other gross negative consequences following the government's announcement of its war on drugs.
2. Promote educational campaigns about drugs and drug use that provide comprehensive and factual information. This will result in a well-informed public and will not cause drug users to be reviled and discriminated against by society.
3. Rescind any law or policy that violates or leads to the violation of drug users' human rights, such as mandatory HIV-antibody testing, exclusion from antiretroviral therapy access for HIV-positive drug users, etc.
4. Urgently implement programs that aim to reduce the dangers associated with drug use, and provide information to prevent the spread of HIV among drug users. Establish programs to make clean needles and syringes

available, which will reduce the spread of HIV and hepatitis among injectors.

5. Cover the costs related to prevention, care, and treatment for drug users, including rehabilitation, detoxification, and substitution therapy, under the national health care plan.

6. Involve both active and former drug users at all levels to address drug-related problems in Thailand, including policy development.

At the Government House, TDN representatives met with four officials from the Thai National Task Force on Drugs, including one representative from the Narcotics Control Bureau. They discussed their concerns for an hour, and the government officials agreed to explore opportunities to address TDN's demands and recommendations at the national level. Following the demonstration in front of the Government House, TDN representatives walked to the Parliament building, where they, along with a few supportive Senators, held a briefing and press conference on the drug war crisis and the urgent need to investigate and cease government support for violent means of suppression. TDN also seized the opportunity to demand the implementation of harm-reduction approaches (e.g., syringe exchange), which remain virtually non-existent in Thailand.

Recognizing the importance of international support, TDN also called on its international partners to support their June 12 action and organized an "International Day of Action" in protest of the Thai drug war (*Drug War Chronicle*, 2003) (Figure 1.2). This day of action involved a letter-writing campaign to deplore the prime minister's drug policies and protests in various countries, including the United Kingdom, Canada, South Africa, Japan, the United States, Nepal, Australia, and Russia. In each country, individuals marched to their respective Thai embassies, presented TDN's demands in writing, prompting media outlets around the world to cover the events.

TDN became increasingly recognized as a voice for drug users that could not be ignored. In light of this, TDN increased their efforts to engage officials from various institutions and agencies. For example, in the wake of the June 12, 2003, action, in August 2003, TDN representatives presented at a meeting of the Office of Narcotics Control Board (ONCB). The goal of this meeting was to develop a working collaboration between TDN and ONCB. During the meeting, TDN representatives shared information about their organization

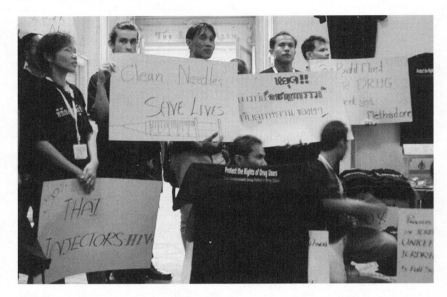

Figure 1.2. A member of TDN participates in a silent protest during the International Conference on the Reduction of Drug-related Harm (Chiang Mai). *Source*: Thai Drug Users' Network, Karyn Kaplan

and again expressed their concerns regarding the need for effective responses to the health and human rights situation facing drug users. TDN's participation in national and international task forces continued to grow when the U.N. Office of Drugs and Crime's Task Force on Drugs and HIV invited TDN to become a permanent member of the strategic planning group that same year. Since this time, TDN has continued to attend these task force meetings as drug user representatives.

Despite their efforts to promote harm-reduction approaches and greater recognition of the drug users' right to health, TDN realized that change would be slow coming and more would have to be done in the short term to address the harmful consequences of the drug war. In the light of this, TDN continued to seek opportunities to develop capacity within its organization to deliver and advocate for harm-reduction programming. This was accomplished through a series of training sessions in harm reduction and human rights for its members that were funded through various sources including the International Harm Reduction Association, the Open Society Institute, and UNAIDS. However, to promote these approaches among other stakeholders, TDN also frequently involved government employees, such as representatives from the Ministry of Public Health, in these training sessions. Through these activities, which involved organizations such as the Thai AIDS Treatment Action Group (TTAG) and the Center for AIDS Rights, TDN members increased their knowledge of human rights and harm-reduction approaches, and in the months following, an increasing number of TDN members would speak publicly at demonstrations and to the media about the need for greater recognition of the rights of drug users as well as the need for harm-reduction approaches within Thailand. The importance of TDN's ongoing media work was underscored by the fact that Prime Minister Shinawatra retained his ownership over many major Thai outlets after being elected, and in doing so was able to hide many of the worst aspects of the drug war.

On December 3, 2003, two days before the king of Thailand's birthday, Prime Minister Shinawatra declared victory in the drug war, calling the campaign a major success (BBC News, 2003). TDN was, however, well prepared for this announcement and on December 4, 2003, again engaged in direct action to protest the ongoing drug war. On this day, TDN and its allies gathered at Thammasat University in Bangkok to perform "a ceremony" in honor of King Bhumibol Adulyadej's birthday. Wearing bright yellow T-shirts, carrying bright yellow banners and signs, TDN sang songs for the king and later issued a letter saying, "We have resolved to reduce or quit our drug use and to give our loving support to our friends who still struggle with drug use; to express our love and loyalty to our King . . . on his birthday; and to demonstrate our own commitment to solving drug-related problems." These messages were delicately crafted as the Thai public has historically only received negative messages about drugs (e.g., "drugs and drug users are bad," "abstinence is the only solution"). Discussing drugs in relation to the king was a sensitive matter and therefore the message had to be expressed carefully to avoid alienating the public who adore their king. TDN also requested that the king of Thailand intervene in the government's drug war to "reverse the . . . failed campaign of violence and suppression" and promote the rights of drug users, and also referred to their members' direct experience of the adverse effects of the drug war. In undertaking this action on the day before the king's birthday, TDN hoped that the king would, in his annual public birthday speech, which is televised across the country, denounce the drug war. Despite the declaration made by the prime minister, the king did make reference to the drug war during his address and the called on the prime minister to take responsibility for the associated killings and conduct appropriate investigations, simultaneously abhorring the prime minister's "arrogance" vis-à-vis local and international concern over domestic crises such as the drug war (Cohen, 2004).

Although the prime minister of Thailand declared "victory" in the ten-month drug war, this government campaign continued, leading TDN to continue its efforts to highlight the human rights violations associated with the drug war. During April and May 2004, TDN assisted researchers from Human Rights Watch (New York) in investigating human rights violations associated with the drug war. This led to the release of a comprehensive report titled "Not Enough Graves" that documented an array of human rights violations, including discrimination against drug users by police and within health care settings, arbitrary arrest and blacklisting, breaches of due process, intimidation, violence, coerced or mandatory drug treatment, and exclusion from essential health care including government sponsored HIV/AIDS treatment programs (Cohen, 2004). The report also contained a series of recommendations for the government of Thailand and the United Nations, as well as international donors to Thailand. Included was a call to end human rights violations associated with the war on drugs and calls for appropriate harm reduction and HIV prevention services for drug users in community and prison settings.

In July 2004 the International AIDS Society (IAS) Conference took place in Bangkok. TDN then seized opportunities throughout the IAS meeting to mobilize their membership and allies in an effort to raise awareness of Thailand's drug war and the health issues facing drug users. In the days leading up to the conference, members of TDN managed to meet face to face with the prime minister and raised concerns regarding the lack of appropriate health care and harm-reduction programming for drug users. During the conference TDN also made efforts to "shame" the U.N. Office of Drugs and Crime, the World Health Organization, and UNAIDS for their lack of leadership in promoting best practices in HIV prevention and treatment for IDUs, and for failing to criticize the Thai government for continuing the drug war. Several initiatives were organized around this conference, including a public demonstration on July 11, 2004, in which TDN members, their international allies, and representatives from the Thai Network of People Living with HIV/AIDS (TNP+), demanded greater recognition of the health and human rights issues facing drug users. For this demonstration, TDN members wore T-shirts displaying the words "Clean needles, Methadone, and AIDS Treatment for Drug Users-No More Drug War." These T-shirts, like previous TDN T-shirts, were immensely popular and were purchased by conference delegates from around the world. As well, during the conference TDN distributed 10,000 pins that said "Stop the War on Drug Users" and distributed 10,000 sterile syringes as a means of advocating for the establishment of syringe distribution programs in Thailand and elsewhere. The sterile syringe kits also included information about the HIV and human rights crisis among IDUs internationally, and called on individuals and organizations to demand that methadone and buprenorphine be added to the World Health Organization's Essential Drugs List.

Following the International AIDS Conference, TDN continued its advocacy and activism in an effort to address the health and human rights situation facing drug users. In addition to ongoing training in harm reduction and human rights for its memberships, TDN continued to raise money to further its work locally and internationally and continued to raise awareness of the drug war and the need for harm-reduction programs through regular presentations, including presentations to the Vietnam government, the Centers for Disease Control Global AIDS Project in Cambodia, and presentations at the International Conference on Drug-related Harm. TDN also garnered greater attention for its work, and was invited on a regular basis to join various policy-making initiatives and task forces specific to drug and HIV/AIDS policy. Despite the fact that TDN became increasingly involved in more formal policy-making initiatives, the organization did not lose sight of its grassroots origins and did not cease from engaging in direct actions relevant to their mission. One of the more notable events occurred in October 2004, when TDN mobilized more than 130 drug users and persons living with HIV/AIDS and protested outside the board meeting for GFATM taking place in Chiang Mai. TDN made several demands, including that the GFATM board give serious attention to TDN's proposal that was then being considered for funding. The GFATM Secretariat's screening committee had approved TDN's proposal for consideration by the Technical Review Panel, which subsequently recommended that the application be approved by the GFATM Board (Kerr et al., 2004). Following the GFATM's third-round review, the GFATM Board bravely approved the application despite the lack of support from Thailand's CCM, and despite the fact that the application failed to clearly meet any of the GFATM non-CCM exemption criteria described above (Kerr et al., 2004). Because the GFATM approved TDN's non-CCM application from Thailand, but did so outside its stated criteria, the GFATM Board has since asked the GFATM Secretariat to re-examine its non-CCM criteria and generate options and recommendations that can be applied for future rounds of the GFATM (Kerr et al., 2004). Collectively the actions of TDN served to expose the limitations associated with the GFATM CCM criteria, which are amplified in circumstances where those with HIV or at risk for HIV are highly marginalized within their own country (Kerr et al., 2004). This was clearly the case in Thailand, where despite the existence of an established CCM, much needed public health interventions were not implemented because they were highly incongruent with national government policies. In recognition of their efforts to address the drug war, in 2004, TDN was given the International Award for Action on HIV/AIDS and Human Rights by Human Rights Watch and the Canadian HIV/AIDS Legal Network (Canadian HIV/AIDS Legal Network, 2004).

Looking Ahead

Thailand's drug war illustrates the severe human rights violations and health-related harms that can result from enforcement-based approaches to illegal drug use. The story of TDN on the other hand provides a powerful illustration of how affected communities can mobilize and counter the horrific effects of such drug enforcement. Despite the growing body of evidence showing the harms resulting from these approaches, the dominant response to illegal drug use in both developed and developing countries has, as in Thailand, been to intensify law enforcement in an effort to limit the supply and use of drugs (Drucker, 1999; Knutsson, 2000; Wodak, 2001; Kerr et al., 2004). The use of law enforcement as an isolated intervention has, however, become increasingly controversial because a rapidly growing body of research has demonstrated that these approaches often produce an array of physical, social, and behavioral effects that result in the exacerbation of health-related harms and the violation of internationally established human rights (Burris et al., 2004).

Aside from the obvious direct harms (e.g., beatings, killings), many additional direct and indirect health consequences are associated with aggressive forms of enforcement aimed at illicit drug users. For instance, in creating a climate of fear and discrimination, drug users may be discouraged from accessing essential health care, including HIV prevention and addiction treatment services. Numerous studies have now demonstrated that IDUs are often reluctant to access syringe exchanges or carry syringes on their person out of fear of arrest or harsher sentences (Grund et al., 1992a, 1995; Zule, 1992; Koester, 1994; Gleghorn et al., 1995; Bluthenthal et al., 1997; Bourgois, 1998; Weinstein et al., 1998; Bluthenthal, 1999; Diaz et al., 1999; Bastos and Strathdee, 2000; Rhodes et al., 2003). This has resulted in observations of lower syringe access during periods of intense enforcement (Grund et al., 1992b; Maher and Dixon, 1999; Aitken et al., 2002; Wood et al., 2003; Cohen, 2004; Davis et al., in press), an effect that is particularly worrisome given that low access to sterile syringes due to enforcement pressure has been associated with elevated rates of syringe sharing among IDUs (Maher and Dixon, 1999; Aitken, et al. 2002; Rhodes et al., 2003). Also, when discrimination against drug users is widely promoted within society, drug users are less likely to disclose their drug use to their social support networks and health care providers, which in turn can lead to lower uptake of addiction treatment and health services for various medical conditions, and poor health in general due to reduced social support (Rhodes et al., 2005).

Considerable health-related harms can also result from the physical displacement of IDUs into remote and hidden locations. The classic example of this type of displacement observed in North America is the "shooting gallery" (Des Jarlais and Friedman, 1990). Whereas various environments where drug users hide and consume drugs have been described, most are hidden indoor locations where drug dealing and high-risk behaviors flourish. Included are settings where drug users share syringes (Neaigus et al., 1994), store syringes for future use (Rhodes et al., 2003), or receive injections from professional dealers/injectors who use the same syringe to inject several customers (Ball et al., 1998). The use of such shooting galleries has been repeatedly attributed to fear of arrest (Celentano et al., 1991; Schneider, 1998) and has been associated with increased reuse and/or sharing of syringes (Latkin et al., 1994; Lachance et al., 1996). Consequently, shooting gallery attendance has been associated with increased risk for HIV infection (Chaisson et al., 1987; Battjes et al., 1994; Zolopa et al., 1994).

Intense enforcement campaigns can also prompt changes in injection behavior that exacerbate risk for adverse health outcomes. IDUs are known to rush during the injection process to avoid being caught by police while in possession of illicit drugs (Maher and Dixon, 1999, 2001; Aitken et al., 2002; Dixon and Maher, 2002; Small et al., in press). In turn, rushing during the injection process can lead to several harms. For example, IDUs are more likely to skip important steps in the preparation of drug solutions (Maher and Dixon, 1999; Broadhead et al., 2002). Similarly, when injecting in a hurry, IDUs may be less likely to clean injection sites before injection or dress wounds afterward (Broadhead et al., 2002), and risk of vascular damage increases as syringes are inserted in a hurried manner (Maher and Dixon, 2001). These practices substantially increase risks for abscesses and bacterial infections (Murphy et al., 2001). Evidence has also indicated that IDUs are also more likely to engage in indirect sharing of injection equipment during the preparation of drug solutions as a result of hurried injection (Maher and Dixon, 2001). Rushing may also increase risk for overdose when drugs, in particular, opiates, are injected quickly and not first tested for strength (Maher and Dixon, 2001; Broadhead et al., 2002).

Further health-related harms likely resulted from the widespread incarceration of drug users during intense periods of enforcement. Although IDUs typically inject less frequently in prisons (Shewan et al., 1994; Dolan et al., 1996), studies have demonstrated that the injections that occur tend to be carried out in a more "high-risk" fashion than injections in community settings, due in large part to a lack of sterile syringes in prisons (Darke et al., 1998; Malliori et al., 1998). Studies from Thailand have indicated that up to 16 percent of IDUs incarcerated admitted injecting drugs in jail (Beyrer et al., 2003), and incarceration has been associated with HIV incidence among drug users in various settings (Rich et al., 1999; Choopanya et al., 2002; Buavirat et al., 2003; Tyndall et al., 2003).

The Thai Drug Users' Network (TDN) formed in December 2002, and soon after the drug war was launched, TDN mobilized its membership and allies in response to this government-led campaign. Like drug user organizations in other settings, TDN has repeatedly undertaken various forms of activism, advocacy, and public education in an effort to demonstrate the links between health and human rights. Since its earliest actions, TDN repeatedly employed human rights methods and discourses to raise awareness of the health issues facing drug users and the severe harms caused by the Thai government's drug war.

TDN was created in response to the findings of a local human rights docu-

mentation project, and consistent with TDN's future efforts, this project resulted from an effective collaboration between Thai and non-Thai organizations. By documenting and presenting the horrific health and human rights
conditions faced by Thai IDUs, TDN, like other drug user organizations, gave
voice to a highly marginalized population with few opportunities to speak for
itself. These early efforts served to quickly mobilize its membership and allies,
who subsequently took swift and courageous action rooted in human rights
discourses. TDN's work with Human Rights Watch ensures that the links between human rights, health, and the drug war remain evident to observers
throughout the world.

Like many of the more powerful responses to the AIDS epidemic, which
were not based on expert-driven interventions but on mobilizing affected
communities to resist oppression (Epstein, 1996; Stoller, 1998), TDN repeatedly voiced the concerns of drug users in various arenas, countered dominant constructions of drug users, and increased awareness of the need for
harm-reduction programs in Thailand. In taking the courageous step of publicly presenting themselves as current and former drug users, TDN countered
stereotypical constructions of "the drug user," creating what Castells (1997)
referred to as "project identities" that serve to redefine positions in society and
transform larger social structures (Castells, 1996). This transformation was
evident in TDN's increasing recognition as a legitimate voice for drug users
and their increasing participation in policy-making initiatives and decisions
that affect them. Humanizing "drug users" in this context proved to be of immense importance given the efforts of the Thai government to portray drug
users as evil threats to Thai society.

A further key to the success of TDN was the ongoing and constant development of coalitions within and outside of Thailand. The leaders of the organization attended national and international meetings to make others aware
of the situation facing Thai drug users, and garnered additional support from
their allies by drawing attention to the drug war. TDN also balanced its direct action efforts with participation in formal policy development initiatives,
which in turn increased the profile and credibility of the organization. This
growing recognition led to TDN eventually obtaining funding to develop its
own peer-driven interventions from GFATM. In obtaining this funding, TDN
not only enhanced HIV prevention and care in Thailand, but also exposed serious limitations in the policies of GFATM.

Throughout its work, TDN also continually developed the capacity of its membership. TDN members received extensive and ongoing training in human rights methods and harm-reduction approaches, and were continually informed of emerging research evidence and policy development related to drug use and HIV/AIDS in Thailand and internationally. These training sessions and sharing of information serve to empower TDN members to articulate their concerns and needs in various arenas, including policy-making environments and when addressing politicians and the public through the media.

Drug user organizations throughout the world have demonstrated that they can organize themselves to resist oppression and advocate for the recognition of their right to health (Kerr, in press). TDN worked tirelessly to build coalitions, increase public awareness, and counter state-sponsored messages concerning drug users and the severe health effects of Thailand's brutal drug war. This experience demonstrates the powerful role that affected communities can play in addressing their own immediate health and human rights concerns, and highlights the importance of incorporating the activities of these communities into existing public health, education, and policy-making frameworks.

References

Adams, B. 2003. Thailand's crackdown: drug war kills democracy too. *International Herald Tribune*, April 24, 2003, 8.

Aitken, C., Moore, D., Higgs, P., Kelsall, J., and Kerger, M. 2002. The impact of a police crackdown on a street drug scene: evidence from the street. *International Journal of Drug Policy* 13:189–98.

Amnesty International. 2003. *Thailand: grave developments: killings and other abuses*, AI Index ASA 39/008/03 (November 2003). Wanchai: Amnesty International..

Asia Times. 2003. Thailand's drug war gets messy. February 14.

Ball, A. L., Rana, S., and Dehne, K. L. 1998. HIV prevention among injecting drug users: responses in developing and transitional countries. *Public Health Reports* 113:170–81.

Bastos, F. I., and Strathdee, S. A. 2000. Evaluating effectiveness of syringe exchange programmes: current issues and future prospects. *Social Science and Medicine* 51:1771–82.

Battjes, R. J., Pickens, R. W., Haverkos, H. W., and Sloboda, Z. 1994. HIV risk factors among injecting drug users in five US cities. *AIDS* 8:681–87.

BBC News. 2003. Thailand's bloody drug war. February 24.

Beyrer, C., Jittiwutikarn, J., Teokul, W., Razak, M. H., Suriyanon, V., et al. 2003. Drug use, increasing incarceration rates, and prison-associated HIV risks in Thailand. *AIDS Behavior* 7:153–61.

Beyrer, C., Razak, M. H., Jittiwutikarn, J., Suriyanon, V., Vongchak, T., et al. 2004. Methamphetamine users in northern Thailand: changing demographics and risks for HIV and STD among treatment-seeking substance abusers. *International Journal of STD and AIDS* 15:697–704.

Bluthenthal, R. N., Kral, A. H., Lorvick, J., and Watters, J. K. 1997. Impact of law enforcement on syringe exchange programs: a look at Oakland and San Francisco. *Medical Anthropology* 18:61–83.

Bluthenthal, R. N., Lorvick, J., Kral, A., Erringer, E. A., and Kahn, J. G. 1999. Collateral damage in the war on drugs: HIV risk behaviors among injection drug users. *International Journal of Drug Policy* 10:25–38.

Bourgois, P. 1998. The moral economics of homeless heroin addicts: confronting ethnography, HIV risk, and everyday violence in San Francisco shooting encampments. *Substance Use and Misuse* 33:2323–51.

Broadhead, R. S., Kerr, T. H., Grund, J.-P. C, and Altice, F. L. 2002. Safer injection facilities in North America: their place in public policy and health initiatives. *Journal of Drug Issues* 32:329–55.

Buavirat, A., Page-Shafer, K., van Griensven, G. J., Mandel, J. S., Evans, J., et al. 2003. Risk of prevalent HIV infection associated with incarceration among injecting drug users in Bangkok, Thailand: case-control study. *British Medical Journal* 326:308.

Burris, S., Blankenship, K. M., and Donoghoe, M. 2004. Addressing the "risk environment" for injection drug users: The mysterious case of the missing cop. *Milbank Quarterly* 82:125–56.

Canadian HIV/AIDS Legal Network. 2004. Thai Drug Users Network receives human rights award. *HIV/AIDS Policy & Law Review* 9:37.

Castells, M. 1996. *The power of identity.* Oxford: Blackwell Publishers.

Celentano, D. D. 2003. HIV prevention among drug users: an international perspective from Thailand. *Journal of Urban Health* 80 (iii):97–105.

Celentano, D. D., Hodge, M. J., Razak, M. H., Beyrer, C., Kawichai, S., et al. 1999. HIV-1 incidence among opiate users in northern Thailand. *American Journal of Epidemiology* 149:558–64.

Celentano, D. D., Vlahov, D., Cohn, S., Anthony, J. C., Solomon, L., and Nelson, K. E. 1991. Risk factors for shooting gallery use and cessation among intravenous drug users. *American Journal of Public Health* 81:1291–95.

Chaisson, R. E., Moss, A. R., Onishi, R., Osmond, D., and Carlson, J. R. 1987. Human immunodeficiency virus infection in heterosexual intravenous drug users in San Francisco. *American Journal of Public Health* 77:169–72.

Choopanya, K., Des Jarlais, D.C., Vanichseni, S., Kitayaporn, D., Mock, P. A., et al. 2002. Incarceration and risk for HIV infection among injection drug users in Bangkok. *Journal of Acquired Immune Deficiency Syndrome* 29:86–94.

Cohen, J. 2004. *Not enough graves. Human Rights Watch*, 16 (8). http://hrw.org/reports/2004/thailand0704.

Darke, S., Kaye, S., and Finlay-Jones, R. 1998. Drug use and injection risk-taking among prison methadone maintenance patients. *Addiction* 93:1169–75.

Davis, C. B. S., Metzger, D., Becher, J., and Lynch, K. In press. Effects of an intensive street-level police intervention on syringe exchange program utilization: Philadelphia, Pennsylvania. *American Journal of Public Health.*

Des Jarlais, D. C., and Friedman, S. R. 1990. Shooting galleries and AIDS: infection probabilities and 'tough' policies. *American Journal of Public Health* 80:142–44.

Diaz, T., Vlahov, D., Hadden, B., and Edwards, V. 1999. Needle and syringe acquisition among young injection drug users in Harlem, New York City. *National HIV Prevention Conference* 654.

Dixon, D., and Maher, L. 2002. Anh Hai: Policing, culture and social exclusion in a street heroin market. *Policing and Society* 12:93–110.

Dolan, K., Hall, W., and Wodak, A. 1996. Methadone maintenance reduces injecting in prison. *British Medical Journal* 312:1162.

Drucker, E. 1999. Drug prohibition and public health: twenty-five years of evidence. *Public Health Reports* 114:14–29.

Drug War Chronicle. 2003. Stop the murder of Thai drug users—International Day of Action. June 12.

Ehrlich, R. S. 2003. Thailand's drug war leaves a bloody trail. *Washington Times.* February 21.

Epstein, S. 1996. *Impure science: AIDS, activism and the politics of knowledge.* Berkeley: University of California Press.

Gleghorn, A. A., Jones, T. S., Doherty, M. C., Celentano, D. D., and Vlahov, D. 1995. Acquisition and use of needles and syringes by injecting drug users in Baltimore, Maryland. *Journal of Acquired Immune Deficiency Syndrome and Human Retrovirology* 10:97–103.

Government of Thailand. 2003. A fight to overcome drugs. Order of the Prime Minister's Office no. 29/B.E. 2546.

Grund, J. P., Blanken, P., Adriaans, N. F., Kaplan, C. D., Barendregt, C., and Meeuwsen, M. 1992a. Reaching the unreached: targeting hidden IDU populations with clean needles via known user groups. *Journal of Psychoactive Drugs* 24:41–47.

Grund, J. P., Heckathorn, D. D., Broadhead, R. S., and Anthony, D. L. 1995. In eastern Connecticut, IDUs purchase syringes from pharmacies but don't carry syringes. *Journal of Acquired Immune Deficiency Syndrome and Human Retrovirology* 10: 104–5.

Grund, J. P., Stern, L. S., Kaplan, C. D., Adriaans, N. F., and Drucker, E. 1992b. Drug use contexts and HIV-consequences: the effect of drug policy on patterns of everyday drug use in Rotterdam and the Bronx. *British Journal of Addiction* 87: 381–92.

Kaplan, K., and Suwannawong, P. 2002. *The AIDS and human rights crisis among injecting drug users in Thailand.* Presented at The XIV International AIDS Conference, Barcelona.

Kerr, T., Ishida, T., Suwannawong, P., and Panitchakdi, P. 2003. *Global Fund third round proposal: Preventing HIV/AIDS and increasing care and support for injection drug users in Thailand.* Bangkok: Raks Thai Foundation.

Kerr, T., Kaplan, K., Suwannawong, P., Jurgens, R., and Wood, E. 2004. The Global Fund to Fight AIDS, Tuberculosis and Malaria: Funding for unpopular public-health programmes. *The Lancet* 364:11–12.

Kerr, T., Small, W., Peeace, W., Douglas, D., Pierre, A., and Wood, E. 2006. Harm reduction by a "user-run" organization: A case study of the Vancouver Area Network of Drug Users (VANDU). *International Journal of Drug Policy* 17 (2):61–69.

Knutsson, J. 2000. Swedish drug markets and drugs policy. In *Illegal drug markets: from research to policy*, ed. M. Hough and M. Natarajan, 179–202. Monsey, NJ: Criminal Justice Press.

Koester, S. K. 1994. Copping, running, and paraphernalia laws: Contextual variables and needle risk behavior among injection drug users in Denver. *Human Organization* 53:287–95.

Lachance, N., Lamothe, F., Bruneau, J., Franco, E., Vincelette, J., and Soto, J. 1996. Injecting and sharing IV equipment in different cities: a potential risk for HIV dissemination. Abstract. *International Conference on AIDS* 11:351.

Latkin, C., Mandell, W., Vlahov, D., Oziemkowska, M., Knowlton, A., and Celentano, D. 1994. My place, your place, and no place: Behavior settings as a risk factor for HIV-related injection practices of drug users in Baltimore, Maryland. *American Journal of Community Psychology* 22:415–30.

Maher, L., and Dixon, D. 1999. Policing and public health: Law enforcement and harm minimization in a street-level drug market. *British Journal of Criminology* 39:488–512.

Maher, L., and Dixon, D. 2001. The cost of crackdowns: Policing Cabramatta's heroin market. *Current Issues in Criminal Justice* 13:5–22.

Malliori, M., Sypsa, V., Psichogiou, M., Touloumi, G., Skoutelis, A., et al. 1998. A survey of bloodborne viruses and associated risk behaviours in Greek prisons. *Addiction* 93:243–51.

Mastro, T. D., Kitayaporn, D., Weniger, B. G., Vanichseni, S., Laosunthorn, V., et al. 1994. Estimating the number of HIV-infected injection drug users in Bangkok: a capture–recapture method [see comments]. *American Journal of Public Health* 84:1094–99.

Murphy, E. L., DeVita, D., Liu, H., Vittinghoff, E., Leung, P., et al. 2001. Risk factors for skin and soft-tissue abscesses among injection drug users: a case-control study. *Clinical Infectious Diseases* 33:35–40.

Neaigus, A., Friedman, S. R., Curtis, R., Des Jarlais, D. C., Furst, R. T., et al. 1994. The relevance of drug injectors' social and risk networks for understanding and preventing HIV infection. *Social Science and Medicine* 38:67–78.

Razak, M. H., Jittiwutikarn, J., Suriyanon, V., Vongchak, T., Srirak, N., et al. 2003. HIV prevalence and risks among injection and noninjection drug users in northern Thailand: Need for comprehensive HIV prevention programs. *Journal of Acquired Immune Deficiency Syndromes* 33:259–66.

Rhodes, T., Mikhailova, L., Sarang, A., Lowndes, C. M., Rylkov, A., et al. 2003. Situational factors influencing drug injecting, risk reduction and syringe exchange in Togliatti City, Russian Federation: a qualitative study of micro risk environment. *Social Science and Medicine* 57:39–54.

Rhodes, T., Singer, M., Bourgois, P., Friedman, S. R., and Strathdee, S. A. 2005. The social structural production of HIV risk among injecting drug users. *Social Science and Medicine* 61:1026–44.

Rich, J. D., Dickinson, B. P., Macalino, G., Flanigan, T. P., Towe, C. W., et al. 1999. Prevalence and incidence of HIV among incarcerated and reincarcerated women in Rhode Island. *Journal of Acquired Immune Deficiency Syndromes* 22:161–66.

Schneider, C. L. 1998. Racism, drug policy and AIDS. *Political Science Quarterly* 113:427–46.

Shewan, D., Gemmell, M., and Davies, J. B. 1994. Behavioural change amongst drug injectors in Scottish prisons. *Social Science and Medicine* 39:1585–86.

Small, W., Kerr, T., Charette, J., Wood, E., Schechter, M. T., and Spittal, P. M. 2006. Impact of intensified police activity upon injection drug users in Vancouver's Downtown Eastside: Evidence from an ethnographic investigation. *International Journal of Drug Policy* 17 (2):85–95.

Srirak, N., Kawichai, S., Vongchak, T., Razak, M. H., Jittiwuttikarn, J., et al. 2005. HIV infection among female drug users in Northern Thailand. *Drug and Alcohol Dependence* 78:141–45.

Srisurapanont, M., Ali, R., Marsden, J., Sunga, A., Wada, K., and Monteiro, M. 2003. Psychotic symptoms in methamphetamine psychotic in-patients. *International Journal of Neuropsychopharmacology* 6:347–52.

Stoller, N. 1998. *Less from the damned: queers, whores, and junkies respond to AIDS.* New York: Routledge.

Tyndall, M. W., Currie, S., Spittal, P., Li, K., Wood, E., et al. 2003. Intensive injection cocaine use as the primary risk factor in the Vancouver HIV-1 epidemic. *AIDS* 17:887–93.

Valdimarsson, O. 2003. *Harm reduction conference opens with call for better treatment.* Geneva: Red Cross Red Crescent.

Vanichseni, S., Kitayaporn, D., Mastro, T. D., Mock, P. A., Raktham, S., et al. 2001. Continued high HIV-1 incidence in a vaccine trial preparatory cohort of injection drug users in Bangkok, Thailand. *AIDS* 15:397–405.

Weinstein, B., Toce, P., Katz, D., and Ryan, L. L. 1998. Peer education of pharmacists and supplying pharmacies with IDU packets to increase injection drug users' access to sterile syringes in Connecticut. *Journal of Acquired Immune Deficiency Syndrome and Human Retrovirology* 18 (Suppl. 1):S146–47.

Wodak, A. 2001. Drug laws. War on drugs does more harm than good. *British Medical Journal* 323:866.

Wood, E., Kerr, T., Small, W., Jones, J., Schechter, M. T., and Tyndall, M. W. 2003. The impact of police presence on access to needle exchange programs. *Journal of Acquired Immune Deficiency Syndromes* 34:116–18.

Zolopa, A. R., Hahn, J. A., Gorter, R., Miranda, J., Wlodarczyk, D., et al. 1994. HIV and tuberculosis infection in San Francisco's homeless adults. Prevalence and risk factors in a representative sample. *Journal of the American Medical Association* 272:455–61.

Zule, W. A. 1992. Risk and reciprocity: HIV and the injection drug user. *Journal of Psychoactive Drugs* 24:243–49.

2

The Impact of Human Rights Violations on Health among Internally Displaced Persons in Conflict Zones

Burma

Thomas J. Lee, M.D., M.H.S., Luke C. Mullany, Ph.D., M.H.S.,
Adam K. Richards, M.D., M.P.H., Cynthia Maung, M.B.B.S.,
Htee Moo, and Mahn Mahn

The makeshift hut in an eastern Burma[1] rain forest is filled with mostly women and children, who have been waiting. Although they will wait, sitting quietly on woven mats, for only a few hours today, in reality this community has been waiting for months. Saw Htoo, an ethnic Karen health worker and refugee, has at last arrived. After a treacherous three weeks clandestinely crossing the Thai-Burma border, fording rivers, traversing mountain passes, evading military patrols and landmines, and carrying six months of medical supplies to serve his charge of roughly 2,000 people, his team has reached this community and their wait is temporarily over. Saw Htoo is part of the Backpack Health Worker Team, a network of ethnically diverse, indigenous health workers who travel their war-torn land to serve largely internally displaced persons who would otherwise have no access to formal health care. He will spend several days in this village treating malaria, respiratory infections, diarrhea, and anemia, administering vitamin A supplements and deworming medicine, encouraging breastfeeding and bed nets, and collecting health information. He would stay longer, but, as he explained, "The villagers must eventually report our presence or risk punishment from military authorities. However, they give us advance notice so we have enough time to escape."

The Four Cuts Policy and the Black Zones of Eastern Burma

Saw Htoo must escape the troops of the Burmese military junta, the State Peace and Development Council (SPDC). The regime's Four Cuts Policy is a counterinsurgency campaign executed against civilians since 1962 which aims to cut the four crucial links between "insurgents" and local villages: food, funds, recruits, and information. The cornerstones of this policy include detention, torture, rape, and execution of villagers in resistance areas; systematic destruction of crops, food supplies, and livestock; forced labor and military conscription (including children); and forced relocation (Karen Human Rights Group, 2000; U.S. Department of Labor, 2000; Norwegian Refugee Council, 2003; International Labour Organization, 2004; Shan Human Rights Foundation, 2002). The Karen, Karenni, and Mon ethnic peoples living between the military-controlled central plains and the mountainous Thai-Burma border are a subset of those targeted by this campaign. They survive in what the junta designates "black zones," where international assistance is prohibited and an estimated 600,000 to 1,000,000 people have been displaced (Burmese Border Consortium, 2002).

Within these black zones, the military regime ruling Burma has not allowed access to international relief organizations, effectively shielding from scrutiny the health-related effects of this decades-long conflict. "No one comes to count our births and deaths," note local health workers. No one, in fact, has come to document the births and deaths of more than a generation of people, many of whom have lived their entire lives during the Four Cuts policy. Despite $47 million provided by U.N. agencies in 2000, 11 million euros by the European Union from 1996 to 2002, and 30 international nongovernmental organizations (NGOs) providing $7 million per year in humanitarian aid (United Nations, 2005), no SPDC-sponsored or international nongovernmental health activities originating from within Burma have been reported in these zones.

Consequently, information on the health effect of the SPDC military regime's Four Cuts policy and the health status of these populations has been nonexistent. Recent national statistics underestimate the true magnitude of this situation because they depend on surveys that generally do not access black zone populations (United Nations Children's Fund [UNICEF], 2005). Even the World Food Program, which feeds more than 1 percent of Burma, reported that, although one-third of the children in Burma are suffering from malnutrition, they "were being prevented by the junta from assessing a true national figure of those in need, which was likely to be much higher" (World Food Program, 2004). The junta policies limiting access by agencies operating within Burma became so restrictive in 2005 that the Global Fund to Fight Aids, Tuberculosis and Malaria, in a moment of clarity, terminated $98 million in grant agreements.

Access is also restricted from the Thai side of the border, a situation that highlights the contrast between refugee and internally displaced person (IDP) resource allocation. Although 130,000 refugees in Thailand receive roughly $20 million of annual direct humanitarian assistance from a consortium of agencies, the much larger number of IDPs across the border in Burma receive no support from these sources. Organizations providing support for refugees are not permitted by Thai authorities to provide cross-border relief, in observance of international borders, and reflecting Thai concern for SPDC relations.

Continuing human rights violations, restriction of humanitarian aid, grave health status, enormous gaps in health information, and an imbalance in resource distribution are not unique to the IDPs of eastern Burma. While individuals who cross an international border can claim protection and assistance under the 1951 refugee convention as refugees, those who remain within their home country have no similar recourse. Because of international law's long-standing principle of national sovereignty, IDPs are often forced to rely on protection and assistance mediated by their governments. In some settings, this aid is prevented by the passive neglect of incompetent or underfunded ministries of health; in others, such as Burma, the active oppression by the ruling body is the cause of the displacement. Even when a local government is supportive, active conflict, lack of security, poor infrastructure, and overriding economic and political incentives prevent the effective delivery of health services and other relief. As a result, the 21.3 million IDPs worldwide received vastly less attention than the 11.5 million refugees (U.S. Committee for Refugees, 2005), despite their far greater numbers. Population-based interventions that would normally be provided via the channels appropriate for refugee settings are generally lacking for IDPs (Norwegian Refugee Council, 2004).

Unlike large international relief organizations, indigenous health workers who live and work within the displaced communities have a unique opportunity to penetrate the black zones. Mobile teams of indigenous Karen, Karenni, and Mon health workers in eastern Burma have recently organized to better coordinate health care delivery and documentation efforts. Despite poor security, population mobility, and lack of resources, they have succeeded in conducting a series of surveys demonstrating mortality rates that are the highest in Southeast Asia, and comparable to the countries with the worst mortality rates in Sub-Saharan Africa. Data collected by these mobile teams demonstrate the much poorer health status of IDP populations in eastern Burma, the high proportion of deaths due to preventable illness, landmines, and other violent causes, and the impact of military regime policies and widespread abuses of human rights.

Much of the progress in measuring the health status of these IDP communities in eastern Burma has been possible through a partnership between ethnic minority health leaders along the Thai-Burma border and our group, Global Health Access Program (GHAP; www.ghap.org). GHAP is a nonprofit organization working to improve the well-being of communities in crisis through the provision of health and public health services, capacity building, and resource enhancement. We have had a long-term, close working relationship with border health groups, including the mobile medical teams, since 1998 and have emphasized the development of skills, knowledge, and local resources that are essential for capacity building and sustainability. Our volunteers have provided technical support for medical and public health programs, health worker training, and health information systems, and advocated on behalf of border groups through fundraising, grant writing, and raising awareness through the media. In this chapter, we report on our collaborative efforts with the cross-border health programs to describe the effect of ongoing conflict and human rights violations in eastern Burma on the health status of internally displaced communities.

Penetrating the Black Zones: Health Care and Information

Although the ethnic groups along the Thai-Burma border have a long history of lay health workers, the indigenous health movement was given a dramatic boost by the arrival of Dr. Cynthia Maung. A physician and refugee herself, she fled Burma following the military regime's brutal response to the 1988 prodemocracy uprising and established the Mae Tao Clinic (MTC) to address the health needs of displaced persons on the Thai-Burma border. Over the ensuing 17 years, the MTC has grown to its current capacity, with more than 100,000 patient-care visits in 2004, and has trained hundreds of health workers. For this work, Dr. Maung and health workers received the Jonathan Mann (1999) and Ramon Magsaysay awards (2002).

When it became clear, however, that the MTC was unable to reach the neediest inside Burma, Dr. Maung teamed with local ethnic leaders to form the Backpack Health Worker Team (BPHWT). This multiethnic organization of mobile medical teams conducts health activities for a population of approximately 140,000 IDPs living largely in black zones in Karen, Karenni, and Mon territories. Since its inception, the program has expanded to seventy teams of three to five health workers ("backpack medics") plus essential support staff members, who travel on foot, carrying backpacks of medical supplies, educational materials, and data-collection instruments. Working in cooperation with community leaders, the health workers provide curative and preventative services, and deliver educational messages on a variety of public health topics such as water and sanitation, family planning, malaria prevention, landmine awareness, and others.

The target population is dispersed throughout nine townships (all seven Karen townships, southern Karenni, and northern Mon), varying in size between 5,000 and 25,000 people. There are more than 600 villages with a median size of 200 people. Each township is subdivided into "village tracts" supervised by a senior health worker who is responsible for coordinating the teams in his/her area. The medics in each team travel between as many villages as possible in their assigned village tract, which includes anywhere from three to twelve villages, in addition to numerous small temporary communities "hiding" from SPDC soldiers. A schematic diagram of worker movement is shown in Figure 2.1.

The teams carry medical supplies designed to serve a population of 2,000

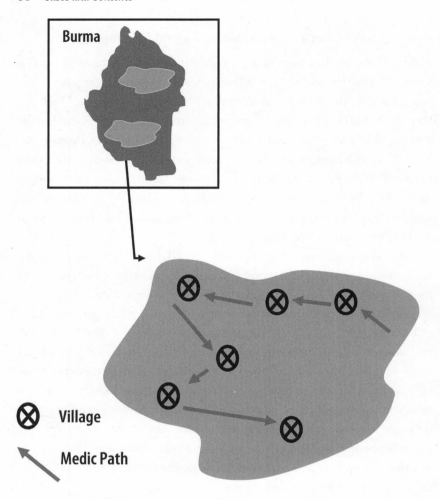

Figure 2.1. Schematic diagram of village tract and movement of medics through the target population. *Source*: Backpack Health Worker Team

for six months, but they often encounter larger populations and supplies can run out before the six-month period is completed. Different lengths of time are spent with each community, depending on the movement of communities and the need to avoid ongoing conflict or SPDC forces, with some communities becoming inaccessible if the route becomes too dangerous. Although security is poor, the health workers are familiar with the local terrain, are highly mobile, and navigate the ongoing conflict to access these previously unreachable populations.

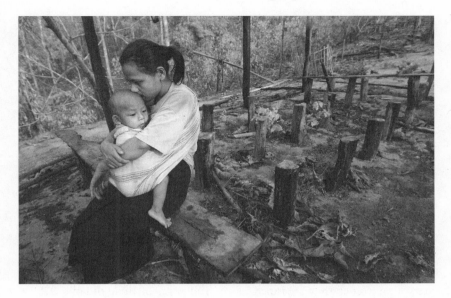

Figure 2.2. A Karen woman sits in the pews of a burned church, evidence of Burma regime terror tactics. Photo: Dang Ngo

In response to the lack of knowledge on the health status and needs of this population, BPHWT developed a health information system (HIS) to inform program decision making. They began working in the back room of a ramshackle "safe house" in Thailand, with initial data consisting of case counts handwritten into notebooks. In mid-1999 a new class of health worker trainees at MTC spent a week in a camp of 5,000 IDPs to complete a survey of all households. This camp, similar to many others, was perched just on the Burmese side of the border so that people could run to the relative safety of Thailand at the first sign of conflict. It was the first such survey attempted by the border health organizations, and the resulting unusable pile of long and partially completed questionnaires was a minor disaster (the major disaster occurred when the camp was burned down by SPDC troops two weeks later) (Figure 2.2).

These initial attempts resulted in a request to GHAP for more formal training, initiating what has become an extended series of workshops in monitoring and evaluation, computer training, epidemiology, survey design, and data management and analysis. Through ongoing collaboration with GHAP, leaders of the BPHWT have developed substantial internal capacity to manage their information infrastructure. As one senior health worker affirms, "One day we will return to our villages and coordinate our own health departments."

Major Barriers

In the black zones, carrying backpacks full of medicine and collecting health and demographic information is dangerous work. Since the inception of the program six health workers have died because of landmines or attacks by SPDC soldiers, who actively target health workers. Such attacks are in direct violation of the principles of protection offered to medical personnel of both established and mobile units under the first Geneva Convention. Village heads, schoolteachers, and others who help organize health care such as "Vitamin A and Deworming Day" are at risk as well. Health workers note that "most village heads are old women—if they are men they are killed, and if they are young women they are raped." Even traditional birth attendants (TBAs), who are generally elderly women, are subject to abuse by soldiers. One health worker reported that two TBAs had bags tied over their heads before they were beaten and thrown into a river, and one TBA had been shot and killed. Health information activities are especially risky, as any evidence of data collection arouses suspicion. Carrying even paper and pen can be dangerous; in the words of one worker, "it would be safer to count using pebbles."

Health worker mobility is severely restricted by security concerns. Existing roads and bridges are patrolled by soldiers, making it necessary for some health workers to walk as long as one month through jungle terrain to reach a primarily rural and widely dispersed population. Not infrequently, health workers transport medicines across rivers using bamboo rafts while swimming beside them; one BPHWT worker has drowned in the process. Even in Thailand, travel is fraught with perils. Each meeting is notable for the absence of health workers who cannot return from Burma. Ironically, health workers who have walked for weeks evading soldiers and landmines in an active conflict area sometimes cannot cross the border and travel the final few kilometers in peaceful Thailand. Human rights groups have documented numerous abuses by Thai border authorities against Burmese migrants; and specific reports maintain that Dr. Maung and health workers remain at risk for arrest and deportation (Human Rights Watch, 2003).

Population displacement within Burma is an enormous hurdle; BPHWT data show that 35–50 percent of households were forcibly displaced at least once each year (2000–2002). The majority do not relocate to identifiable displacement camps, making it difficult to maintain data on the size and location of the population served. Under these conditions, health workers need to update population and demographic information frequently, a formidable challenge only possible with the assistance of village heads and other community leaders.

Because of these extraordinary obstacles, BPHWT was compelled to develop and apply a number of different and innovative methods for their health information system. The system needed to address these major barriers, while meeting minimum requirements to produce methodologically sound population-level indicators including valid measures of morbidity and mortality. These requirements included: the ability to establish population denominators; the ability to address population fluidity and health worker mobility; the use of health workers, villagers, and TBAs as data collectors; twice-a-year contact and training with a subset of health workers; and, finally, a system that would not overly burden health workers. We describe four separate health-monitoring activities, each context-specific and designed with these requirements in mind. Each activity illustrates the continuing impact of the ongoing conflict on population-level health status.

Methods

The BPHWT surveillance system of morbidities and demographics provides program leaders with quantitative information on health outcomes (e.g., malaria, diarrhea, and pneumonia), target population changes, and human rights abuses (e.g., landmine injuries, forced labor, gunshot wounds) related to the conflict.

Estimating Morbidity Rates

Organizing and reporting of the vast quantities of information collected by the field workers has improved steadily since August 1998. Medics collect demographic information by village and village tract to be included in each backpack team's report, and monthly case counts by age and sex for specific morbidities. Other information includes a brief description of health education efforts, an overall report on the security situation in the village tract, a rough map depicting the route traveled by backpack workers, a medical inventory form, and photographs of their work. At each six-monthly meeting, team leaders are responsible for collecting and organizing this information into a presentable form for program leaders. These team-level reports are then combined into a single document that describes both quantitatively and qualitatively the activities and progress of the BPHWT program.

During initial stages of the program, case counts were collected with limited connection to the source population. The surveillance system components consisted only of case counts for the wide variety of treated illnesses, and thus could only describe the relative proportions of each illness, and resource needs. Program leaders required indicators that would account for both varying population size and time periods, which would allow for standardized comparisons across subgroups of the target populations. An incidence rate that included a quantitative description of the population and time frame for morbid events would provide this needed flexibility. The primary challenge with developing these rates was the mobility of health workers, and the mobility and changing size of the population that could access the health workers.

The first step was to estimate the target populations. Mobile medics conducted a census of each village tract that included sex and age groups. Although this information was essential for conducting cluster surveys (see below), incidence rates required a more accurate measure reflecting the movement of medics through the tract and the constraints on movement due to security. A new data-collection instrument enabled the mobile medics to record their path through the village tract, which included the name of each village, date of entry and exit, and current population (≤ 5 and > 5 years). The population of individual villages was determined in most cases by consultation with the village head or by direct head count.

Next, a measure of the population with access to the backpack medics working in a given village (called an "access population") was formulated. During each six-month term, workers construct a rudimentary map of the visited area, showing the location of villages, and landmarks such as rivers, roads, and mountains. When medics pass through a village, depending on distance, topography, and security, people from nearby villages may or may not be able to access the medics. For each village, using hand-drawn maps and consulting with area leaders, an estimate of the access population size was made for each village. Figure 2.3, containing hypothetical villages A–I, illustrates BPHWT efforts to determine access populations. For example, when

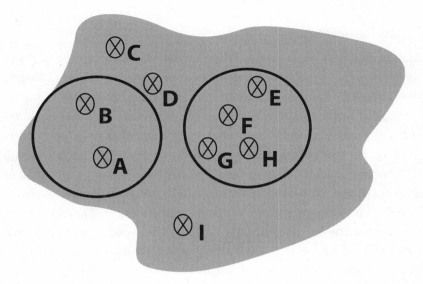

Figure 2.3. Estimating the size of the access population as mobile medics move through the village tracts. This hypothetical village tract has nine villages, labeled A through I. Based on maps and reports from field leaders, we can define the access population of any given village X as the sum of the populations of villages that have access to the medic when working in village X.

working in village A, persons in village B also come to receive care, but those from villages C to I do not. Thus, the combined population of villages A and B is the access population for when the health worker team works in village A. Similarly, the access population while the team is in village G equals the sum of populations in villages E, F, G, and H. These access populations often change over time, as the security situation fluctuates and individual communities are displaced due to the conflict.

The access population for each village where the health worker team works is multiplied by the number of days spent working there to produce a person-days denominator, allowing the calculation of a rate for a given condition within each access population area. In practice, however, person-time is summed over access populations and over village tracts to create summary rate measures for each of the administrative areas. These summary measures are then compared between areas so program leaders can prioritize health needs between areas, adjust resource flows to each area based on need, and monitor changes over time.

Methodological Issues

Maintaining tight quality control mechanisms remains a difficult challenge for BPHWT due largely to security issues. Constraints on movement of medics, field leaders, and program administrators limit direct observation of medics during their work to monitor performance and ensure consistent case definitions. Incomplete information is common because data may be lost, not recorded, or intentionally destroyed to avoid discovery during encounters with military personnel. Restrictions on movement make accurate recording of frequent population displacement difficult, and some areas may be completely cut off from contact. Similarly, often only a limited number of field leaders are able to return to Mae Sot for regular meetings, increasing dependency on the training-of-trainers model, and delaying communication between program administrators, field leaders, and primary data collectors in the field.

Because the vast majority of communities within the BPHWT target area have no secondary sources of health care, the arrival of the medics in a village is often treated as an event of great importance. As the overall burden of morbidity from both chronic and infectious conditions is high, many community members present prevalent cases to the backpack medics on the first day. Thus, the case counts incorporated into estimated summary measures include nonincident cases, and overestimate true incidence. Bias due to this "first day effect" is greatest for nonacute conditions, and thus limits external comparisons. The summary measures, however, are normally used for internal comparisons between areas and over time.

The access population size for any particular location also differs for some conditions. For example, landmine injuries are considerably more life threatening than other conditions. In this case, community members are more likely to travel longer distances to bring the victim to see the medic. Thus, for landmines the entire village tract can be considered the access area.

Sample Results

Despite these problems, the morbidity and demographic surveillance work has produced useful data. For example, the basic demographic information illustrates a direct result of the ongoing conflict: reduced male-to-female ratio. It is common in conflict and postconflict settings to find male-to-female ratios less than 1, due to increased male mortality from fighting or male absence due

Table 2.1. Male-to-female ratios (males per 100 females) among 15- to 45-year-olds in the BPHWT target population, by year and by township, 2004

Year	Male-to-female ratio	Township (2004)	Male-to-female ratio (2004)
1999	88.8	Kayah	99.7
2000	88.0	Taungoo	97.5
2001	93.8	Kler Lwee Tu	91.5
2002	91.9	Tha Ton	87.6
2003	92.1	Pa Pun	99.8
2004	94.2	Pa An	86.4
		Du Pla Ya	95.1
		Mergue	96.8
		Mon State	94.9

to conscription. For example, the male-to-female ratio was 88:100 among Afghan refugees in Pakistan (Yusaf, 1990) and 80:100 among families of former rebels in Angola (Grein, 2003). Similarly, in this population, BPHWT has consistently measured the male-to-female ratio among 15- to 45-year-olds between 88 and 94 per 100 females, presented in Table 2.1. These ratios illustrate the severity of armed conflict, and the notable differences by area. These estimates from the surveillance data have been validated by population-based cluster surveys finding similar ratios (89 in 2002, 92 in 2003).

Similarly, using the morbidity surveillance system, the BPHWT has tracked landmine injuries and gunshot wounds. Summary measures annualized from 2002 to 2004 are presented in Figure 2.4 for each area. The annualized rate for the entire BPHWT surveillance area from 2002 to 2004 was 11.3 per 10,000 per year, illustrating the significant toll of landmines on this population. Both the military regime and the armed ethnic groups have used landmines throughout the period of internal conflict. The ruling junta has actively used landmines against civilians, laying mines in villages and crop fields to prevent return after forcibly evicting villagers during counterinsurgency campaigns. In addition, there have been frequent reports of "atrocity demining": forcing civilians to walk ahead of soldiers to detonate landmines (Landmine Monitor, 2004) (Figure 2.5).

The constant movement reflected in the morbidity surveillance system precluded the accurate estimate of mortality rates, as deaths are relatively rare events compared with illness and unlikely to occur during a short stay by medics in a given village. As basic mortality rates (crude, under-five, infant,

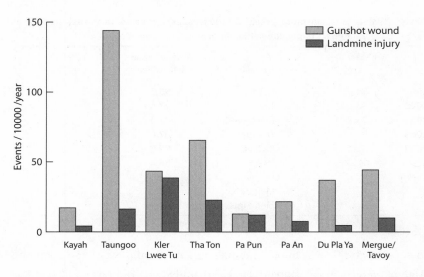

Figure 2.4. Summary measures (events/10,000/year) for gunshot wounds and landmine injuries in the BPHWT target population (by township, annualized 2002–2004)

maternal, and neonatal) are fundamental health indicators, BPHWT immediately saw the need to consider other data-collection methods to enable the collection of vital event data. One of the first attempts to improve the collection of vital event data, including births and deaths in the community, was the development of a data-collection instrument that the health workers gave to local community leaders. These individuals received basic training from the health worker on how to record vital events, which the health worker later retrieved. Initiation date and form pickup date then defined the surveillance period, and vital events during the period were combined over all surveyed areas to estimate mortality and birth rates.

While in some areas, this system produced good-quality data, the collection processes were insufficiently consistent to produce estimates for the region. Also, in many communities no appropriate individual was identified. Community members expressed concern regarding the risk of collecting data without the permission of the SPDC. Other problems included literacy issues, difficulty with retention of instructions, and loss of data forms during displacement.

Traditional birth attendants (TBAs), although mostly illiterate, are widely present in almost all of the target communities. Because of the TBA train-

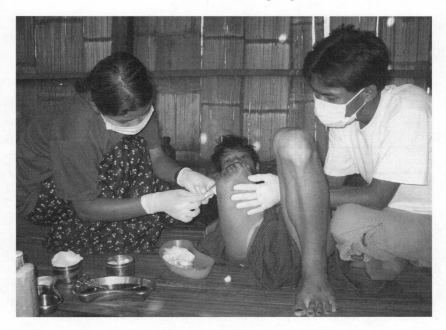

Figure 2.5. Medics care for a patient with a landmine injury. *Source*: Backpack Health Worker Team

ing program of the BPHWT, TBAs can be provided more structured training on data-collection responsibilities than other community members. Finally, TBAs also have much better access to female members of the target population, and are generally aware of all pregnancies, deliveries, maternal and neonatal deaths, even those occurring within a few hours of birth. We designed a simple, pictorial data-collection instrument designed to collect only this information, and enabled recording of many pregnancies and outcomes on a single sheet. Although we wanted to measure infant and child mortality, deaths beyond the neonatal period would not necessarily be known by TBAs, and prior attempts at TBA data collection had taught us that more complicated data forms would not be completed correctly. The form currently in use by the TBAs was initiated in January 2002 and is now being used by BPHWT and other border health organizations with TBA training programs. A section of the form illustrating the potential outcomes is shown in Figure 2.6.

During field training workshops, TBAs receive instruction on form completion. Each pregnant woman whom they assist is indicated by circling a picture

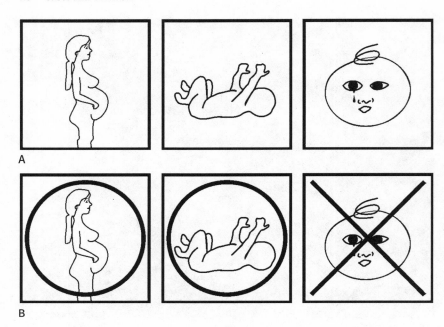

Figure 2.6. Data-collection form used by traditional birth attendants (TBAs) by BPH-WTs and other border health organizations. (*A*) TBAs use drawings of a pregnant woman, a baby at delivery, and a one-month-old baby to record maternal and neonatal outcomes for pregnancies. (*B*) TBAs record a neonatal death by circling the pregnant woman, circling the baby at delivery (i.e., live birth), and crossing out the one-month-old baby (i.e., infant died before reaching postneonatal age). *Source*: Backpack Health Worker Team

of the pregnant woman, the first picture in the set of three. The middle picture is used for counting live births; if the infant is born alive the TBA draws a circle around the baby, while stillbirths are indicated with an "X." The final picture in the set of three is designed to reflect the vital status at the end of the neonatal period. The period of 28 days was explained as either one month, four weeks, or one complete lunar cycle. If the child is alive at the end of this period, the TBA will circle the final picture in the set of three; if not, the TBA will record an "X."

The unstable security situation presents major difficulties. In many situations, the TBAs receive training and forms, only to find that they cannot return to the next follow-up field workshop for review training and form exchange because security concerns prevent their safe movement. Likewise, the efforts of TBA trainers to resupply TBAs with safe birth kits and collect the data forms at regular times are thwarted when access to some TBAs' communities becomes impossible. The mostly female TBAs are also more vulnerable than the male health workers to violence and sexual assault. Because they are usually elderly, they have greater ties to the community and are also less mobile, hindering evasion of hostile forces. These additional factors compound the difficulties inherent in estimating neonatal mortality through pictorial data collection by minimally literate TBAs.

Despite the security issues and methodological challenges, the TBAs have produced remarkably consistent neonatal and maternal mortality rates over time, and with acceptably narrow confidence intervals. For example, estimates for neonatal mortality rates (NMRs) from data collected in 2002 by TBAs from BPHWT and other border health organizations are shown in Figure 2.7. The use of TBAs as data collectors allowed the collection of more than 1,500 live births per year, far more than would have been possible using a more traditional rapid-survey method. With a crude birth rate of 40 per 1,000 population, BPHWT health workers would have had to survey almost 7,000 households to obtain the same number of live births. The high number of live births allows for more accurate estimates and narrower confidence intervals. Access to a large number of pregnancies and live births is especially important for estimating maternal mortality, which is still a relatively rare event even in regions where the maternal mortality ratio (MMR) is very high. Because the NMR and MMR are ratios with live births as the denominator, estimation does not require knowing the exact access population of the TBAs, although potential differences between communities with and without access to these TBAs limits generalization of these results to the wider IDP population in eastern Burma.

The extremely high maternal mortality ratio (1000–1200 per 100,000 live births) is in particular a key indicator of health disparity, because of the strong association between maternal deaths and lack of health services. The oppressive policies of the military regime, combined with minimal expenditure on health services, results in virtually no access to skilled assistance at birth, a key requirement for reducing maternal death (UNFPA, 2003). This lack of access to reproductive health services is likely a substantial contributor to high maternal mortality. Approximately 5 percent of deliveries in BPHWT areas

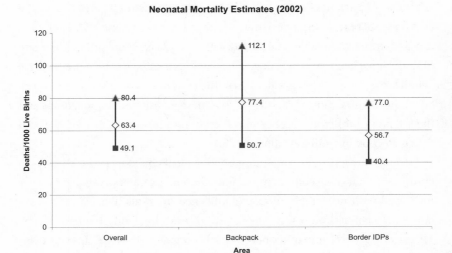

Figure 2.7. Neonatal mortality rates (neonatal deaths/1,000 live births) in BPHWT and other border health organization areas estimated by TBAs using the pictorial data form, 2002

occur in the jungle and 78 percent at home, and only 4 percent of women have access to emergency obstetric care (BPHWT, 2003). The striking contrast with neighboring Thailand (MMR 44) highlights the effect of this lack of access to reproductive health care.

Rapid-Assessment Population-wide Surveys

Since 2000, BPHWT has conducted a series of population-wide rapid-assessment surveys for various indicators of morbidity and mortality as well as for needs assessments for a variety of health programs. These assessments addressed weaknesses of prior methods, which relied on a more constant presence of a data collector and/or required the training of nonbackpack personnel. Although the training of villagers had the potential to reduce the workload of backpack health workers and to improve community involvement in the process, the training took valuable time, increased error, introduced problems with literacy, and created potential security issues for villagers. Rapid-assessment surveys were more suitable for the mobile health workers, but also presented a variety of limitations requiring modification of standard methods. In addition, implementing other methods of data collection enabled validation of results collected by using different methods.

A village-based cluster-sampling method was deemed the best way to effectively represent the BPHWT population while maintaining a survey design that was logistically feasible, given the widely dispersed villages, travel on foot over mountainous terrain, and security concerns that force circuitous and irregular travel. In general, BPHWT was able to follow standard methods for conducting cluster-sample surveys (Bennett, 1991), with slight modifications. For example, we selected smaller cluster sizes (20 households versus the standard 30), so that no single mobile team was overburdened by data collection. We also increased the numbers of clusters to account for low-response rates in the early years of the surveys. The chosen sampling frame for all surveys since 2001 has consisted of the entire population served by BPHWT. The census data from the morbidity surveillance system (see Sample Results) were used to randomly select clusters proportionate to village population size. Within each cluster, households were selected with an interval-sampling method, randomly choosing a direction from the approximate center of the village and then visiting every nth household, where n equals the number of village households divided by twenty.

Security issues and the unique operational method of the mobile backpack team resulted in important constraints to implementation. For example, interviewers could often spend only a few days in each village, limiting the length of the survey. And, the current household surveys conducted by BPHWT are limited to two-sides of one page, with a corresponding increase in data quality and response rate. In addition, if the head of household was unavailable, the next nearest household was selected, as spending time to return for follow-up visits would have created security concerns. Although these types of substitutions were not ideal, they were practical necessities given security and time constraints.

Ideally, these types of rapid-assessment surveys would be completed in as short a time frame as possible. This was not logistically feasible for backpack health workers, and surveys by necessity were conducted when health workers reach preselected clusters (villages) in the course of their usual work over approximately a three-month period. The extended time frame resulted in temporally different recall periods for households across the target area, introducing potential biases if health indicators were changing significantly during the data-collection period. We did not, however, expect mortality rates or other basic indicators would fluctuate widely over three months unless influenced by a major event, such as a major military offensive.

The inclusion of potentially dangerous areas was necessary to reduce bias from limiting data collection to more secure areas. In addition, excluding such areas in advance would have been difficult due to the fluidity of the security situation. If an entire village had been displaced and moved essentially intact (which is not uncommon, as villagers often attempt to stay together), the medic attempted to locate the villagers and conduct the interval-sampling process. If displaced villagers could not be accessed because of security reasons, then the nearest accessible village was selected. BPHWT leaders stressed, however, that health workers should never take greater risks simply for the collection of data.

The workshops conducted with the BPHWT administration team and the health workers responsible for the survey were a critical and challenging part of the process. Because the health workers could only spend a limited amount of time in Thailand, the workshops for survey training were intensive and short, lasting only 4 to 5 days. GHAP provided training regarding interview techniques, sampling methods, survey questions, and relevant case definitions. In addition, because only supervisory health workers could return to Thailand and were not able to visit all clusters themselves, they were required to train other health workers in the field and to assist them in completion of the survey. Thus field training documents were created to assist with field workshops for this purpose, akin to a training-of-trainers method.

The administrative team receives more advanced training in survey methods, basic epidemiology, data management and entry, and analysis and interpretation. Field workers returning from the field for a short time deliver completed survey forms to this team and interact closely to quickly resolve any concerns regarding confusing or incomplete information. Forms are catalogued, reviewed, and entered, and brief analyses are completed to root out questions for field staff members and to present preliminary results. More complete results are presented and discussed when the field staff returns for the next workshop. These activities reflect the ultimate goal of the process: to enable the border health organizations to eventually manage their own health information systems.

Surveys conducted since 2000 have included nutrition, water and sanita-

Table 2.2. Survey profile, demographic data, and mortality rates (95% CI) in the BPHWT target population

	2002	2003
Total population	123,680	134,981
Households sampled	1,290	1,609
Coverage (percent returned)	65%	80%
Population sampled	7,496	9,083
Population <5 years old	1,382 (18.4%)	1,858 (20.4%)
Males per 100 females	89	92
IMR (per 1,000 live births)	135 (72–197)	122 (70–175)
U5MR (per 1,000 live births)	291 (208–374)	276 (190–361)
CMR (per 1,000 persons/year)	25 (18–32)	21 (15–27)

Notes: IMR, ratio of infant deaths (<1 year old) to live births; U5MR (under five mortality rate), ratio of child deaths (<5 years old) to live births; CMR (crude mortality rate), ratio of all deaths to midyear population.

tion, malaria, and reproductive health. Mortality surveys have been done in conjunction with these surveys on an annual basis since 2001. Selected results for mortality from 2002 to 2003 are presented in Table 2.2. The infant (infant mortality rate [IMR] = 91–135) and child (under age 5 mortality rate [U5MR] = 221–291) mortality rates calculated in these samples are significantly higher than estimates for Burma as a whole (IMR = 76, U5MR = 107; 2003 data). Although higher peak mortality rates have been reported from other areas of the world, the rates from this displaced population in eastern Burma are striking; based on 2003 estimates, only Sierra Leone had a higher countrywide under-five mortality rate (UNICEF, 2005). In the context of Southeast Asia, Cambodia reported 140 as the highest U5MR among ASEAN countries, and adjacent Thailand reported a U5MR of 26 (UNICEF, 2005). Despite wide confidence intervals, the IMR and U5MR have been remarkably consistent. In addition, the quality of the data and the response rate has improved each year.

In 2002–2003, landmines and other violent causes accounted for more than 5 percent of all deaths, highlighting the presence of ongoing conflict. More impressively, the most commonly reported causes of death were malaria (>40%), diarrhea (>15%), and, among adult females, pregnancy-related causes (>20%). These findings emphasize how the conflict has created conditions for the predominance of these preventable causes of death.

A population pyramid for 2003 is shown in Figure 2.8, from a total estimated midyear population of 8,989 persons. Nearly 50 percent of the popu-

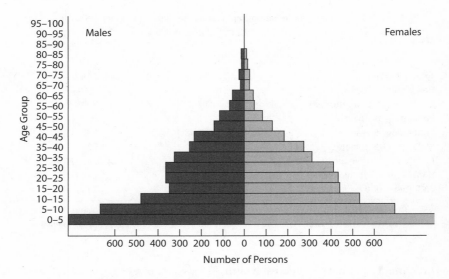

Figure 2.8. Population pyramid for a population-based sample of households from the BPHWT program area, 2003

lation is less than 15 years old (compared with 33% reported by Burma), similar to the world's least-developed nations (United Nations, 2001). There was a surplus of females over males in the 15- to 45-years age group (92 males for every 100 females), consistent with conflict-related mortality, and in line with estimates based on the BPHWT morbidity surveillance.

Linking Human Rights with Health Indicators

The BPHWT health information system was not initially intended for advocacy purposes. The initial *modus operandi* of BPHWT was to work "below the radar" to avoid retribution by the SPDC. However, violence directed against health workers and villagers who participated in health activities made it clear that they were already targets. In addition, BPHWT leaders have come to realize that advocacy offers one of the most effective means for them to improve the health of their population. They perceive that the most important determinants of health in eastern Burma are the civil conflict and the human rights abuses perpetrated by the military. Approaches to disease and malnutrition that target the downstream effects of war and poverty will do little to provide sustainable gains in population health until the upstream determinants are improved. As one field worker explained, "What is the point of building latrines and clean water systems if the people will be forced to move?"

In 2003, after receiving some basic human rights training, BPHWT leaders and health workers expressed interest in documenting human rights violations and the effect on health status. Focus groups were conducted in 2003 with health workers and backpack leaders to determine the most common and/or significant abuses. Among a wide variety, the most significant and common included forced displacement, food insecurity (defined as the taxation, theft, or destruction of food supply, crops, or livestock), forced labor, soldier violence, landmine injuries, obstruction of access to health care, and rape.

Human rights documentation based on qualitative interviews with a relatively small number of respondents can produce detailed, insightful, and often powerful descriptions of human rights violations. "License to Rape" (Shan Human Rights Foundation, 2002), for example, was widely disseminated and had a major effect on the international recognition of sexual violence committed by SPDC soldiers. A limitation of qualitative methods, however, is that it can be difficult to make assertions about the widespread or systematic occurrence of human rights violations at a population level.

BPHWT and GHAP had a different approach in mind, with two specific goals. First, we wanted to assess the prevalence of these human rights violations at a population level using epidemiological methods from public health. Second, we wanted to document the effect of these human rights violations on health status, again at a population level. This would quantitatively document the direct association between human rights violations and health indicators.

The rapid-survey methodology used in previous years represented the most appropriate context-specific strategy to reach these goals, and was a method of human rights documentation more fitting to the BPHWT method of operation: they could not spend a long time in a given village conducting detailed interviews, and they could not undergo the more extensive training required for qualitative interviews. BPHWT health workers were already trained and accustomed to doing population-wide cluster surveys. In 2004, BPHWT adapted their previous mortality survey instrument to include eight questions addressing the human rights violations identified during focus group discussions. The key mortality and morbidity indicators from prior surveys were included so that specific links between human rights violations and household

**Table 2.3. Proportion of households among the BPHWT target population
reporting selected human rights violations, 2004 (%)**

Township	Forced labor	Soldier violence	Landmine injury	Forced relocation	Food insecurity
Kayah	47.7	0.0	0.0	0.0	0.0
Taungoo	5.7	2.1	1.4	45.4	71.6
Kler Lwee Tu	0.0	1.7	1.7	60.5	18.5
Tha Ton	33.8	3.8	2.9	0.0	27.5
Pa Pun	36.2	0.5	0.0	4.1	12.6
Pa An	74.1	0.3	0.0	0.0	17.3
Du Pla Ya	11.9	1.8	0.2	0.6	30.2
Mergue	37.3	7.5	0.8	14.2	33.9
Total	32.9	1.9	0.7	9.1	26.0

health status could be assessed, enabling a description of the population-level prevalence and impact of human rights violations.

Of 2000 households sampled in eight of the nine townships covered by BPHWT, 1834 (91.7%) were completed. The proportion of households reporting selected human rights violations is shown in Table 2.3. Overall prevalence of forced labor (32.9%) and food insecurity (26.0%) was high, and almost 2 percent of households reported soldier violence (being shot at, stabbed, or beaten). The estimated landmine injury rate was 13/10,000 persons/year. The overall prevalence of forced displacement was much lower than in previous years (35–50% in 2000–2002). The time of this survey, September to November 2004, occurred during a widespread unofficial cease-fire in BPHWT areas, and except for two areas (02 and 03), much less conflict was reported. Of note, there was a wide variance in the prevalence of human rights violations between townships. Interviews with the health workers provided illuminating reasons for this, and were consistent with health workers' perception of human rights violations in their townships. People living in townships characterized by high levels of armed conflict (Taungoo, Kler Lwee Tu) were more likely to be the victims of forced relocation and landmine injuries, whereas in areas with less conflict (Kayah, Tha Ton, Pa Pun Pa An, Du Pla Ya, Mergue) forced labor was commonly reported (11.9–74.1%). This suggests that as areas become more stable, some human rights violations may decrease, but others are likely to take their place. Measuring multiple human rights violations at a population level over time will permit direct assessment of this hypothesis. Of note, in Kayah, a Karenni cease-fire area, nearly half the

Table 2.4. Odds ratios (with 95% CI) for selected human rights violations and health outcomes in the BPHWT target population, 2004

Outcome	Forced relocation	Forced labor	Food insecurity
Child death	2.8 (1.2–6.4)	1.5 (0.9–2.5)	1.6 (1.0–2.6)
Adult death	1.6 (0.8–2.9)	1.7 (1.1–2.5)	1.7 (1.2–2.4)
Severe malnutrition	0.7 (0.1–6.0)	1.5 (0.3–6.4)	6.0 (3.9–9.2)
Landmine injury	5.2 (1.4–20.1)	3.5 (0.9–13.3)	4.6 (1.3–15.5)
Parasitemia	1.3 (0.8–2.1)	1.5 (1.0–2.1)	1.7 (1.2–2.4)

population reported forced labor, demonstrating that the resolution of armed conflict between ethnic minorities and the SPDC did not result in an end to human rights violations. From these observations, one can see how repeated implementation of this type of survey could be used to monitor the prevalence of human rights violations as "human rights indicators," with many uses, such as the evaluation of the effect of cease-fire agreements on human rights violations, and monitoring compliance with international treaties on forced labor.

The occurrence of human rights violations was associated with specific health indicators (Table 2.4). For example, forced displacement due to military activities was associated with increased odds of child death (odds ratio [OR] = 2.8) and landmine injury (OR = 5.2). Similarly, when households reported loss of food supply due to taxation, destruction, or theft by military personnel, the odds of child (OR = 1.6) and adult (OR = 1.7) death were increased, as were odds of a positive malaria parasitemia test (OR = 1.7), severe malnutrition in children (OR = 6.0), and landmine injury (OR = 4.6). These unique data collected by BPHWT demonstrate and quantify the prevalence of systematic human rights violations and their profound impact on the health status of this population.

Summary of Methods

Over the past seven years, the collaboration between BPHWT and GHAP has enabled development of a number of innovative methods for collecting information and taking action on health and human rights within the context of ongoing conflict. The availability of multiple methods has allowed for cross-validation, especially important in a setting where close monitoring of worker performance and adherence to protocols is challenging. For example, annualized landmine injury rates (11.3/10,000/year) estimated through the morbidity surveillance program match closely with the rapid-assessment population-based surveys (13.1/10,000/year). Maternal mortality measured by TBAs (1,000–1,200) also agreed with the rapid-assessment survey (1,100), and neonatal mortality measured by TBAs is consistent with what would be expected given the infant mortality measured by rapid assessment. The proportion of infant mortality that occurs during the neonatal period according to these two separate data-collection activities was approximately 57 percent, which is comparable to an expected proportion of 40–50 percent in high-mortality settings (Lawn et al., 2005). The consistency in results between methods supports their validity.

Ideally, these health status indicators and human rights data would be validated by external sources. Although population-based data collection in eastern Burma is extremely limited, the Burma Border Consortium, despite using different methods and accessing a somewhat different population of IDPs in eastern Burma, conducted an extensive survey in 2004 that produced a remarkably similar child mortality rate of 286 under age 5 deaths per 1,000 live births (Thailand Burma Border Consortium, 2004). We hope that efforts such as this continue to add to the small but growing body of information coming out of the black zones within Burma.

Taking Action

A public health and human rights perspective not only illuminates relationships between exposures and health outcomes, but also provides an imperative to take direct action to promote the right to health. Beyond the data, the BPHWT health information system has helped to identify partners and leverage resources; to improve and expand specific programs; and to generate information for advocacy on a local and international level. The first rapid-assessment survey conducted in 2000 demonstrated widespread malnutrition among children. Using the World Health Organization's recommended cutoffs for severe and moderate malnutrition, one can see that 11.4 percent were malnourished. Vitamin A deficiency appeared to be a major problem, with low access to meat products or nonanimal sources of vitamin A and a high prevalence of Bitot spots, precursors for corneal damage potentially leading to blindness. These data allowed BPHWT and GHAP to raise awareness and acquire donated medicines to initiate a community-wide vitamin A supplementation and deworming program. BPHWT continues to monitor

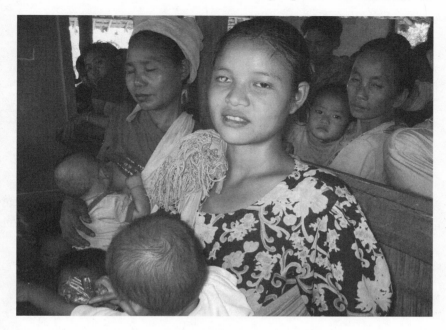

Figure 2.9. A mother waits with her child for vitamin A—too late for her with a corneal scar. *Source*: Backpack Health Worker Team

vitamin A coverage, night blindness, and middle upper arm circumference to assess the effect of this program (Figure 2.9).

Data on malaria collected through both rapid surveys and morbidity surveillance have also led to improvements in cross-border malaria activities. BPHWT has been treating more than 20,000 cases of malaria yearly, with more than half of the entire population acquiring malaria each year in some areas, and with malaria causing nearly 40 percent of all child deaths. This led to the implementation of a pilot integrated malaria control program that applied internationally recognized principles and state-of-the art technology, including rapid diagnostic tests, regionally approved artesunate combination therapies, long-lasting insecticide-treated nets, and community-based monitoring systems. Using annual survey methods and morbidity surveillance, health workers were able to demonstrate dramatic decreases in malaria point prevalence and incidence, and improved knowledge and practices among villagers. After a two-year pilot phase among 2,000 IDPs, the pilot was expanded in 2005 to include more than 10,000 IDPs in 16 village areas (Figure 2.10).

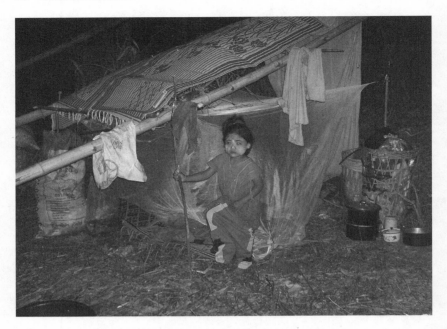

Figure 2.10. An insecticide-treated net protects a displaced child living in a temporary shelter. *Source*: Backpack Health Worker Team

Similarly, BPHWT data describing extremely poor reproductive health conditions have led to initiation of the largest health program to date targeting reproductive health needs within IDP communities in eastern Burma. Maternal mortality data, with a significant proportion of deaths from postpartum hemorrhage and sepsis, and other BPHWT reproductive health data were presented to the Gates Institute for Population and Reproductive Health. This resulted in subsequent support for a program to establish mobile reproductive health centers within IDP communities to serve a dual purpose: to train health workers to provide basic emergency obstetric care, family planning, antenatal care, and TBA training, and to serve as referral centers for these same services.

In addition to health programs, representatives from BPHWT, GHAP, and other supporters have presented BPHWT health information in a variety of reports, news media, and other settings to raise awareness and influence policy. For example, data linking nutritional status of children and forced displacement were included in a report on the effect of food insecurity and internal displacement on malnutrition in children (Burmese Border Consortium, 2003). BPHWT data have also been presented at numerous international conferences, universities, and government meetings, including the Thai parliament and the U.S. Congress. These activities raise awareness and stimulate broader discussion of the impact of human rights on health status. In addition, given the dearth of data from conflicted areas of Burma, this information plays a potentially important role in policy decisions on key issues affecting refugees and IDPs. What is the effect of internationally funded development projects such as proposed pipelines or dams on the human rights situation or health status in these areas? What should be the policy of governments toward foreign aid to Burma given the health status in these areas and the impact of systematic human rights abuses? Are these areas ready to tolerate repatriation of refugees? This information serves to illuminate the black zones so that policy makers can make decisions with some degree of understanding.

Looking Ahead

The work of the BPHWT provides an example of how indigenous groups can collect sound information on both health status and human rights, in a highly unstable conflict zone despite mobile populations, poor security, rural infrastructure, and minimal capital resources. Future efforts to measure health status, human rights, and their interrelationships may draw on this work. Although such settings are complex and will ultimately vary widely in terms of infrastructure, political and military realities, and international involvement, some basic principles may be translatable.

The capability of displaced populations to measure and affect their own condition should be acknowledged. Successful participatory models of disease surveillance and control in this IDP setting provide a basis for a shift in perspective: from one of helpless victim to resourceful agent. A similar paradigm shift recently occurred in relation to antiretroviral treatment, as people living with HIV in poverty forced the international community to recognize their capability to treat themselves. The work of the BPHWT provides an example of the capacity of IDPs to track health status and affect the transmission of disease in their areas. The international community should support the dissemination of other successful interventions in the IDP setting, and should provide resources and training to IDPs to manage and measure the effect of their own health programs.

The use of indigenous workers is indispensable, especially in settings where other persons have poor access or would place themselves and the target population at risk. For example, in eastern Burma only trusted and respected persons such as health workers from within the community could traverse the difficult terrain, avoid detection by military troops, and collect sensitive health and human rights information. Even illiterate or seemingly less capable persons, such as elderly TBAs, can be helpful depending on the type of data collected. Although we recognize that the use of local people carries the potential for bias, rigorous data-collection methods can minimize this, and internal validation of estimates generated by multiple methods can strengthen credibility.

Novel methods to enhance indigenous capacity to collect health and human rights information should continue to be developed, applied, and evaluated. These methods should account for characteristics of displaced and vulnerable populations, such as mobility, illiteracy, and insecurity. Such characteristics are typical for the populations that have the highest need and are typically the most ignored because of the inability to acquire information. Adaptation of standard methodologies to accommodate practical or logistical constraints must not, however, sacrifice basic epidemiological and demographic principles, even in settings where monitoring is limited.

These adapted methods should be integrated into already existing health program activities. In low-resource settings, integration is imperative to avoid overburdening already strained health information systems. The BPHWT information system carefully accounts for factors such as the normal work and movement pattern of the medics, the security implications, and the time for training and completion for data instruments. Although an externally managed system may reduce the chance of bias, in situations without sufficient resources to conduct separate investigation, the alternative may be the absence of information.

We hope that this work inspires future endeavors investigating the devastating impact of human rights violations on health status. The integration of human rights data into health information systems provides a unique method to measure human rights violations at a population level, and their association with mortality and other major health indicators. This potentially provides the means to collect powerful evidence for critical questions that continue to plague the international community: how widespread are human rights violations by a rogue government, military regime, or rebel army? Are the abuses systematic or sporadic occurrences? How significant and extensive are the impacts? In an era in which the international community still hesitates to intervene in the face of ethnic cleansing or even genocide, this type of information will, it is to be hoped, prompt action to intervene and prevent unnecessary loss of life.

Acknowledgments
The authors wish to thank the dedicated health workers who were involved in the collection of this information.

Notes
1. Burma is also known as Myanmar. We use *Burma* throughout this chapter in accordance with the preference of the 1990 General Elector winner, the National League for Democracy.

References
Backpack Health Worker Team. 2003. Annual Report.

Bennett, S., Woods, T., Liyanage, W. M., and Smith, D. L. 1991. A simplified general method for cluster-sample surveys of health in developing countries. *World Health Statistics Quarterly* 44 (3):98–106.

Burmese Border Consortium. 2002. *Internally displaced people and relocation sites in Eastern Burma.*

Burmese Border Consortium. 2003. *Reclaiming the right to rice: Food security and internal displacement in eastern Burma.*

Grein, T., Checchi, F., Escribà, J. M., et al. 2003. Mortality among displaced former UNITA members and their families in Angola: A retrospective cluster survey. *British Medical Journal* 327 (7416):650.

Human Rights Watch. 2003. Human Rights Watch Press Release. www.hrw.org/press/2003/10/thailand100303.htm (accessed November 21, 2005).

International Labour Office. 2004. Developments concerning the question of the observance by the Government of Myanmar of the Forced Labour Convention, 1930 (No. 29). www.ilo.org/public/english/standards/relm/gb/docs/gb297/pdf/gb-8-1.pdf (accessed November 21, 2005).

Karen Human Rights Group. 2000. *Suffering in silence.* Universal Publishers, Parkland, FL.

Landmine Monitor. 2004. *Landmine Monitor Report: Burma.* www.icbl.org/lm/2004/burma#fn7042 (accessed November 21, 2005).

Lawn, J., Cousens, S., and Zupan, J. 2005. Four million neonatal deaths: When? Where? Why? *Lancet* 365 (9462):891–900.

Norwegian Refugee Council. 2003. *Profile of internal displacement: Myanmar (Burma).*

Norwegian Refugee Council. 2004. *Internal displacement: Global overviews of trends and developments.* Global IDP Project, Norwegian Refugee Council, Geneva.

Roberts, L., Riyadh, L., et al. 2004. Mortality before and after the 2003 invasion of Iraq: Cluster sample survey. *The Lancet Online.* http://image.thelancet.com/extras/04art10342web.pdf (accessed November 21, 2005).

Shan Human Rights Foundation. 2002. *License to rape.* www.shanland.org/resources/bookspub/humanrights/LtoR/ (accessed November 21, 2005).

Thailand Burma Border Consortium. 2004. *Internal displacement and vulnerability in eastern Burma.*

United Nations. 2001. United Nations Development Programme, *Human development indicators,* Human Development Report, 156. New York: Oxford University Press.

United Nations. 2003. Service Office - Burma. *Humanitarian assistance to Burma.* December 2002 (published, March 2003). New York: United Nations.

United Nations Population Fund (UNFPA). 2003. *Maternal mortality update 2002— A focus on emergency obstetric care.* New York: UNFPA.

United Nations Children's Fund (UNICEF). 2005. *The state of world's children.* New York: UNICEF.

U.S. Committee for Refugees. 2005. Key statistics. *World Refugee Survey 2005.* www.refugees.org/uploadedFiles/Investigate/Publications_&_Archives/WRS_Archives/2005/key_statistics.pdf.

U.S. Department of Labor. 2000. *Report on labor practices in Burma.* Washington, DC: Bureau of International Labor Affairs.

World Food Program. 2004. Annual Report.

Yusaf, F. 1990. Size and demographic characteristics of the Afghan refugee population in Pakistan. *Journal of Biosocial Science* 22 (3):269–79.

Consequences of a Stalled Response

Iatrogenic Epidemic among Blood Donors in

Central China

Wan Yanhai and Li Xiaorong, Ph.D.

In 1996 Dr. Gao Yaojie, a 76-year-old retired professor of obstetrics and gynecology at Henan University, became alarmed when some of her past patients came to her seeking help for a complex array of symptoms, which she gradually realized could be caused only by AIDS. Dr. Gao went to the villages where she had served in the Henan countryside to see for herself. She visited rural districts in the southern Henan Province and found villages with a startlingly high number of young adults who were ill and dying. Even without the laboratory capability to do blood testing for HIV, she came to the conclusion that these people probably had AIDS. One village particularly hard hit was Wen Lou, where she estimated that perhaps 40 percent of the adults were infected with HIV. Dr. Gao conducted careful interviews and took detailed medical histories. She learned that they all shared a common story. The villagers had been targeted by blood-collection agencies and had sold their blood for cash. Her investigation also revealed that these enterprises had been reusing the blood-collecting equipment without adequately sterilizing it and reinfusing blood cells taken from one donor into other donors. This was a staggeringly substandard and dangerous medical practice, and it appeared that an epidemic of blood-borne pathogens, including HIV, was under way.

Dr. Gao insisted that medical care be provided for these patients and that the investigation of the outbreak be widened. Local authorities told her to cease her activities and barred her from entering affected villages. They pressured the villagers not to meet with her. When Dr. Gao persisted, her adult children lost their jobs. When she tried to take her case to the national authorities in Beijing, she was detained and put under house arrest by the local police in Henan.

Meanwhile, the government tried to prevent journalists and advocacy groups from entering the "AIDS villages" of Henan. Investigators who made it to the villages affected were threatened and detained and their cameras confiscated. Infected villagers and family members who wanted to speak with journalists were interrogated and imprisoned. Local villagers and activists who tried going to Beijing to petition the central government were prevented from boarding trains and in some instances detained by police. Eventually, a few limited programs for care and counseling were set up in Wen Lou, but when villagers came from neighboring areas for medical care, they were forcibly turned away and told, "China is poor—we can afford only one Wen Lou."

Epidemic and Scandal in Central China

Fully accurate prevalence figures still are not available for the epidemic of infectious diseases among China's rural blood donors. Based on the most reliable data available to date, it appears that China's AIDS epidemic remains limited in scope compared with the vast population. The number of people infected with HIV probably is fewer than 1 in 1,000 adults. By comparison, in Cambodia it is more like 40 per 1,000 adults and in Botswana it is roughly 380 per 1,000 adults. China's situation might be best understood as a series of unlinked epidemics in which the virus remains localized within distinct geographic and population pockets. As of 2002, intravenous drug users and their sexual contacts, concentrated primarily in Yunnan, Guangxi, Sichuan, and Xinjiang Provinces, accounted for an estimated 500,000 to 1.2 million cumulative HIV infections (Zhang, 2002). A similar number of HIV-infected individuals, primarily sex workers and men who have sex with men, live in

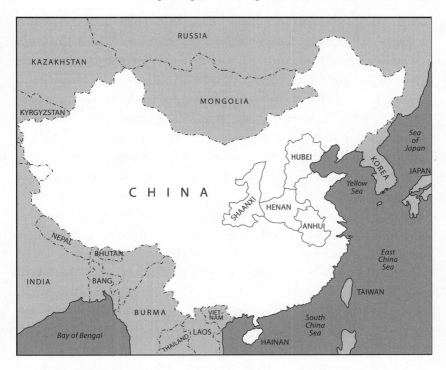

Figure 3.1. In Henan, Anhui, Shaanxi, and Hubei provinces, unscrupulous blood donor companies spread HIV/AIDS and other infectious diseases. After map from the
University of Texas at Austin Libraries, Perry-Castañeda Library (available at
www.lib.utexas.edu/maps/middle_east_and_asia/china_rel01.jpg)

cities along the coast (Zhang, 2002). Another pocket of HIV/AIDS—the one
most poorly documented because of the scandal and cover-up—is the epidemic in at least four provinces of central China, which was first discovered
by Dr. Gao (Fig. 3.1).

Since AIDS was first noted in China about two decades ago, the government's response has been notably inconsistent. At first there was official denial. The news media called AIDS a disease of Western decadence, and in
China the government controls the media. Indeed, the official media are organs of the party apparatus of the People's Republic. Throughout the 1980s
and 1990s, the official position was that Asian cultural values and socialist
ideology would prevent China from having a significant AIDS epidemic. In
the past few years, this has changed substantially, although inconsistencies

remain. The government now puts out more realistic public health prevention messages and in some districts has even established methadone treatment and harm-reduction programs (Zunyou, 2005). Still, China's health system is poor by the standards of developed nations. There is no universal health care, and the cost of antiretroviral medications is far beyond what the ordinary person can afford, even at heavily subsidized prices. During the tightly controlled years of Mao's communism, all public mention of sexuality was forbidden. This is changing slowly, mostly in major metropolitan areas along the eastern seaboard, but open discussion and display of sexuality still makes many Chinese squeamish.

The blood donor scandal uncovered by Dr. Gao was the result of corruption and negligence at both the local and national level. In China, government corruption and negligence are widespread and that includes the public health system. In this epidemic numerous government officials in Henan had been directly involved in the profit-making blood-collection enterprises. Meanwhile, advocacy and deviance from the official line is rarely tolerated in China's one-party political system. The rural poor, ethnic minorities, and the millions of poor rural migrants to the ballooning urban centers have little political voice and few safeguards to protect them. This is the context that allowed the blood donor profit-making schemes to flourish and that permitted the state-sponsored attempts to cover up the epidemic they caused. So not only were rural villagers the victims of gross medical negligence, but the whistleblowers who recognized the epidemic and brought it to public attention were harassed and imprisoned. This is a human rights disgrace on multiple levels, each caused by government corruption, conflict of interest, and the use of the state police apparatus to cover up and intimidate.

Donors were not told about the potential risks of giving blood and not offered even the most rudimentary opportunity to provide informed consent. In their desire to maximize profits, the blood-collection enterprises engaged in grossly negligent medical practices including multiple reuse of collection equipment without sterilization, inadequate education and counseling of donors, and reinfusion of packed red blood cells in pooled fashion without adequate screening and sterilization of blood components; they were allowed to continue doing so well after government officials were told of the dangers. Official oversight of the blood-collecting schemes was wholly absent, because of weak regulatory setups and because high-level officials were profiting from their activities. In fact, the cover-up continues with little serious effort to fully document who was infected and when, to gauge the effect of failing to react promptly to halt the enterprise, and to bring charges against those responsible. And beyond the donors, there is no full understanding of who may have been infected secondarily through contact with an infected blood donor or among the potentially hundreds of thousands of recipients of infected units. Dr. Gao focused on the transmission of HIV, but there are numerous other pathogens that can be transmitted via infected blood, such as hepatitis B and C, malaria, cytomegalovirus, syphilis, and tetanus. Denial and cover-up continue.

Dr. Gao's story eventually reached Elizabeth Rosenthal at the *New York Times*'s Beijing Bureau. She produced a groundbreaking series of articles that appeared between 2000 and 2002. In these articles, she described the epidemic and the harassment of Dr. Gao. In 2001, Dr. Gao was awarded the Jonathan Mann Prize in Health and Human Rights by the Global Council for International Health. The Chinese government's reaction was to deny her a passport to travel to Washington to receive the award. Kofi Annan, Secretary General of the United Nations, accepted it on her behalf. For a while, international recognition pressured Beijing to put the brakes on the local officials in Henan that were threatening Dr. Gao. Still, when a high-level U.S. AIDS research team met with China's leaders in November 2002 and tried to meet with Dr. Gao, she was again put under house arrest and prevented from meeting the international researchers.

Soon after making her discovery public, Dr. Gao was joined by others who also met with police harassment and intimidation by the authorities.. In 1999, Dr. Gui Xien, an epidemiologist at a Wuhan hospital in Hubei Province, reported AIDS cases in Hubei. The local authorities silenced him and did nothing to inform or assist the individuals affected.

A worse fate met Dr. Wan Yanhai, a psychologist and activist, who in 1994 had started an AIDS awareness group in Beijing. Dr. Wan already had run afoul of the government by advocating for human rights, AIDS awareness, and gay and lesbian issues. In response to publishing information on the Internet about the Henan scandal, in August 2002 the government banned his organization, AIDS Action Project, which had been receiving financial support from overseas organizations such as the Ford and Elizabeth Taylor AIDS Foundations. For several days, "three large men" in a black Volkswagon followed him. On August 24, 2002, after attending a gay and lesbian film screening he was detained by Chinese authorities. On August 31, Amnesty International called for his release and activists protested on his behalf outside the Chinese liaison office in Hong Kong. The most immediate reason for his detention was that his organization had published on its website the names of local officials in Henan that had participated in the blood-collecting enterprises. Henan officials, including the Provincial Vice Minister of Health, had met with him earlier that spring and offered him a deal: remove the names from his organization's website and he could collect evidence in Henan. He refused, and in August was taken into custody and charged with sharing state secrets (Marquand, 2002). After 6 weeks of detention, he was released, apparently to preserve China's application to the U.N.-backed new Global Fund for AIDS, Malaria, and Tuberculosis. Dr. Wan also publicly admitted guilt and contrition.

In August of the same year, Ma Shiwen, the deputy director of the Center for Disease Control of Henan's provincial health department, was arrested. According to Human Rights Watch, his crime was to use his computer to send out information on the blood-collection scandal to Chinese AIDS activists. The person responsible for the arrest was reported to be Liu Quansi, former director of the Henan health department, who was being blamed for presiding over the scandal and had been directly involved in the blood-collection business. In 1993–94 he led a delegation to the United States that tried to sell blood products. As part of their sales pitch, Liu claimed there was no HIV in Henan (Pomfret, 2003).

Chinese activist Li Dan also was harassed and arrested. He had helped establish The Orchid School, an alternative boarding school for children in Henan whose parents contracted HIV. In July 2004 police were sent to shut the school and return the children to their villages. They were met by protests from the staff. The police returned a few days later and detained an HIV-positive couple, Wang Guofeng and Li Suzhi, who had been acting as community liaisons for the school. Li Dan began a campaign on his website for their release and was arrested. After a month, Wang Guofeng and Li Suzhi were released, but on Li's release from detention he was beaten by, "a group of thugs who warned him to stop making trouble." At the time the Henan authorities closed at least three facilities for children affected by HIV/AIDS and routinely harassed and arrested activists (Davis, 2004).

In the spring of 2002, a French TV station produced a story on the plight of China's AIDS orphans. These are children who lost one or both parents to AIDS, or whose parents are living with HIV/AIDS and unable to care for them. The crew interviewed and filmed eight Henan villagers who had traveled to Beijing to petition the authorities and two were children whose parents had died of AIDS. It was the first international exposure to the problem of China's AIDS orphans. Typically, the children live in extreme poverty and suffer neglect, discrimination, and isolation. Because a good HIV surveillance study of the population in central China still has not been done, reliable numbers are not yet available to know how many AIDS orphans there are as a result of the blood donor epidemic. There are some preliminary reports from AIDS activist organizations. For example, in Shangcai County, Henan, 3,000 children are thought to have lost one or both parents to AIDS and 82 of the school-age children have been forced out of school for financial reasons and because of social stigma. AIDS orphans leave school to take care of their family and because the parents of other children are afraid they will spread HIV. Some AIDS orphans live alone or are shipped to orphanages, because relatives are afraid of contracting infection. It has been estimated that there will be 1.5 children left behind for each parent that dies of AIDS (Gao, 2002). The Chinese government now acknowledges the problem of AIDS orphans, but as yet has done little to help them. Much of the effort has been taken up by private charities through arrangements set up by local governments and some schools have reduced or eliminated tuition for AIDS orphans. Still, until late 2002 there were reports of local officials preventing the distribution of donations from charities to AIDS orphans. Social stigma and poverty remain a problem for these children.

In February 2002, proof of official government participation in the blood donor scheme appeared in the form of videotape sent to the United Nations, the PRC Ministry of Health, and the news media. It showed 20 villagers' blood donor cards that had been issued by the Henan Ministry of Health and that the individuals had been allowed to be repeat donors. It was not until March 2004 that the national Ministry of Health acknowledged that transmission of HIV had occurred in the 1990s via blood collection (Agence France Presse, 2004). In all it appears there was a 7-year delay between the time the government knew, or should have known, about the contaminated blood-collection practice and when the information was made public.

Is it fair to say the Chinese government should have known better and reacted more forcefully and in line with what other governments had done in similar situations? Before this time, epidemics of contaminated blood-replacement products had occurred in France and Japan. These were situations in which blood-replacement factors had been manufactured for people with hemophilia and recipients of the products became infected with HIV. It was recognized that high-level government officials either knew or should have known the products were unsafe, and were culpable for permitting them to remain in use.

In France, the events occurred in the mid-1980s when perhaps 4,000 individuals, mostly hemophiliacs and many who later died, received tainted blood-replacement factors to prevent uncontrolled bleeding. Three French officials were charged: the former Premier, Laurent Fabius; his superior at the time, the Social Affairs Minister Georgina Dufoix; and the Health Minister responsible for oversight, Edmond Herve. At the core of the scandal was the allegation that the three had delayed introducing a U.S. blood-screening test into France until a rival French product was ready to go on the market. Only Herve was convicted of negligence, specifically for the HIV infection acquired by two recipients of the products. Declaring Herve had not benefited from a presumption of innocence during the long scandal, the judge declined to hand down punishment. Still, at least there was public recognition of official responsibility (BBC News, 1999).

A Japanese scandal also occurred in the mid-1980s over tainted blood products manufactured for people with hemophilia. About 1,400 hemophiliacs were exposed to HIV and at least 500 died as a result. Based on that he should have known and acted, a Tokyo court gave Akihito Matsumara a suspended one-year sentence for his failure to prevent the death of a patient who in 1986 contracted AIDS from a contaminated transfusion. Matsumara had been the head of the government ministry responsible for handling blood and blood products. At the time heat treatment had been known to sterilize HIV blood-replacement products. In the United States the procedure had been in place for two years, but had not been implemented in Japanese blood banks. The scandal in Japan raised a national outcry as to whether its bureaucracy was too tied to the pharmaceutical industry and thereby put profits over people (BBC News, 2001). As yet no Chinese officials have been made publicly or legally responsible for the avoidable blood donor epidemic in Henan, Anhui, Shaanxi, and Hubei provinces.

Assessing the Health Effects

Because paying donors is known to increase the chance of contaminating products, most developed nations rely on voluntary systems to obtain blood for medical use. In China, blood donation is relatively new and often thought of with suspicion. The traditional view is that blood is a precious and vital body component and losing it through donation is a threat to health. Voluntary donation and blood drives are limited. Maintaining an adequate supply of blood and blood products is a challenge to modern Chinese medical practice. The demand for blood-replacement products ballooned as China's affluent classes expanded and its medical infrastructure improved. Combined with government corruption and a weak oversight system for blood banking, this was an ideal setup for unscrupulous entrepreneurs in the 1990s. In and around Henan they started enterprises in the early 1990s and continued operating at least until 1996. The scheme worked by encouraging villagers to sell their blood, which was then broken down into component parts and resold to pharmaceutical and biotechnology companies. The provinces of Henan, Anhui, Shaanxi, and Hubei, the areas where the companies operated, are not just poor. They are off the beaten track of China's rapidly modernizing coastal region. And the companies deliberately worked in rural villages and smaller cities where the vast majority of people are not well educated, and would have no sophisticated understanding of modern blood-banking practices and infectious diseases. And they are poor. They are in great need of cash. They were easy targets. A person selling blood would receive about 45 RMB yen for every 400 to 800 cc of blood. Although this is only about $5, it is a substantial sum of free cash to a peasant in rural China.

At least 300 legal and illegal blood-collecting stations were active in southeastern Henan province between 1993 and 1996. Donors were not screened for HIV or other infectious agents and equipment routinely was reused, often repeatedly, without proper sterilization. It is estimated that hundreds of thousands of villagers were exposed to HIV (Tyler, 1997). Compounding the problem was the use of an additional cost-cutting measure, in which blood taken from one individual was transfused into another individual to get more blood donations. This was done because giving blood frequently can produce anemia by depleting body iron and reducing the concentration of circulating red blood cells. Some people were donating blood 25 times or more in a year. This kind of recurrent bloodletting, in general, is not easily tolerated without experiencing fatigue, exercise intolerance, weakness, rapid heart rate, shortness of breath, and other unpleasant, possibly even fatal symptoms. In numerous villages, high proportions of young men and women were selling blood. To keep the donors coming in, the blood-collection agencies mitigated the symptoms of anemia by taking donated blood, separating the red cells, and reinfusing them into other donors (Zhang, 2004b). They further exacerbated the risks by pooling red blood cells from several different donors and then infusing the combined product into others. Even if done in a sterile fashion, this would be a dangerous and unacceptable medical practice. In China the companies were paying no attention whatsoever to mitigating the risks.

The consequences of the government's delay in shutting down the blood-collection agencies are still not well documented and will not be known until there is a full epidemiological investigation. Because of the staggering demographics, the problem could be enormous. The population of Henan province is 92,560,000, or about 1 of 70 of all humans on earth. Another 36 million people live in Shaanxi Province, 55–60 million in Anhui, and about 57 million in Hubei Province. The total is more than 240 million, or more than the population of all of Western Europe and about equal to the population of Indonesia, the world's fourth most populated nation. According to one estimate there may be a million HIV infections in the southern half of Henan province (Wan, 2002a, 2002b). Should the rest of the province be similarly affected, a figure of 1.5–2 million infections is not unreasonable. In 2002 a study by the Beijing AIDS Education and Research Institute found that in Shangcai County, located in central Henan Province, approximately 34,000 people tested HIV-positive, and more than 3,000 AIDS-related deaths were reported in a total population of 1.3 million, including 1.2 million rural residents. Eighty of 510 Shangcai villages surveyed had more than 100 individuals that tested positive for HIV and more than 10 AIDS-related deaths. For example, in Houyang village 160 people of a total population of about 4,000 had died of AIDS during the preceding five years. For reported HIV/AIDS-related deaths in Henan, 80.7 percent were male and 18 percent were female, and there are a few cases in which the gender was not known; 53.6 percent were between the ages of 20 and 29, the age group most likely to travel from village to town to sell blood. The rate of infection among those who sold blood is estimated between 45 and 50 percent. For rural families, this means that the household economic providers form a "sandwich generation," leaving behind infected spouses, elderly parents, and young children. Their economic difficulties are enormous. China does not have a strong government-sponsored social safety net. At least nine prefectures or townships in Henan were hard hit (Wan, 2002a). All these numbers should be considered preliminary estimates until a full scientific study is done.

It also is important to be mindful that it can take a decade to go from HIV infection to the symptoms of full-blown AIDS. During this time, only blood testing will uncover whether an individual is carrying HIV and hence capable of transmitting it to others. Individuals also can carry for years other infectious agents that were acquired via faulty blood without showing major symptoms and can pass the infections on to others through intimate and even household contact. Because the majority of people who gave blood numerous times were in their sexually active and reproductive years, the underpinnings for a long-lasting epidemic are in place.

At the U.S.-China summit on AIDS in November 2002, China's Center for Disease Control announced that a joint Sino-U.S. team would begin a research study into the blood donor epidemic. This was something of a breakthrough for Chinese investigators. However, the study remains restricted to Shaanxi province where it seems the blood-collection agencies were truly private so the provincial governments probably were not directly involved. Some researchers believe that Shaanxi's problem is less severe than in Anhui, Hubei, and Henan. If that is the case, data from Shaanxi might well not be representative of the situation in more hard-hit locales.

To date, none of the provincial officials involved in Henan, Hubei, or Anhui has lost a position and no criminal charges have been filed against individuals in the industry. While the companies involved in the scandal are no longer active, the entrepreneurs have been allowed to keep their profits. In 1995, China passed tough legislation to control blood-banking procedures, but enforcement was lacking then in Henan and may still be inadequate.

Were China to fully respond, a range of research, prevention, care, and support programs would be undertaken immediately. Research would include a population-based epidemiological assessment of the prevalence and risk factors of blood-borne pathogens, especially HIV, hepatitis C virus, HBV, and syphilis, across the affected provinces. This would require a sampling frame that includes all of the known and suspected geographic and socioeconomic populations. These data would correlate the prevalence of disease with risk factors such as history, frequency, and duration of blood donation, sexual history, and drug use, as risks for HIV infection and primary partner and family member impact. A second research agenda would be to look more broadly to do a recipient study by tracing through existing records and the blood-transfusion system to determine what happened to recipients of infected blood and blood products. If such data were not available from records, a study of blood donor recipients could still be designed based on procedure and diagnosis at medical facilities known to have purchased blood and blood products from the companies known to have participated in these schemes. So, for example, researchers would look to determine the rate of hepatitis C virus infection in people who received blood for cardiac surgery at hospitals where these products were used on the dates when the products were on the market. On the prevention front, widespread voluntary counseling and testing programs are needed: good-quality counseling for risks about sexual transmission to partners, condom promotion and distribution, services for prevention of mother-to-child transmission, and health education.

The government should consider the people affected by this iatrogenic epidemic as a special group entitled to free, expedited access to antiretroviral therapy as it becomes available in China. Most are poor. They should be first, not last. This would require a substantial investment in outreach on the part of the Chinese government, in expanding clinical and laboratory infrastructure, and providing training and support for providers such as physicians, nurses, and pharmacists so that effective antiretroviral therapy becomes a reality in the largely rural and poor affected communities. On the human rights and policy levels a widespread educational effort is needed to reduce the social stigma felt by the victims, especially AIDS infants and orphans, and their surviving family members.

A full, independent, and transparent investigation is needed of the criminal negligence on the part of the public officials and company management that perpetrated the disaster and participated in its cover-up. These individuals must be brought to justice. This is where a true public health response to the disaster also is a human rights response. Given that financial greed was abetted by government involvement, a full public accounting would go a long way to help restore trust in the blood-banking system. That trust and transparency that comes from a full investigation and judicial accounting will facilitate and make acceptable voluntary blood donation among the general population. Scientific data from around the world show that low-risk voluntary blood donation is the best way to maintain the safety of the blood supply, and China should move quickly in that direction.

Intersecting Rights and Health

The epidemic in central China should be seen in the plain-sight context of rights and health, in which government corruption and negligence flourished, the state police apparatus was employed to intimidate and cover up, and the victims and whistleblowers were ignored, harassed, and even jailed. Its victims were the poor and poorly educated, and the most vulnerable. Hundreds of millions of peasants are living in the countryside of China at subsistence level. Their living standard and political influence are not benefiting from China's progress toward modernization. China's ethnic minorities remain disadvantaged economically, socially, and politically in comparison with the overwhelmingly large Han majority population. Yet, the epidemic in central China occurred among poor and rural Han who also have neither political influence nor access to modern health care services. In the 1990s among the first cases of HIV/AIDS that China openly reported were in ethnic minority intravenous drug users living along the southwestern China-Burma border zone of Yunnan Province. Early on there also were case reports of HIV infection among gay and bisexual men living along the eastern seaboard. Intravenous drug use continues to produce new cases of HIV infection, especially in Yunnan, Guangxi, and Sichuan Provinces (Zheng et al., 1994). The rights and health point here is that all these groups live well outside the mainstream of Chinese society.

Since the first case was reported in China in 1985, it is estimated that between 100,000 and 120,000 people have died of AIDS. The Joint United Nations Program on HIV/AIDS (UNAIDS) 2002 report, "HIV/AIDS: China's Titanic Peril," estimates that more than one million Chinese are living with HIV and that the number could grow to 10 million by 2010, with 100,000 individuals each year developing the full-blown AIDS. The Ministry of Health and UNAIDS now identify four trends in China's epidemic: a low national prevalence that is high among specific populations and in certain regions; an increasing number of AIDS patients and AIDS related deaths; an epidemic that is spreading from high-risk populations to the general population; and that risk factors are in place to create a more generalized epidemic. Currently the hardest hit provinces for HIV infection are Henan, Yunnan, the Xinjiang Uygur Autonomous Region, the Guangxi Zhuang Autonomous Region, Anhui, Sichuan, Guangdong, Jiangxi, and Shanghai, and Beijing (UNAIDS, 2002b). Add the population of China's fastest growing province, Guangdong, which increased by about 37 percent over the past 10 years and now is about 70 million, plus that of the Shanghai (16.7 million) and Beijing (13.8 million) municipalities, and Jiangxi Province (41 million), to the approximately 240 million in the four central China provinces of the blood donor scandal, and one sees the potential for what could happen if AIDS is not checked.

Meanwhile, China's public health infrastructure is rudimentary, stigmatization of groups outside the mainstream continues, and protections for vulnerable populations available elsewhere are either not in place or not enforced. After symptoms of HIV/AIDS were first confirmed in Henan villages in the mid-1990s, most people were reluctant to be tested. They were afraid of being outcast and prosecuted and of receiving the brunt of an economic backlash. China has tough laws against drug use and prostitution (Gao, 2002). Seeking testing and care for HIV/AIDS may mean losing employment, having a child expelled from school, being evicted from your home, and even being denied care in a hospital. Chinese leaders have pledged to fight the stigmatizing, to use international funds to educate health care workers about HIV/AIDS, and to establish voluntary prevention and treatment programs. But progress remains slow, the country is huge, and what happens in the rural countryside lags far behind the more modern metropolitan areas.

Chinese law still permits quarantining people being tested or receiving treatment. This adds to the stigma problem and sends out a false message that HIV/AIDS can be transmitted through casual contact. The law also prohibits people with an infection from using public baths or swimming pools, and this can be applied to people with HIV, which does not spread by such casual contact (Chengdu Municipal Government, 2003; Jilin Provincial Government, 2003). Article 16 of the PRC Law on Infectious Diseases prohibits individuals with communicable diseases from continuing to work, and this has been applied incorrectly to people with HIV, especially in the service sector. This occurred in Zhejiang (Zhejiang Province Government, 2003; People's Republic of China, 2004). Despite Article 7 protection in the revised PRC Marriage Law (2001), people with HIV/AIDS can still be refused a marriage license on medical grounds. Articles 8 and 39 of the 1995 PRC Law on Maternal and Infant Health Care require postponing marriage and childbearing until couples infected with infectious and sexually transmitted disease, including HIV/AIDS, are treated. Article 2 of the "Regulations Concerning the Monitoring and Control of AIDS" contains language that requires "monitoring and control" of AIDS patients, persons infected with HIV, and suspected AIDS patients and people in close contact with people with HIV/AIDS. There still is broad language in the law to permit mandatory testing, isolation, and restricting movement. Articles 15, 16, and 17 require the reporting of HIV/AIDS cases by law enforcement, judicial, medical, and public health officials. Health professionals are required to report HIV/AIDS cases, but they are not required to maintain the confidentiality of names and other identifying information of patients. Beijing Municipal regulations require prostitutes and "any person suspected of spreading the AIDS virus" to undergo mandatory testing. Sometimes AIDS is treated as a state security matter (Beijing Municipal Government, 2003; International Federation for Human Rights, 2005). These laws and practices violate the International Guidelines on HIV/AIDS and Human Rights, which require that "public health legislation shall ensure that HIV testing is only carried out with the informed consent of those concerned" (World Health Organization, 2000). Prostitutes and drug users fear being identified through tests or by carrying condoms. Once identified, they may face detention, criminal charges, and mandatory rehabilitation (UN-AIDS, 2002b). Too often the media still portray AIDS as a disease of immoral people, criminals, and prostitutes. These are all health and rights issues that must be addressed.

Meanwhile, the rapid increase in recent years in the number of sexually transmitted diseases (STDs) in China outpaces public health programs for education, prevention, and treatment (Kaufman and Jing, 2002). For the most part, access to modern medical services remains available only to the relatively wealthy in the major cities. AIDS programs for voluntary counseling and testing are rare. Public health protections are insufficiently enforced, especially for the poor in the countryside and for the rapidly expanding population of migrants from the countryside looking for work in the cities. A 1998

Regulation on Blood Collection that was enacted to protect donors has not been implemented efficiently. It took another two years before the Ministry of Health officially banned the unsafe procedures of pooling blood and reusing syringes in hospitals. On the positive side, in 2001 the government acknowledged the spread of HIV/AIDS through unsanitary blood collection when it drafted the Second Plan for the Prevention and Control of AIDS.

Anti-AIDS retroviral medications are just coming to China. In March 2003 the government announced the CARES emergency pilot program designed to distribute free antiretroviral medication in 51 of China's worst-affected areas. It also is designed to reduce high-risk behavior, reduce mother-child transmission, and provide financial assistance to people with AIDS (Xinhua News Agency, 2004). The program is just getting started; only a fraction of those infected with HIV have been identified and a small number receive comprehensive antiretroviral regimens.

Looking Ahead

We still do not know the full story regarding the epidemic among blood donors in central China. The government cannot excuse itself for failing to provide vigorous oversight of the blood-collecting enterprises and preventing local officials from participating in these schemes. It should have acted quickly and decisively when Dr. Gao first made her observations public. By that time, the world was at least 15 years into the AIDS pandemic. There was ready testing for HIV in blood and blood products, well-documented blood-banking procedures for ensuring the safety of donors and recipients, and it was fully understood that contaminated blood and products are lethal. The prosecution of officials in France and Japan for failing to ensure the safety of the blood system had made international headlines well before. On the one hand, the Chinese authorities have reacted excessively against individuals in high-risk groups and then with callous disregard for vulnerable populations. From the human rights and public health perspective, this approach is contradictory to all we know now about HIV/AIDS and protecting the health of populations. (See Box 3.1.)

Chinese public health and government officials eventually were held responsible for their initial cover-up of the severe adult respiratory syndrome (SARS) outbreak, so there is precedent in China for requiring official accountability. Unfortunately, this has not occurred in the aftermath of the central

China blood donor epidemic. In 2003 Human Rights Watch hypothesized that economic concerns were the primary reason for the difference between the government's response to SARS and AIDS. Another reason is one more directly linked to human rights. The Chinese government still considers AIDS to be a disease primarily of "expendable" people in their march toward modernization (Human Rights Watch, 2003). Still there are hopeful signs, especially in the nongovernmental sectors. Since the late 1990s, an increasing number of nongovernmental organizations (NGOs) operating in China deal with HIV/AIDS, even though they sometimes work under restrictive governmental regulations. These organizations bring input from the outside and implement AIDS prevention activities that would be too sensitive for the Chinese government to carry out. This includes, for example, the Beijing AIZHIXING Education Institute and the Children Psychology Research Center, which helps AIDS orphans. Another hopeful sign is the diverse institutions that are incorporating HIV messages and information into their ongoing activities, as well as a number of academic institutions that have become active in AIDS prevention. These include NGOs supported by overseas philanthropies such as the Ford Foundation, Save the Children-UK, the Australian Red Cross, Marie Stopes International, Médecins sans Frontières, the Salvation Army, Oxfam-HK, and others. A number of telephone hotlines are now operating throughout the country for disseminating individualized AIDS prevention information. And there are more community-based groups that target vulnerable populations (UNAIDS, 2002b).

Officials in some areas, such as Henan, continue to harass independent NGOs and interfere with their work in assisting HIV/AIDS patients and individuals in high-risk groups. Officials at the Ministry of Health recently disclosed that they were drafting regulations to hold responsible the officials who cover up HIV/AIDS. The government is adopting new policies about the rights of people living with HIV/AIDS. Time will tell if they are passed into law and, more important, if they are enforced. In September 2002, authorities in Suzhou, a touristy city in the province of Zhejiang, adopted regulations prohibiting discrimination against persons living with HIV. In June 2003, Sichuan Province in Southwestern China announced steps to reverse its discriminatory laws banning persons living with HIV/AIDS from obtaining marriage licenses. In 2003 China applied to the Global Fund for funds to finance the care and treatment, including antiretroviral drugs, of 50,000 persons living with HIV/

Box 3.1. Health and rights timeline: an iatrogenic blood donor epidemic in China

1985   In an effort to prevent the transmission of HIV, the Chinese government bans importing blood and blood products. This creates demand for unscrupulous blood-collection schemes. The *Guangming Daily* urges the central government to ban homosexuality and require blood testing of all foreigners.

1986   *The China Daily* reports four Chinese confirmed HIV positive after "being injected with imported medication" due to blood products imported from the United States. To prevent the spread of AIDS, the official press calls for a crackdown on sexual liberalization and homosexuality.

1987   Port officials in Dailan say they found 60,000 units of gamma globulin imported in 1985 that test positive for HIV. The government officially denies any cases of AIDS transmitted in China.

1988   The Chinese Academy of Preventive Medicine declares all blood products manufactured by the Changchun Institute of Biological Products in Jilin province are free of HIV and 3,700 potential donors tested are free of the AIDS virus.

1989   The *Nanfang Daily* reports that a blood product manufactured in Spain and brought into China from Macao tested positive for HIV.

1990 to   Starting in the early 1990s and continuing at least through 1996, for-profit
1996   agencies collect blood in rural districts of densely populated Shaanxi, Henan, Hebei, and Anhui provinces. They employ high-risk procedures: paying donors, reusing unsterile equipment, and reinfusing pooled cells back into donors. In many instances, provincial officials own these enterprises in whole or in part, and except for the collections programs in Anhui they are largely private.

1992   Shanghai begins testing blood products.

1993   Warnings appear that China is behind in protecting its blood system: there is no nationwide system to test for HIV in blood donors and disposable syringes are still not in common use. French AIDS expert Christian Policard of Sanofi-Diagnostics-Pasteur recommends China test foreigners and high-risk groups such as prostitutes, homosexuals, and drug users for AIDS. Beijing has 45 registered HIV-positive persons with no reports of infection via blood transfusion.

1994   Experts attending an international AIDS symposium in Beijing recommend that China test all blood products for AIDS. So far, testing is performed only in Beijing, Shanghai, Guangzhou, and Yunnan. The *Beijing Youth Daily* reports that three blood donors in Beijing and Shanghai were HIV positive. Wan Yanhai forms an organization in Beijing to advocate for human rights, AIDS awareness, and gay and lesbian issues.

1995   Police in Tianjin find a group forcing kidnapped children to give blood and misleading peasants into donating blood and selling it to state-owned blood banks. The victims are promised good jobs, food, and accommodations. The United Press International reports that China has no system for voluntary

continued

blood donation and does not routinely screen donors for AIDS and hepatitis; hospitals pay anyone willing to sell their blood. The Chinese government reports that at the end of 1994 there were 1,775 cases of AIDS and "some patients were infected during blood transfusions." The Ministry of Health publicly admits the country has a blood-for-cash system with only limited HIV screening. The WHO warns that paying blood donors attracts high-risk groups.

1996   Dr. Gao Yaojie, a 76-year-old retired professor of obstetrics and gynecology at Henan University, becomes alarmed when she realizes her former patients have symptoms of AIDS. She will come to realize these infections are linked to faulty blood-collecting practices. About 90 percent of blood in China comes from paid donors. The *New York Times* reports that blood products manufactured by a Guangzhou Military Region enterprise and sold in Guangdong and Hong Kong tested positive for HIV. After its official denials, the government admits there are contaminated blood products, but still says no one has been infected and none of the products were exported. Premier Li Peng announces new regulations for blood banking and suggests there be new laws banning paid blood donation and meting out punishment for blood dealers. Chinese between age 18 and 55 should donate blood.

1998   The central government publishes the "Medium and Long Term Plan for AIDS Prevention and Control," which bans unsafe blood-collecting practices and calls for prevention, health education, and prevention of HIV transmission through the blood supply by 2002.

2000   On October 28, Elizabeth Rosenthal focuses attention to the iatrogenic blood scandal in an article published in the *New York Times*, "In Rural China, a Steep Price of Poverty: Dying of AIDS."

2001   For the first time, Chinese officials publicly acknowledge sending health experts to rural villages in Henan province to investigate reports of the blood donor scandal. In June they publish the "China Plan of Action to Contain, Prevent and Control HIV/AIDS (2001–2005)," which calls for testing blood for HIV and that more than 85 percent of blood for clinical use is to be provided by nonprofit blood centers (the rest supplied by authorized hospitals for their own use). Meanwhile, local Chinese officials block Dr. Gao Yaojie's application for a passport to visit the United States to accept a human rights award for her anti-AIDS work.

2002   Wan Yanhai meets with provincial Chinese officials associated with the iatrogenic blood epidemic. Chinese authorities detain him after the meeting.

2003   Wen Jiabao is the first Chinese premier to publicly shake hands with an HIV-positive person. The government announces a program to provide the "four frees": free anti-HIV drugs to rural AIDS patients and low-income persons, free voluntary counseling and testing, free drugs to prevent maternal-child transmission, and free schooling for AIDS orphans. By now, HIV cases related to blood or plasma donation are reported in all provinces, autonomous regions, and municipalities, except Tibet. The number of infected persons is

continued

Box 3.1. Health and rights timeline: an iatrogenic blood donor epidemic in China,
continued

	unknown. Despite supposed new official openness, Ma Shiwen, deputy director of the Center for Disease Control in Henan province, is detained, allegedly for making public a classified document that the Chinese government was aware of and hid the exploding AIDS epidemic in the countryside.
2004	In July, Henan provincial officials close down the Orchid School, an alternative boarding school for children whose parents have AIDS. In response to advocating for these children, police arrest Wang Guofeng and Li Suzhi, an HIV-positive couple. Li Dan posts messages of support for Wang and Li on his website. He is arrested. After being released, he is beaten and warned to stop making trouble.
2006	The Chinese government, WHO, and UNAIDS estimate that 650,000 people are living with HIV in China, and approximately 70,000 new HIV infections and 25,000 AIDS deaths occurred in 2005. AIDS and human rights activist Hu Jia is put under home arrest and beaten in Henan province for trying to help children orphaned by AIDS. In March, Li Dan is given a Reebok Human Rights Award for AIDS activism. Implementing the "Four Frees and One Care" policy continues to be uneven. In China the majority of HIV-positive individuals are unaware of their status.

Source: Adapted in part from www.casy.org/chron/BloodSupply.htm

AIDS in some of its hardest-hit areas. In its application, China acknowledged that HIV had spread through unsafe blood-collection centers beyond Henan, into six additional provinces. The application also admitted that "stigma has hampered the social and political response" to HIV/AIDS, including a government survey which showed that AIDS and other serious health problems contributed to poverty in rural areas, where the health care system is the weakest. In December 2003, the government launched the "Four Free and One Care" policy: free HIV testing, free antiretroviral drugs, free school fees for orphans, free preventives from mother-child transmission, and relief (care) for HIV patients living under hardship. The policy was intended for victims in rural Henan Province (Zhang, 2004b). This is a start, but even if implemented, the plan is not adequate to meet the needs of the people affected. Corruption and lack of political will on the local level is compromising its implementation. In February 2004, the State Council created the Working Committee on AIDS to coordinate and implement the government's AIDS policy. In April 2005, authorities amended the law on infectious diseases, removing AIDS from the list of diseases requiring mandatory quarantine.

These are signs of openness. But the real test is whether the government will end all discriminatory laws and practices, allow public debate on prevention and treatment policy, permit civil society advocacy groups to provide assistance to victims, and allow greater freedom of information and of the press regarding the epidemic. Opportunities exist for creative and thoughtful responses; there is a chance to learn from the experiences of the international community and individual countries about how they deal with the stigmatization and discrimination against people with HIV/AIDS and their families. The Chinese government could elevate the HIV/AIDS campaign to the highest level of political commitment and broaden their narrow focus, implementing programs that target social, economic, and political challenge as a matter of human rights protection instead of seeing HIV/AIDS as a "medical condition." This would, of course, include people living with HIV/AIDS, their families, and AIDS orphans. It also would include expanding rural health care, state-subsidized primary care, and home care, all of which would be costly. In addition, people living with HIV/AIDS and civil society groups outside of the official government must be encouraged to participate in this policy making.

References

Agence France Presse. 2004. Officials say most Chinese provinces may have AIDS from selling blood. March 3.

BBC News. 1999. World: Europe blood scandal ministers walk free. March 9.

BBC News. 2001. Japan blood scandal official convicted. September 28.

Beijing Municipal Government. Adopted 14 September 1990, amended 2 November 2003. *Regulations of Beijing municipality for the implementation of the control and monitoring of AIDS.*

Bureau for Disease Control, Ministry of Health. 1995. Guiding opinions in regard to reinforcing the prevention and control of AIDS. 21st Notice of the State Council. In *Collected documents of the administration of AIDS/HIV prevention and treatment.*

Bureau for Disease Control, Ministry of Health. 1999. Guiding opinions for the management of people infected with HIV and AIDS patients. In *Collected documents of the administration of AIDS/HIV prevention and treatment.*

Chang, L. 2002. China to provide free drugs to AIDS-stricken villagers. *Wall Street Journal.* October 18.

Chengdu Municipal Government. Adopted 30 November 2000, amended 2 November 2003. Article 9, *Regulations of the municipality of Chengdu on the containment, prevention and control of sexually transmitted diseases.*

Coram, T., P. Aggleton, R. Parker, and M. Maluwa. June 2002. HIV/AIDS related stigma and discrimination: Foundation and framework for action. UNAIDS.

Davis, S. 2004. Hold Beijing to account for its AIDS coverup. *International Herald Tribune*. August 25.

Gao, Y. 2002. Save AIDS orphans. *Ren yu Renquan* (*Humanity and Human Rights*, an online Chinese journal). May 17.

Human Rights Watch. 2003. *Locked doors: The human rights of people living with HIV/ AIDS in China*, August.

International Federation for Human Rights. 2005. *China at a critical stage: Violations of the right to health in the context of the fight against AIDS*. April.

Jilin Provincial Government. Adopted 7 November 1992, amended November 2003. Article 9. *Regulations of the province of Jilin on the containment, prevention and control of sexually transmitted diseases*.

Joint United Nations Programme on HIV/AIDS (UNAIDS). 1999. *Handbook for legislators on HIV/AIDS, law and human rights: Action to combat HIV/AIDS in view of its devastating human, economic and social impact*.

Joint United Nations Programme on HIV/AIDS (UNAIDS). 2002a. Global crisis, global action, adopted at the UNAIDS Conference, June 27, 2002.

Joint United Nations Programme on HIV/AIDS (UNAIDS). 2002b. *HIV/AIDS: China's titanic peril*, Beijing.

Kaufman, J., and Jing, J. 2002. China and AIDS: The time to act is now. *Science* 296:2339–40.

Marquand, R. 2002. China AIDS activist riled officials. *Christian Science Monitor.* September 3.

People's Republic of China. Adopted 21 February 1989, amended on 28 August 2004. *Law on infectious diseases*.

Pomfret, J. 2003. China detains health official for publicizing AIDS coverup. *Washington Post Foreign Service*. October 8.

PRC Med and Long Term Plan for AIDS Prevention and Control, 1998–2010. 1998. In *Collected documents of the administration of AIDS/HIV prevention and treatment*. Bureau for Disease Control, Ministry of Health, People's Republic of China. Tyler, P. 1997. China concedes blood serum contained AIDS virus. *New York Times.* October 25.

Wan, Y. 2002a. An analysis of HIV/AIDS epidemic in Shangcai County, Henan Province. *Ren yu Renquan.* September 19.

Wan, Y. 2002b. China's AIDS orphans need care. *Ren yu Renquan.* May 17.

World Health Organization (WHO). 2000. *Guidelines for second generation HIV surveillance*. Accessed at www.who.int/hiv/pub/epidemiology/pub3/en/ (accessed November 14, 2005).

Xinhua News Agency. 2004. Health ministry announces 51 AIDS pilot zones. April 6.

Yu, E. H. S., Xie, Q., Zhang, K., Lu, P., and Chan, L. L. 1996. HIV infection and AIDS in China, 1985 through 1994. *American Journal of Public Health* 86:1116–22.

Zhang, K. 2002. Epidemiology of HIV in China. *British Medical Journal* 324:803–4.

Zhang, F. 2004a. *Progress of the China National Free Antiretroviral Therapy Program.* Chinese Center for Disease Control and Prevention, National Center for AIDS/STD Prevention and Control. January 12.

Zhang, K. 2004b. Report on the five year inquiry into AIDS in Henan. Cited in International Federation for Human Rights. 2005. China at a critical stage: Violations of the right to health in the context of the fight against AIDS. April.

Zhejiang Province Government. 2003. *Methods of Zhejiang Province for the prevention and control of AIDS and sexually transmitted diseases.* Adopted 29 December 2003.

Zheng, X., Tian, C., Choi, K-H., Zhang, J., Cheng, H., Yang, X., Li, D., Lin, J., Qu, S., Sun, X., Hall, T., Mandel, J., and Hearst, N. 1994. Injecting drug use and HIV infection in southwest China. *AIDS* 8:1141–47.

Zunyou, W. 2005. Plenary presentation at the 17th International Conference on Harm Reduction. March, Belfast, UK.

4

Women's Health and Women's Rights

Selling Sex in Moscow

Julie Stachowiak, Ph.D., and Alena Peryshkina

The burgeoning Russian sex industry is marked by widespread violations of the rights to health, dignity, and life itself. The exploitation of tens of thousands of women and girls in this industry by those who run it, profit from it, and use it is both a context of rights violations and a public health disaster in the making. Because Russia is undergoing linked epidemics of substance use, sexually transmitted infections (STIs), HIV, and hepatitis C virus, the nexus of sex for sale has the potential to markedly worsen these epidemics among the women who sell sex for a living, their clients, and their clients' other partners. While male clients are at the center of potential epidemic spread of STIs and HIV beyond the sex work core, it is the women on the Russian streets who face discrimination, harassment, and violence. And because post-Soviet Russia is marked by widening disparities in income and employment between Moscow and a few other large cities, and the vast and impoverished regions that remain in the Russian Federation, the supply of women willing to work in this industry, especially in Moscow, remains enormous.

When the Soviet Union collapsed in 1991, along with it went a police state and a puritanical society that had quite tightly controlled some forms of sexuality, including prostitution, although even in Soviet times sex workers could be found soliciting foreign tourists in the large hotels. With the end of state subsidies for an array of enterprises, unemployment soared across the Russian Federation. In a short time, women in Moscow and major cities across the former Soviet Union were selling sex on the streets, at truck stops, in international hotel lobbies, and through escort services. Today there are pickup locations all along the highway that leads from Moscow's Sheremetyevo Airport to the city, where women and their pimps, called *sutenyorsha*, congregate at *tochkas* (literally, "spots") at highway off-ramps to sell sex. Men drive up—sometimes three to five in a single car—and select one or more women. The women get into the cars and are driven off and serve the men. It is in this street-based scene that our organization, AIDS Infoshare, has been providing outreach, education, condoms, and conversation to these women for the past decade.

We have learned a great deal from the women on the airport road, about the interactions of sexual health and rights, about the way this harsh industry functions, about relationships with the police, and about what these young women want. Selling sex on the Moscow streets is dangerous and degrading, and many aspects of the work are somewhat specific to Russia's capitol and to the car-based highway scene, but this is just one component of a much larger industry. Russian and Former Soviet Republic women are selling sex in many cities in the Russian Federation, but also in Western Europe, Israel, India, Thailand, and the United States (Atlani et al., 2000). By elucidating here some aspects of the Russian sex industry at its heart, we hope that the work AIDS Infoshare has been doing may be of wider use to these women and to those seeking to help them.

Moscow sex work draws from an enormous population and a wide geographic area. In addition to Muscovites selling sex, there are women from other regions of Russia, and women from the many former Soviet Republics, especially Ukraine, Moldova, Belarus, and Lithuania (Stachowiak et al., 2005). Most live illegally in the Moscow area. In a throwback to Soviet days, it takes a special permit to relocate residence in Russia. Within a few days, every new entrant to the city must register with the police by presenting a valid visa, work permit, hotel permit, or affidavit from a legal Moscow resident they are staying with. The difficulties women selling sex face in Moscow are a special irony in that the prostitution itself is not illegal and the exploitation to a great extent comes from the fact they are living illegally in the city (Moscow City Ordinance No. 33, July 9, 1997). In effect, the women are stateless in their own country and confederation. Without legal residency, they do not qualify for public, social, and medical services; they can be shaken down at any time by the police. Pimps, the police, and anyone else who realizes they are living without legal status exploit them. The outcomes of this illegal status are not only the potential for exploitation, but poor health outcomes. In our study of sex worker risk for HIV and STI (done in collaboration with investigators from Johns Hopkins University), we found that women who reported being unable to see a physician were twice as likely to have a current STI as were women who did have medical access (Stachowiak et al., 2005). Indeed, lack of access to health care was the only risk factor that remained independently associated with having an active STI among these women after controlling for age, educational level, and other demographic factors.

The health threats involved in sex work in Moscow, and in Russia in general, are occurring in a crucially important wider health context. The overall health status of Russians, and the state of public health efforts overall, have been in marked by sharp declines in the post-Soviet era. Russians are succumbing to epidemics of obesity, alcohol and tobacco abuse, heart disease, and reemergent tuberculosis. The lifespan of a boy born today in Russia is 58 years, equal to and lower than in some of the world's poorest nations. To put this in perspective, male life expectancy in Bangladesh is 60 years, in Vietnam 67 years, and in the United Kingdom 75 years. Meanwhile, Russian women have some of the lowest fertility rates in the world (People Facts and Figures, www.os-connect.com/pop). If current trends continue, demographers predict that by the year 2050 there will be approximately 100 million Russians or about 50 million fewer than when communism imploded. Over the next 5 to 20 years, the number of women between age 20 and 29 will decline by half. Over the next decade the relatively nascent and contained HIV/AIDS epidemic could ravage the nation. The World Bank estimates that by 2020 there will be at least 5 million HIV-positive Russians, but without aggressive prevention and public awareness efforts that number could be much larger. The demographic prediction is that without a large migration into the country, over the next generation there likely will be 5 million fewer Russians in the workforce and 30 percent fewer in school. The demographer Murray Feshbach pointed out that while HIV/AIDS epidemics have occurred in many developing country settings with young populations and high fertility rates, HIV is spreading in Russia in a population already in sharp demographic decline—a heretofore unprecedented situation and one that may make the demographic effect of AIDS in Russia all the more severe (Feshbach, 2003).

The other context for understanding the explosion of women selling sex in Russia and the former Soviet Republic is the economic collapse that befell the country when the communist system abruptly ended. In a few years the average Russian had less than half the savings than he or she had under the old system. There were massive layoffs as the government unloaded inefficient industries. And it failed to collect taxes; so many workers that were still employed by the state were not paid. Public employees like teachers and health care workers received barely enough to get by. Pensioners suffered as the ruble plummeted in value and the old state subsidies on basic products vanished. The state-sponsored youth and sports clubs that were the pride of Soviet communism disbanded for lack of funds. There was a stock market crash and many lost their investments in the newly privatized market. Mafia-like organized crime syndicates took over. The "black market" became "the market." A new group of Russians that could afford imported goods became conspicuous consumers of automobiles, blue jeans, and CDs. The crime syndicates trafficked primarily in narcotics, weapons, and prostitution. By the beginning of 2000, it is estimated there were more than 10,000 organized crime groups with 60,000 members operating in Russia. These events are part of the backdrop for understanding why so many educated Russian women started selling sex for a living. When AIDS Infoshare asked about motivations for entering the sex trade, nearly all said it was to provide something better for their children or their families.

AIDS Infoshare

Under communism, public health had been a state function. Nonstate actors had no role in health, in general, and no role in public health, in particular. As normal life fell apart in the post-Soviet 1990s and the commercial sex industry expanded quickly, openly, and transnationally, a small group of Russian and American AIDS advocates organized AIDS Infoshare as a nongovernmental organization. We began in 1993. Our goal was to bring awareness to Russians about AIDS and to provide both the medical and general information that was emerging about AIDS worldwide in Russian-language versions and at little or no cost; hence, AIDS Infoshare. In 1996, as the epidemic began to emerge among sex workers, AIDS Infoshare began a concerted effort to reach women in the sex industry. AIDS Infoshare has been in continuous operation since it was founded.

When we started working with the women selling sex, researchers and advocates knew little about them. We began by doing simple street outreach. Staff members would spend evenings climbing into vans and speaking with the shivering girls who were waiting for clients. We visited the apartments they shared and got to know pimps, called *sutenyori* in Russian. Many of the women we met were educated mothers sending money home. That initial outreach work generated a large-scale National Institutes of Health (NIH)-funded epidemiological study to investigate the changing risks for acquiring HIV, hepatitis B and C, and STIs. Since 1997, Russia has been experiencing epidemics of syphilis and HIV; HIV is still most closely associated with intravenous drug use. However, the recent trend seems to be that an increasing number of women engaged in commercial sex are injecting drugs and acquiring HIV, so these epidemics may be overlapping. For example, in a sample of 200 sex workers in Moscow, 36 percent admitted using drugs and 79 percent of them said they were injecting (AIDS Infoshare, 1999). If this pattern follows what has occurred elsewhere in the world, HIV will be increasingly transmitted by sexual contact and this spread will likely involve both commercial and noncommercial sex.

To meet the critical need for outreach education, prevention, and treatment of STIs, including HIV, AIDS Infoshare established an innovative research collaboration that includes SANAM, a Moscow-based nongovernmental organization (NGO) with a clinical and services focus, the Ivanovsky Institute of Virology of Moscow University, and the Departments of Epidemiology and International Health of the Johns Hopkins University School of Public Health. The Ivanovsky Institute of Virology is a branch of the Russian Academy of Medical Sciences. It trains scientists in virology and immunology and its Immunochemistry Group is the first in Russia to be capable of subtyping HIV isolates. With these partners, AIDS Infoshare developed a novel approach that combines street outreach, testing, counseling, and medical services with a population-based research program grounded in a health and human rights perspective.

The research plan looks for social and structural factors that affect the lives of women selling sex, such as their day-to-day work conditions, the violence and intimidation they face, homelessness, and the overall human rights context, including onerous laws. We are attempting to relate social, legal, and structural factors to definable risks for acquiring and transmitting diseases such as HIV, hepatitis B and C, syphilis, gonorrhea, *Chlamydia trachomatis*, herpes simplex virus type 2, bacterial infections, and unplanned pregnancy. In addition to doing standard laboratory analyses for diagnosing STI, the research design includes doing sophisticated molecular subtyping to track the epidemiology of STIs, especially HIV-1 among Moscow-based sex workers. By sequencing the HIV-1 isolates found during the cross-sectional and cohort feasibility phases of the study, we hope that it will be possible to track disease patterns and, in particular, compare the subtypes found in drug-injecting and noninjecting commercial sex workers.

An essential arm of the research protocol is to conduct open-ended, indepth interviews with sex workers. The surveys are designed to learn about their knowledge and experiences in three broad subject areas: (1) sexual risk behavior, (2) injection drug use behavior, and (3) other factors or behaviors that increase vulnerability to HIV and STIs. These interviews are performed multiple times in an iterative process to build on, validate, and explore themes that appear in prior interviews. AIDS Infoshare started by recruiting from a pool of women we already knew. That familiarity created trust needed for the women to be open and honest. We also interviewed pimps, police, and crime officials, and the medical specialists that treat this population. The interviews with medical specialists were designed to assess their knowledge of and attitudes about the Russian epidemics of STIs, such as hepatitis B and C and HIV, and their more general understanding of the conditions faced by commercial sex workers. Our study is also designed to assess the effect of legislation and policies on public health and commercial sex workers. We worked with experts to review and analyze the 1993 Constitution of the Russian Federation and Fundamental Legislation on Public Health of Citizens of the Russian Federation, the 1998 Russian Federal Law on Drugs and Psychotropic Substances, the 1995 Law on Prevention of the Spread of HIV Infection in the Russian Federation; the 1993 Optimization of Control over STIs; Order 286 of the Ministry of Health of the Russian Federation; the 1991 Law on Medical Insurance of the Citizens of the Russian Federation; the 1985 instruction manual for the serodiagnosis of syphilis, Order 1161 of the Ministry of Health of the USSR; the 1993 treatment and prevention of syphilis, recommended methods; the 1994 National AIDS Prevention and Control Programme; the 1997 Order 1570 of the Ministry of Health of the USSR on improving the detection of patients with gonorrhea and trichomoniasis and the 1997 Criminal Code of the Russian Federation. The legal reviews informed later efforts in working with the police and security authorities and helped us understand the legal- and rights-related aspects of health risks faced by sex workers.

Moscow's Commercial Sex Industry

Women who sell sex in Moscow come from Moscow and the former Soviet Union and Eastern Bloc. More than 90 percent of the women fall into the category of "migrant" workers (Montgomery, 2000). Estimates of the number of women in the sex industry vary widely. Media reports range between 13,000 and 30,000 sex workers in greater Moscow, police claims of several million, and 70,000 is widely accepted and reported by the Ministries of Health and Internal Affairs (Platt, 1998; Dehne, 1999). None of these numbers is likely to be accurate. It is an underground, fluid life. Our work has found that many women work 3 to 6 months and then stop sex work temporarily or permanently. Most start working before age 25, usually between ages 16 and 17. In Russia 17 is the legal age of majority, but we have heard of girls as young as age 8 in prostitution (AIDS Infoshare, 1999). The women receive money and/or drugs in exchange for sexual acts with men. AIDS Infoshare has identified subgroups of women that have differing pay scales and risks. The largest number are street-based and/or working at truck stops and train stations. They are paid less and their lives are more dangerous than the women who work the international hotels and escort agencies. Age and drug use, including use of alcohol, methamphetamines, and the increasingly common club drug ecstasy apparently play a role in pay and safety. The women who come to Moscow without money and legal residency depend on pimps for housing until they earn enough money to rent their own room or apartment, shifting the power balance away from women and limiting their ability to make safer choices with partners and acts.

Economic conditions that are outside a woman's control play a large role in what happens to her. The economic crisis of August 1998 caused prices for sex to fall by 50 percent. At the time, 40 percent of the women we interviewed reported that the amount they could earn was contingent on their willingness to have sex without a condom. Also at the time, about 20 percent said they engaged in anal sex with clients to increase the pay (AIDS Infoshare, 1999).

Physical abuse from clients is common. In 2000, 86 percent of sex workers told AIDS Infoshare they experienced physical abuse from clients "sometimes" or "often" (AIDS Infoshare, 2000). They also described living in a form of indentured servitude. A woman living illegally in Moscow cannot report a crime perpetrated against her to the police. To the extent that such abuses are being caused and aggravated by lack of Moscow residency is a government-sanctioned human rights violation. The police also can be complicit or even perpetrate crimes against the women. They regularly stop single women, and young women with men, and ask for documents. This can occur at any time, but happens most often at night. The women frequently pay money or provide sex for free to the police to avoid arrest and harassment.

From 2001 to 2005, AIDS Infoshare conducted qualitative and quantitative research to learn why and how women go into Moscow's sex industry. The women enter commercial sex through different routes, including trafficking (see also Chapter 7, by Zimmerman and Watts), being lied to and coerced, by having their papers taken, and by being kept in a state of indentured servitude (Chudakov et al., 2002; Beyrer, 2004). Although most said they started sex work voluntarily, they also told us that at the time they started they had no idea how little freedom they would have working for a pimp. The pimp is needed for protection from police and clients. Most said they were financially supporting family members, as others have noted across Russia (*Pacific AIDS Alert Bulletin*, 1996; Gadasina, 1997; Ditmore and Saunders, 1998; Butcher, 2003; Manopaiboon et al., 2003).

Women selling sex in roadside settings are usually hired for a specific price and then taken away by clients in cars. The women are most often not the ones who negotiate the type of sex, the length of time, or the price. The pimp does this. Clients may be told that only certain girls will perform anal sex. A major fear and stress for the women is to be "bought" by one client and taken to a spot where many more men are waiting.

The Network of Sex Work Projects, an organization that links sex worker health programs around the world, found that one of the main requirements for low incidence of HIV and STI among sex workers is for sex workers to have control over their work environment (Ditmore and Saunders, 1998). In

Moscow that often is not the case. Often they cannot demand condom use. In general, the women who work the truck stops, streets, and highways are much less safe than the women who work in brothels, in the international hotels, and for the escort services. The less control she has, the less able she is to protect herself and her clients from STIs (Ditmore and Saunders, 1998; Chan and Reidpath, 2003). Here is a typical description as told to AIDS Infoshare,

> The rules are not as strict as they were at my second spot where we were not allowed to refuse the client. We come here by 11:00 a.m. The mamochkas stand near the highway, and we wait in the bus somewhere farther away—for example, near the garages. The mamochka stops the car and names a price. It can vary from 1500 rubles up to 150 dollars and depends on the girl's appearance. Then the mamochka gets into the client's car and they come to the bus. She enters the bus and says the price. Some of the girls come out from the bus. If nobody pleases the client, then another price is announced and other girls come out. If the client likes any girl then she gets into his car. He pays money to the mamochka, and the girl does not get to his car until he has done this.

Sex workers who are victims of assault cannot go to the police if they do not have legal residency status. Usually nor can the pimps. The common theme we hear is, "There is no one to tell." In Russian settings gender-based violence is far too common. In one study conducted in St. Petersburg 25 percent of adolescent girls said they had experienced sexual violence (Lunin et al., 1995). The Moscow police victimize illegal sex workers through harassment, forced sex, and arbitrary arrest. They use a variety of pretexts in addition to lack of residency documentation, such as allegations of "hooliganism," disorderly behavior, and public drunkenness to conduct raids and arrest sex workers. The women frequently are required by their pimps to participate in "*subbotniki,*" which means to have sex with the police free of charge. It is a form of payment from the pimps to the police that permits them to operate without being bothered (Aral et al., 2003). In what seems to be contradictory, but perhaps shows the depth of their exploitation, some women report enjoying *subbotniki.* Evidently, the women get to know the police and feel the relationship between pimp and police protects them from client violence and being swept up in police raids.

Focus on Sexually Transmitted Infections, especially HIV/AIDS

During the Soviet era, the public health system did little to track and treat sexually transmitted infections. It considered STIs to be a problem for decadent capitalist societies, not virtuous socialist ones. The first case of HIV in the Soviet Union was publicly identified in 1987, but was also downplayed as a serious problem (Ministry of Health of the Russian Federation, 2000). The first AIDS death was reported more than a decade later, in 1998—well after the Soviet Union had ended and the Russian Federation had been born. Officials emphasized that the woman had been a prostitute with many foreign clients, including Africans, since the 1970s. Well after the communist system fell, health officials continued to avoid and downplay HIV/AIDS. Yet, HIV was emerging and its conditions for rapid spread being met. From 1999 to 2000, Russia experienced a 300 percent increase in HIV infections (UNAIDS, 1999), along with an epidemic of syphilis in which cases from 1990 to 1997 increased from 5.44 to 277.3 per 100,000 (Tichonova, 1997).

So far, the steep upward curve of HIV incidence primarily has been attributed to unsafe use of injection drugs, currently estimated at 80–90 percent of people with HIV infection (Rhodes et al., 1999, 2002). Since 2000, there has been increasing concern that HIV is spilling over from intravenous drug users to the "general population." While the data may be questionable, the concern is legitimate because a spread from drug users to the more general population has occurred elsewhere and has been frequently associated with prostitution (Tyndall et al., 2002). The result of this fear has been to further stigmatize commercial sex workers. Estimates of the proportion of sex workers injecting drugs varies from 25 to 80 percent (Lakhumalani, 1999; Atlani et al., 2000; Dehne et al., 2000; Lowndes et al., 2003). The large variation in the statistics is indicative of the lack of a good study as is the reported prevalence of HIV among sex workers injecting drugs: 17 percent in St. Petersburg, 61 percent in Togliatti, and 65 percent in Kaliningrad (Dehne and Kobyshcha Iu, 2000; Dehne et al., 2000; Lowndes et al., 2002). There are reports that in some regions commercial sex workers in Russia account for the majority of HIV-positive women (e.g., 82% of HIV-positive female patients treated at a regional health center in Kaliningrad made their living by selling sex) (Dehne et al., 1999). Whatever the numbers, it is fair to say that women who sell sex are at heightened risk over the general population for acquiring HIV, especially where government-sponsored health education campaigns do not inform the public about safer sex, and condom use. The city of St. Petersburg is one of the few places where public health programs include active outreach, HIV/AIDS education, providing clean needles to drug users, and free or low-cost condoms.

Recent research by AIDS Infoshare and the Centers for Disease Control and Prevention indicates that the overall prevalence of HIV among women selling sex in Moscow is likely to be less than 5 percent, and still highly concentrated among the women who are intravenous drug users. In other words while women in the sex industry have high vulnerability, their rates of infection still are relatively low (*End-year report 2002*, 2002; Kozuharov, 2004; Shakarishvilli et al., 2005; Stachowiak et al., 2005). Sex workers in Russia nevertheless are accused in the media and by policy makers of being important contributors to spreading HIV (Daniszewski, 2002; Kozuharov, 2004). Those who favor punitive measures and those who favor prevention and treatment accuse women that sell sex of being a "bridge" for spreading HIV to the general population and the result is to further stigmatize them.

Looking Ahead

How would a rights and health approach contend with the inequities, violence, and health risks that women face selling sex? It would include focused research that is conducted without bias or stigma.

The qualitative study was conducted among female street sex workers in Moscow, Russia, from October 2002 through March 2003. Sex worker respondents were identified during outreach programs conducted by AIDS Infoshare. In these programs, trained staff members went in pairs to visit various *tochkas*. During each visit, the teams distributed condoms and informational brochures that contain information on safe sex, medical facilities, health education about substance abuse, signs and symptoms of STIs, and so on. The women were given the opportunity to ask questions either in a group or privately of the team members.

All women signed an informed consent agreement and received the ruble equivalent of 20 U.S. dollars. The interviews were conducted using a semi-structured instrument containing questions about: demographics, recruitment into sex work, working conditions, relationships with clients, pimps, family, violence, drugs and alcohol use, condom use, health issues, and plans for the future. Each interview lasted between 45 and 90 minutes and was conducted either at the woman's place of work or in a café. All interviews were audiotaped, transcribed verbatim, and translated from Russian into English.

To assess risk factors and measure prevalence of STIs among female sex workers in Moscow, Russia, we conducted a cross-sectional study among 478 women involved in prostitution. Subjects were recruited in a variety of ways. Although much emphasis was initially placed on outreach activities through AIDS Infoshare's outreach team, it is estimated that only about 10 percent of participants were successfully recruited when approached by the outreach team. Far more successful was the snowball method, whereby women who participated in the study were given cards to distribute to other sex workers. To avoid identification of participants as sex workers if they were stopped by police, as well as by other patients at the clinic, the cards identifying women as study participants named them as members of "Moscow Club for Women's Health."

Women coming to the clinic underwent the complete informed consent procedure. Following the informed consent procedure, participants underwent the following sequence of events at the same visit: (1) a pretest HIV and STI counseling session; (2) blood draw and urine collection (samples were then sent immediately to the laboratory to be tested); (3) physician collection of medical history and symptom report; (4) gynecologic exam; (5) interviewer-administered quantitative survey; (6) post-test HIV and STI counseling session; and (7) follow-up meeting with the physician to discuss positive test results, answer additional questions, provide treatment and referrals, as appropriate. Participants were given ruble equivalent of twenty U.S. dollars, condoms, and literature on HIV and STI prevention. The study physician made a determination of whether treatment was indicated based on reported symptoms and findings during gynecologic examinations and rapid labs. Necessary treatment was provided free of charge.

Another step would be to pass legislation compatible with the 1996 Second International Consultation on HIV/AIDS and Human Rights, which states, "With regard to adult sex work that involves no victimization, criminal law should be reviewed with the aim of decriminalizing, then legally regulating occupational health and safety conditions to protect sex workers and their clients, including support for safe sex during sex work. Criminal law should not impede provision of HIV/AIDS prevention and care services to sex workers and their clients" (Second International Consultation on HIV/AIDS and Human Rights, 2004). In Moscow and elsewhere in Russia, meeting these goals would require changing residency and work laws, or at least changing them for vulnerable groups such as sex workers, but would not require debate about decriminalization of sex work, because prostitution is already legal in Russia. Still passing new legislation alone will not address economic disadvantage and stigma, social attitudes toward women, and make much-needed improvements in public health. It could begin to address the limitations on access to medical services. And this access could include a vastly heightened public commitment to STI prevention and treatment, especially HIV/AIDS; as well as harm reduction, violence prevention, addiction services, and family-planning services. STI and HIV services alone would be unlikely to meet the many needs of women selling sex beyond those directly related to sexual health—and our data suggest these other nonsexual health-related services are more likely to be valued by the women themselves. The good news is the cost of providing these services is relatively modest in comparison with many other modern medical technologies. It is fair to say that Russian girls and women all over the country, and including the ones who sell sex for a living, deserve access to safe and effective reproductive health services nested in primary health care (Overs, 1992; Butcher, 2003; Chan and Reidpath, 2003).

Women selling sex also face stigmatization. Prostitution has been stigmatized throughout human history and most recently blamed for contributing significantly to the HIV epidemic (Salamov and Pokrovskii, 1998). Instead of blame, it would be more helpful for the government to sponsor proven public health prevention programs. Stigma in health care settings may be an additional barrier to seeking needed care, and again, it is critical to reaching the goal of providing services and controlling STI and HIV. A related goal would be to use access to health services to make contact with and assist women who want to stop selling sex, and to do so safely. Clearly, health care is also a important setting in which to promote safer sex strategies like condom use for the women who continue to sell sex for a living (Alexander, 1992; Morgan et al., 1992; Tambashe et al., 2003). Research and prevention programs have done a good job establishing why condoms are not used consistently (Vanwesenbeeck, 2001; Basuki et al., 2002; Vuylsteke et al., 2003).

The reasons women go into sex work are part of a complicated "risk environment" of social, economic, and individual factors. Each affects program planning and execution (Alexander, 1992; Overs, 1992; Rhodes et al., 1999). Looking at only the act of transmitting HIV probably misses information that can help develop more effective programs. It may come as a surprise to people outside of the sex industry that STIs and HIV often are not the primary concern of the sex workers themselves (Wolffers and van Beelen, 2003). In a recent study conducted among inner-city sex workers in the United States, women selling sex identified their main problems to be rape, depression, tuberculosis, and access to health insurance. HIV/AIDS was never mentioned (Baker, Case, and Policicchio, 2003). In a study conducted in South Africa, a country with extremely high HIV prevalence, sex workers clearly stated that violence was a much greater problem for them than HIV (Nairne, 2000). A study conducted in ten regions of Russia found the most frequently mentioned concerns of sex workers to be lack of money, police violence, problems with their pimps, and then STIs and HIV (Bardakova et al., 2004). Our data confirm much the same set of concerns among Moscow women. The point is that effective programs likely are going to have to deal with a range of underlying conditions and include interventions that start from the moment a woman or girl decides to sell sex, to her reaction to situations that put her at risk, and then to interventions that reduce harms to her health. Our research indicates that women in the sex industry need mental health services, including drug and alcohol abuse programs. They also need programs to help them cope with violence. AIDS Infoshare works with the women who sell sex in a collaboration that engages public health professionals, policy makers, law enforcement officials, and scientists and researchers (Mertz, Sushinsky, and Schuklenk, 1996; Wolffers and van Beelen, 2003). A special effort continues in research, in part, because for far too long Russian public health structures have not put emphasis on conducting good epidemiology on its sex industry. Without an accurate picture of reality, the system oscillates between denying that a problem exists and issuing alarmist case reports. Solid population data are needed to determine disease prevalence and patterns of transmission and to target appropriate interventions.

Finally, improving access to health care services for women selling sex, regardless of residency or nationality, would be both sound public health policy and a marked improvement in human rights practice. To continue to deny women medical services, allow the police to profit from the industry, and maintain the social marginalization of these women is to ensure their ongoing exploitation and to aid and abet HIV and other STIs as they threaten the health of Russia. It is hard to imagine a clearer example of where rights-based approaches to public health could be more beneficial—and hard to imagine a country and a historical moment more critical than Russia's in 2007 in which to put such rational and humane policies in place.

References

AIDS Infoshare. 1999. Data on female commercial sex work in Russia (unpublished). Moscow.

AIDS Infoshare. 2000. Preliminary data on 200 female sex workers (unpublished). Moscow.

Alexander, P. 1992. Key issues in sex work-related HIV/AIDS/STD prevention interventions. *AIDS Health Promotion Exchange* (1):4–6.

Aral, S. O., St Lawrence, J. S., Tikhonova, L., Safarova, E., Parker, K. A., Shakarishvili, A., et al. 2003. The social organization of commercial sex work in Moscow, Russia. *Sexually Transmitted Diseases* 30 (1):39–45.

Atlani, L., Carael, M., Brunet, J. B., Frasca, T., and Chaika, N. 2000. Social change and HIV in the former USSR: The making of a new epidemic. *Social Science and Medicine* 50:1547–56.

Baker, A. C. 1994. Issues of human rights and HIV. Guest commentary. *AIDS Link* (25):6.

Baker, L. M., Case, P., and Policicchio, D. L. 2003. General health problems of inner-city sex workers: A pilot study. *Journal of the Medical Library Association* 91 (1):67–71.

Bardakova, L., Stibich, M. A., and Stachowiak, J. A. 2004. Using free list methodology to enhance program activities for street sex workers in ten regions of Russia. *In press.*

Basuki, E., Wolffers, I., Deville, W., Erlaini, N., Luhpuri, D., Hargono, R., et al. 2002. Reasons for not using condoms among female sex workers in Indonesia. *AIDS Education and Prevention* 14 (2):102–16.

Beyrer, C. 2004. Is trafficking a health issue? *The Lancet* 363 (9408):564.

Butcher, K. 2003. Confusion between prostitution and sex trafficking. *The Lancet* 361 (9373):1983.

Chan, K. Y., and Reidpath, D. D. 2003. "Typhoid Mary" and "HIV Jane": Responsibility, agency and disease prevention. *Reproductive Health Matters* 11 (22):40–50.

Chudakov, B., Ilan, K., Belmaker, R. H., and Cwikel, J. 2002. The motivation and mental health of sex workers. *Journal of Sex and Marital Therapy* 28 (4): 305–15.

Daniszewski, J. 2002. Russia sits on edge of an HIV/AIDS epidemic. *Los Angeles Times.* September 9.

Dehne, K. 1999. *The determinants of the AIDS epidemic in Eastern Europe: Monitoring the AIDS pandemic report.* Geneva: UNAIDS.

Dehne, K. L., Khodakevich, L., Hamers, F. F., and Schwartlander, B. 1999. The HIV/

AIDS epidemic in eastern Europe: recent patterns and trends and their implications for policy-making. *AIDS* 13 (7):741–49.

Dehne, K. L., and Kobyshcha Iu, V. 2000. *The HIV epidemic in Central and Eastern Europe: Update 2000.* Geneva: UNAIDS.

Dehne, K. L., Pokrovskii, V. I., Kobyshcha Iu, V., and Schwartlander, B. 2000. Update on the epidemics of HIV and other sexually transmitted infections in the newly independent states of the former Soviet Union. *AIDS* 14 (Suppl. 3):S75–84.

Ditmore, M., and Saunders, P. 1998. Sex work and sex trafficking. *Sex Health Exchange* (1):15.

Feshbach, M. 2003. *Russia's health and demographic crises: Policy implications and consequences.* Washington, D.C.: Chemical and Biological Arms Control Institute.

Gadasina, A. 1997. Struggling to survive in Russia. *Planned Parenthood Challenges* (1–2):40–42.

Geneva: European Centre for the Epidemiological Monitoring of AIDS (EuroHIV). 2002. *End-year report 2002, No. 68.*

Joint United Nations Programme on HIV/AIDS (UNAIDS). 1999. AIDS epidemic update. Geneva: Joint United Nations Programme (UNAIDS) World Health Organization.

Kozuharov, S. 2004. Half of all prostitutes in St. Petersburg have HIV. *St Petersburg Times.* April 22.

Lakhumalani, V. 1999. [The prostitution situation in a number of cities of Russia, Ukraine and Byelarus]. *Zhurnal Mikrobiologii Epidemiologii Immunobiologii* (1):102–4.

Lowndes, C., Rhodes, T., and Judd, A. 2002. Female injection drug users who practice sex work in Togliatti City, Russian Federation: HIV prevalence and risk behavior. Paper presented at the 14th International AIDS Conference, Barcelona, Spain.

Lowndes, C. M., Alary, M., and Platt, L. 2003. Injection drug use, commercial sex work, and the HIV/STI epidemic in the Russian Federation. *Sexually Transmitted Diseases* 30(1):46–48.

Lunin, I., Hall, T. L., Mandel, J. S., Kay, J., and Hearst, N. 1995. Adolescent sexuality in Saint Petersburg, Russia. *AIDS* 9 (Suppl. 1):S53–60.

Manopaiboon, C., Bunnell, R. E., Kilmarx, P. H., Chaikummao, S., Limpakarnjanarat, K., Supawitkul, S., et al. 2003. Leaving sex work: barriers, facilitating factors and consequences for female sex workers in northern Thailand. *AIDS Care* 15 (1):39–52.

Mertz, D., Sushinsky, M. A., and Schuklenk, U. 1996. Women and AIDS: The ethics of exaggerated harm. *Bioethics* 10 (2):93–113.

Ministry of Health of the Russian Federation. 2005. Official HIV/AIDS Statistical Report of the Russian Federation. Moscow: Russian Scientific-Methodological Center for HIV/AIDS Prevention.

Montgomery R. 2000. Outreach activities: A successful HIV/AIDS and STD prevention strategy among female commercial street sex workers in Moscow, Russia. Abstract MoOrD256. Paper presented at the XIII International AIDS Conference 2000, Durban, South Africa.

Morgan-Thomas, R., and Overs, C. 1992. AIDS prevention in the sex industry. *Newsletter Women's Global Network on Reproductive Rights* 38:33–36.

Nairne, D. 2000. We want the power; findings from focus group discussions in Hillbrow, Johannesburg. *Research for Sex Work* 3:3–5.

Overs, C. 1992. Seropositive sex workers and HIV/AIDS prevention: a need for realistic policy development. *AIDS Health Promotion Exchange* 1:1–3.

Platt L. 1998. *Profile of sex workers in Moscow.* Moscow: AIDS Infoshare Russia.

Rapid increase in HIV rates—Orel Oblast, Russian Federation, 1999–2001. 2003. *Morbidity and Mortality Weekly Report* 52 (28):657–60.

Rhodes, T., Ball, A., Stimson, G. V., Kobyshcha, Y., Fitch, C., Pokrovsky, V., et al. 1999. HIV infection associated with drug injecting in the newly independent states, eastern Europe: the social and economic context of epidemics. *Addiction* 94 (9):1323–36.

Rhodes, T., Lowndes, C., Judd, A., Mikhailova, L.A., Sarang, A., Rylkov, A., et al. 2002. Explosive spread and high prevalence of HIV infection among injecting drug users in Togliatti City, Russia. *AIDS* 16 (13):F25–31.

Rhodes, T., Stimson, G. V., Crofts, N., Ball, A., Dehne, K. L., and Khodakevich, L. 1999. Drug injecting, rapid HIV spread and the 'risk environment.' *AIDS* 13 (Suppl. A): S259–69.

Salamov, G. G., and Pokrovskii, V. I. 1998. Moscow sexual workers: AIDS knowledge and sexual practices. Abstract 60224. Paper presented at the 12th International Conference on AIDS, Geneva, Switzerland.

Second International Consultation on HIV/AIDS and Human Rights. 2004. *HIV/AIDS and Human Rights International Guidelines.* Geneva: UNAIDS.

Sex work on the rise. International news. 1996. *Pacific AIDS Alert Bulletin* (12):14.

Shakarishvilli, A., Dubovskaya, L. K., Zohrabyan, L. S., et al. 2005. Sex work, drug use, HIV infections and spread of STI in Moscow, Russian Federation. *The Lancet* 366 (9479):57–60.

Stachowiak, J. A., Sherman, S., Konakova, A., Krushkova, I., Peryshkina, A., Strathdee, S., and Beyrer, C. 2005. Health risks and power among female sex workers in Moscow. *SIECUS Report* 33 (2):18–25.

Tichonova, L., Borisenko, K., Ward, H., Meheus, A., and Renton, A. 1997. Epidemics of syphilis in the Russian Federation: trends, origins, and priorities for control. *The Lancet* 350:210–13.

Tyndall, M. W., Patrick, D., Spittal, P., Li, K., O'Shaughnessy, M. V., and Schechter, M. T. 2002. Risky sexual behaviours among injection drugs users with high HIV prevalence: implications for STD control. *Sexually Transmitted Infections* 78 (Suppl. 1), i170–75.

Vanwesenbeeck, I. 2001. Another decade of social scientific work on sex work: a review of research 1990–2000. *Annual Review of Sex Research* 12:242–89.

Vuylsteke, B. L., Ghys, P. D., Traore, M., Konan, Y., Mah-Bi, G., Maurice, C., et al. 2003. HIV prevalence and risk behavior among clients of female sex workers in Abidjan, Cote d'Ivoire. *AIDS* 17 (11):1691–94.

Wolffers, I., and van Beelen, N. 2003. Public health and the human rights of sex workers. *The Lancet* 361 (9373):1981.

5

Reducing Harm in Prisons

Lessons from the United States and Worldwide

Julie Samia Mair, J.D., M.P.H.

The health and safety of prisoners is the responsibility of the correctional systems and authorities that hold them in custody. Worldwide prison conditions play an important role in transmitting infectious diseases such as HIV, drug-resistant tuberculosis, and hepatitis. Prisoners also are victims of violence and sexual assault that have harmful, often disastrous, health consequences. It is both a health threat and an abuse of their human rights that, as a matter of law and policy, incarcerated individuals are routinely denied proven disease-prevention and harm-reduction strategies and are subject to inmate-on-inmate and guard-on-inmate violence. The consequence of this negligence is that prisons in many settings, including in the United States, too often serve as incubators for the transmission of disease inside the facilities and into the general public when inmates are released. Although still controversial in many countries, an ever-increasing number of correctional systems in diverse nations worldwide offer condoms and safe injection equipment to prevent or limit the spread of infectious diseases. These approaches, generally grouped as harm reduction or harm minimization, have the potential to meet both public health tests for efficacy and human rights goals of providing minimum standards of access to health care. Nevertheless, they have been fraught with political and operational challenges. And while prevention services have often been limited, access to basic health care has also been problematic, most notably in jails and other shorter-term detention settings.

From October 2004 to April 2005, researchers from the District of Columbia Prisoners' Legal Services Project and the Johns Hopkins Bloomberg School of Public Health interviewed 117 women incarcerated at the District of Columbia Jail and adjacent Correctional Treatment Facility. We found serious deficiencies in the health services provided to the female inmates, including unnecessary lags in access to care for chronic illnesses, interruptions in medication delivery, a general failure of the sick call system for acute problems, inadequate care for mental health and substance abuse disorders, and a general need to review and revise procedures for the delivery of health services. Among the most prominent recommendations are the immediate needs to address overcrowding and underfunded mental health services and to implement measures to prevent interruptions in the delivery of medications, especially for HIV antiretrovirals, which must be administered properly to prevent drug resistance. Unfortunately, the problems uncovered in this study are common in prisons elsewhere in the United States and in many countries around the world.

The Right to Health in Prison

Many international human rights instruments apply to prisoners. Some address specifically the right to health care, while others do so less directly. Some agreements are binding on the states that ratify them, while others elaborate general principles that, although not obligatory, should be accepted as the standard for government behavior (Lines et al., 2004; Cornell Law School). Article 5 of the 1948 Universal Declaration of Human Rights (UDHR), which some argue has reached the status of customary international law, states, "No one shall be subjected to torture or cruel, inhuman or degrading treatment or punishment." Having signed on to the 1948 UDHR, states are required to protect persons in custody from rape and other forms of violence and to take reasonable measures to maintain the highest attainable standard of physical and mental health, including the provision of and equal access to preventive, curative, and palliative health services (International Covenant on Economic, Social and Cultural Rights, 1976; Mariner, 2001; Lines et al., 2004). Although the special circumstances of confinement do not always permit the same delivery of care as is available on the outside, it is government's responsibility to make a concerted effort to provide free health services similar to what is available to the general public (Reyes, 2001a; WHO Europe, 2005). Reliance on a community standard does not condone the delivery of inferior health services to prisoners even if health care in the community is poor (Penal Reform International, 2001).

In specific, correctional authorities have a duty to provide safe and healthy living quarters; protection from violence and coercion; adequate health care services and medicines, as far as possible, free of charge; commencing and continuing medical treatments begun on the outside, including those for drug users; information and education about preventive health measures and healthy lifestyles; medical screening, including the detection, prevention, and treatment of sexually transmitted diseases, including HIV/AIDS. There also should be specific protection for vulnerable prisoners, such as individuals who are HIV positive, and adequate counseling should be made available before and after HIV testing. And protective measures should be taken to prevent inmates from acquiring communicable diseases, such as tuberculosis (TB), that are readily spread in confined settings (WHO Europe, 2001).

Infectious Diseases in Prison

Prisoners tend to be less healthy than the general population. Living conditions in prison often exacerbate health problems that existed before incarceration and catalyze new health conditions. Incarcerated individuals thus may have a greater need for health care in prison than on the outside (Reyes, 2001a). Meanwhile, resources are always limited. The consequence is that correctional authorities have to make tough choices among the services offered to prisoners, including trade-offs among health care, counseling, rehabilitation, education, and maintaining and administering prison facilities.

When compared with the general public, prisoners are disproportionately affected by some of the most serious communicable diseases, such as HIV/AIDS, hepatitis, and tuberculosis. In 1996, between 13 and 19 percent of all HIV-infected persons in the United States had served time in U.S. prisons and jails and the estimated prevalence of HIV infection among inmates was 4–10 times higher than in the general U.S. population. Twenty-nine to 32 percent of people infected with hepatitis C virus (HCV) had served time and it was estimated (likely an underestimate) that the prevalence of HCV was 9–10 times higher among inmates than in the general population. And, 12–15 percent of all people in the United States infected with hepatitis B virus (HBV) had served time. Approximately 35 percent of all persons in the United States with TB had been in a U.S. correctional facility, and the prevalence of TB among inmates was estimated to be 4–17 times higher than in the general U.S. population. High numbers of inmates also have sexually transmitted infections (STIs), such as syphilis, chlamydia, and gonorrhea (National Commission on Correctional Health Care, 2002). The United States is not unique in this regard. To varying degrees worldwide, infectious diseases are common problems in correctional settings.

Many individuals enter prisons with compromised health due to socioeconomic factors such as unsanitary living conditions and substandard access to health care and to behaviors such as high-risk sexual conduct and intravenous drug use with unsafe injection practices. Prison conditions, such as overcrowding, poor ventilation, violence, unprotected sex (consensual and nonconsensual), tattooing, psychological stress, poor nutrition, and substandard medical and mental health care, serve to exacerbate existing poor health and expose inmates to new illnesses (Choopanya et al., 1991; Taylor et al., 1995; Dolan and Wodak, 1999; CDC, 2001, 2004; Post et al., 2001; Krebs and Simmons, 2002; Beyrer et al., 2003; O'Sullivan et al., 2003; Baillargeon et al., 2004; Champion et al., 2003; WHO Europe, 2005; Zamani et al., 2005).

Although substandard prison conditions can promote the spread of many infectious agents, we will focus on HIV, hepatitis, and TB. HIV, the virus that causes AIDS, can be transmitted through blood, semen, preseminal fluid, vaginal secretions, and breast milk. In prison the important routes are by anal, vaginal, and oral sexual contact (CDCb, 2006) and by sharing infected needles or injection equipment. At the beginning of every injection, blood is introduced into the needle and syringe so the risk of transmitting HIV is particularly high by this route. Reusing spoons and other containers also can spread HIV through the infected drug solution (CDCd, 2006). Heterosexual transmission of HIV is more likely from men to women than from women to men (Reyes, 2001b). Infection with another sexually transmitted disease greatly increases the efficiency of transmitting HIV whether there are breaks in the skin (e.g., syphilis, herpes) or not (e.g., chlamydia, gonorrhea) (CDCc, 2006). In women, STIs such as genital herpes, chancroid, and syphilis often go undetected if they do not produce symptoms and the lesions are inside the genital tract (Reyes, 2001b). HIV increases the risk of acquiring opportunistic infections, including TB, which is especially dangerous in the prison setting because it can be transmitted via airborne contact such as coughing and sneezing. A person with both HIV and TB is 800 times more likely to develop active TB disease than someone who is HIV negative (CDCe, 2005). Individuals with HIV and AIDS have an increased risk of developing multidrug-resistant TB (CDCf, 1999; CDC, 1992), which can be difficult to treat and fatal.

HCV is transmitted primarily by exposure to infected blood and other bodily fluids. Within 5 years of starting to inject drugs, 50–80 percent of injection drug users (IDUs) become infected with HCV. Most (75–85%) of these individuals become chronically infected, and most of them (70%) develop chronic liver disease, which can progress over a 20- to 30-year period to cirrhosis, liver cancer, and end-stage liver disease. Early on, most people with chronic HCV infection do not know that they are infected and thus can transmit the virus to others without knowing it. HIV speeds up the progression to cirrhosis and liver cancer in people with HCV, and complicates long-term therapy with multiple-drug regimens (CDC, 2002a). Like HCV, hepatitis B virus (HBV) is transmitted by blood and bodily fluids. It is estimated that 50–70 percent of IDUs become infected with HBV within 5 years of beginning to inject. Although only 2–6 percent of people infected with HBV become chronically infected, 60 percent of them go on to develop chronic liver disease, which can progress to cirrhosis, liver cancer, and end-stage liver disease. Again, early on symptoms are mild or nonexistent, so most people with chronic HBV infection are unaware of their infection and can unknowingly transmit the virus to others (CDC, 2002b). Hepatitis A virus (HAV) is transmitted primarily through fecal-oral contact. It is a self-limited disease, and after recovery most people retain lifelong immunity. Most do not go on to chronic infection or long-term liver disease. HAV is relatively common among IDUs, transmitted through fecal contamination of drug equipment. To date, no outbreak of HAV has been reported in U.S. correctional settings even though many inmates use drugs and engage in high-risk sex (Weinbaum et al., 2003).

It is the responsibility of correctional systems to do all that is reasonably possible to prevent the spread of infectious diseases. As we will discuss, this requires a multifaceted approach, including testing where appropriate, immunization (e.g. HBV, HAV), access to proven harm-reduction technologies, and prevention of violence.

Sex in Prison

Reducing the frequency of high-risk sexual behavior in prison is the best strategy for limiting the risk of transmitting all three hepatitis strains, HIV, and other STIs (CDC, 2002b; Weinbaum et al., 2003). Unfortunately, most correctional facilities treat condoms as contraband. Prisoners are not under constant surveillance by the correctional staff, which affords opportunities to engage in prohibited behavior. Rape is all too common in men's prisons, as is unsafe consensual sex. The reported prevalence of consensual sex among inmates varies but apparently is substantial (Koscheski et al., 2002). One study of 150 male inmates in Ohio found that although 77 percent identified themselves as heterosexual, nearly 20 percent reported homosexual activity with another inmate during the prior year; 8.5 percent engaged in sex at least once a week and 7.4 percent admitted to a continuing relationship (Tewksbury, 1989; Koscheski et al., 2002). In a study of inmates in Oklahoma, 80 percent identified themselves as heterosexual, 13 percent as bisexual, and 8 percent as homosexual; 24 percent said they had permitted another man to touch their penis or had touched another man's penis, 23 percent had performed or received oral sex, and 20 percent admitted to participating in anal sex with another inmate (Hensley, 2001; Koscheski et al., 2002). Two studies of homosexuality among female inmates in the United States found at least one-third of women engaged in sexual activity with another inmate (Koscheski et al., 2002). Because the imbalance of power between an inmate and a staff member prevents actual consent, all sexual encounters between staff members and inmates are considered assault.

Sexual assault, defined broadly to include physical force, threats, and coercion, is a significant problem in prisons worldwide (Heilpern, 1998; Mariner, 2001; Reyes, 2001a; Kunselman, 2002). For a variety of reasons, including fear of reporting, the true prevalence of prison sexual assault is unknown (Kunselman et al., 2002). The U.S. Congress conservatively estimates that about 13 percent, or more than 1 million inmates, were sexually assaulted in U.S. correctional facilities over the past 20 years (Prison Rape Elimination

Act; Mair et al., 2003). Often assaults are repeated and involve numerous assailants including other inmates, correctional staff members, and other individuals who have contact with inmates. The victims are women, men, and children in juvenile facilities. Anecdotal reports suggest some male inmates engage in pre-emptive sex to avoid being raped.

Intravenous Drug Use

The reported prevalence of intravenous drug use in prison varies among studies but it appears to be substantial and is an important cause of infectious disease transmission. Contraband drugs are smuggled into prisons by staff members, visitors, and others who have reason to be inside.

In a study of ten Greek prisons, 33.7 percent of 861 responding inmates reported injecting drugs at some time in their lives and 60 percent said they had injected in prison (20.2% of total sample). Of great concern for the spread of infectious diseases, 83 percent of the drug injectors reported sharing injection equipment (Koulierakis et al., 2000). A European Union study found high IDU prevalence rates in 21 prisons in seven European countries: Belgium, France, Germany, Italy, Portugal, Spain, and Sweden. From 9 percent in France to 59 percent in Sweden, inmates reported injecting within 12 months before incarceration and between 25 and 79 percent of them said they had injected while in prison; and 5–15 percent said they began injecting drugs while incarcerated (Jürgens and Bijl, 2001a). Other studies also have found prison to be the place where people start injecting drugs (Lines et al., 2004). Overcrowding, violence and coercion, frustration, and boredom are reasons prisoners inject drugs (Jürgens and Bijl, 2001a; Reyes, 2001a).

Prisoners are more likely than IDUs in general society to engage in unsafe injection practices, such as sharing injection equipment. This greatly increases the potential health harms of injecting drugs (Hellard et al., 2004). A qualitative study of 20 formerly incarcerated male IDUs in British Columbia found that while drugs were available in prison only six to seven syringes were being used among a population of about 200. The frequency of injecting varied with some prisoners reporting injecting several times a day. Injection equipment was a highly valued commodity and kept operational for as long as possible by being repeatedly fixed with parts made from older syringes and pens. Not only would this practice create a risk for transmitting infectious agents, reusing equipment causes scarring and vein damage. And an inmate might not disclose being HIV positive for fear of losing access to used syringes (Small et al., 2005).

Perhaps the first report of HIV spread in prison by injecting drugs occurred in 1993 in Glenochil, Scotland (Taylor et al., 1995). All of the HIV-positive inmates said they had injected drugs while in prison and nearly all (97%) said they had shared needles and syringes. Two of the HIV-positive men had acquired the virus before entering the facility and continued to inject and share equipment. None of the non-IDU prisoners tested was HIV positive. Clearly, injecting drugs was the major culprit. Sharing injection equipment in prison also has been associated with HIV epidemics in Lithuania (Jürgens, 2004) and Australia (Dolan and Wodak, 1999). One U.S. study found that among 33 male inmates that had contracted HIV in prison, 16 (49%) had acquired it by sexual contact with another man and 6 (18%) by intravenous drug use (Krebs and Simmons, 2002). Hepatitis B and C also are transmitted by unsafe injection practices. A 2000–2001 Australian study (O'Sullivan et al., 2003) and a 2004 Scottish study (Champion et al., 2003) both found sharing injection equipment to be the likely cause of outbreaks of HCV.

Harm Reduction

Harm reduction is a general term used to describe strategies for minimizing the adverse effects of unhealthy behaviors that individuals persist in. While a purely criminal justice approach may see drug use as a moral hazard to be stigmatized and punished, harm reduction may be viewed as a set of strategies based on a "disease model" (Fischer, 1995; Marlatt, 1996; Gostin and Lazzarini, 1997). The 2005 WHO Europe *Status Paper on Prisons, Drugs and Harm Reduction* summarizes the evidence on harm reduction related to drugs in prison (WHO Europe, 2005). WHO Europe believes "the public health case for action is strong. Those involved in deciding policies and services for prisons now have the evidence of effectiveness to add to the successful experiences in several countries in Europe and elsewhere. They should conclude that harm-reduction measures can be safely introduced into prisons, that such measures can significantly bolster preventing the transmission of HIV/AIDS in communities, and that action in the interests of public health as a whole is required" (WHO Europe, 2005). Since the early 1990s, several countries have implemented harm reduction and prevention programs in prisons that usually include information, education, and communication; voluntary testing and counseling; condom distribution; making available bleach or other disinfectants; syringe exchange; and substitute drug therapy such as methadone treatment (WHO Europe, 2005). For example, Iran, reported to have the highest rate of heroin addiction in the world, plans to establish 60 centers across the country and add 45 centers in prisons to provide no-cost needle exchange, methadone treatment, condom promotion, HIV testing, and antiretroviral drugs to treat HIV (Srikameswaran, 2005).

Unfortunately, not all states are enthusiastic about harm reduction. In 1995, a public health working group in the United States published recommendations to encourage the Office of National Drug Control Policy to redefine its approach based exclusively on use reduction to a more balanced approach that includes harm reduction (Reuter and Caulkins, 1995). They recommended that "the principal goal for drug policy should instead be to reduce the harms to society arising from the production, consumption, distribution, and control of drugs. Total harm (to users and the rest of society) can be expressed as the product of total use and the average harm per unit of use and thus can be lowered by reducing either component. Attention has been focused on the first; greater attention to the second would be beneficial." Despite recommendations from the public health community, the U.S. government's 2005 *National Drug Control Strategy* makes no mention of harm reduction or any of its components (White House, 2005), and this policy is applied to prisons. A 2003 U.S. federal district court case, *Gibbs v. Martin* (unpublished) illustrates this thinking. Three HIV-positive inmates in the Michigan Department of Correction were ticketed for sexual misconduct and placed in 30 days of punitive confinement and then placed indefinitely in administrative segregation. HIV-negative inmates with the same infraction were released into the general population after 30 days of punitive confinement. In claiming that indefinite administrative segregation was improper, the inmates argued, among other things, that a less-restrictive alternative existed in the form of distributing condoms. The court disagreed, writing that

> prisoners are not supposed to engage in sexual acts with other prisoners. Why should the prison provide condoms, so prisoners can perform what is prohibited? Second, in reality, we are dealing with a prison environment and prisoners are not model citizens. Should we trust that prisoners (some, like Plaintiff Elmer, who are in prison for criminal sexual conduct) will reliably use condoms when perform-

ing prohibited sexual misconduct? Should the prison require that HIV+ prisoners who engage in prohibited, but 'consensual' sex (even with condoms supposedly provided by the prison itself) inform their sexual partners that they are HIV+? This is a prison environment and we believe that we should defer to prison authorities where appropriate. General policies need to be implemented that protect the health and safety of all the inmates. Plaintiffs' request jeopardizes the risks to non-HIV+ prisoners; they, too, have a right to be protected from contracting this fatal and incurable disease.

This reasoning fails to address the fundamental principle of public health that individuals should have the knowledge and ability to maintain and improve their own health (WHO Europe, 2005). Educating prisoners on the risk of transmission of diseases such as HIV, HCV, and HBV and affording them access to condoms and clean injection equipment would satisfy both human rights and promote the health of the prison population and that of the general public. Unfortunately, the views of the Michigan court are not unique. Distributing condoms and safe injection equipment to prisoners has met with fierce resistance in many correctional systems, in large part because sex and drug use are generally prohibited in prison and providing these items is seen as condoning and even encouraging prohibited behavior. Some are also concerned that the products will be misused, for example, made into weapons. The objection to methadone or buprenorphine therapy is that while it may assist individuals to stop injecting drugs it does not necessarily stop them from using drugs even though they are medicines dispensed by and under the supervision of a medical professional (Jürgens and Bijl, 2001b). Recently, both medications were added to the "Complementary List" of the WHO Model List of Essential Medicines as "essential medicines for priority diseases, for which specialized diagnostic or monitoring facilities, and/or specialist medical care, and/or specialist training are needed" (WHO, 2005).

Distribution of Condoms

Each year the number of correctional systems in Europe distributing condoms increases. In 1989, 53 percent made them available, 75 percent in 1992, and 81 percent in 1997; more recent data show they are available in all but four systems (Jürgens, 2004). Condoms are available for some prisoners in other countries including Canada, Australia, and the Ukraine (Stern,

2001; Jürgens, 2004). In Canada, condoms have been distributed in federal prisons since 1992 and are now available in most other systems (Canadian HIV/AIDS Legal Network, 2004/2005b). Seven jurisdictions in the United States distribute condoms to incarcerated populations: five jail systems (Los Angeles County, New York City, Philadelphia, San Francisco, and Washington, D.C.) and two state prison systems (Mississippi and Vermont) (Hammett et al., 1999; Nerenberg, 2002). Condom distribution is most effective when they are "easily and discreetly accessible" (Jürgens and Bijl, 2001b). To date, no system that adopted condom distribution has reversed it (Jürgens, 2004).

Available evidence does not support the concern that distributing condoms condones and encourages prohibited sexual activity, including rape; or that condoms are used as weapons or to hide contraband (May and Williams, 2002; Nerenberg, 2002; Dolan et al., 2004). The first published report on condom distribution in a U.S. correctional facility was based on a 2000–2001 survey of 307 inmates and 100 correctional officers at a Washington, D.C. jail. Interviews with jail administrators and a review of disciplinary reports since the program's inception revealed no incidents of major security infraction involving condoms and no evidence of increased sexual activity. Most inmates (55%) and correctional officers (64%) supported the program (May and Williams, 2002).

Another study looked at the feasibility of distributing condoms to prisoners in New South Wales, Australia and, in particular, whether prisoners would use them during sex. In November 1997, 150 vending machines that distributed condoms free of charge were installed in 23 male correctional facilities housing about 6,220 men. They dispensed a box containing one condom, one packet of lubricant, one sealable disposal bag, and an information card. In March 1998, researchers sent a survey to the entire inmate population and interviews were conducted with 13 senior prison officials and 37 correctional officers. From the inception of the program until September 1998, 294,853 condoms were dispensed averaging 24,571 each month, or the equivalent of each inmate obtaining one condom per week. Although the response to the survey was low (9%), the responding sample was similar to the entire prison population in terms of age, most serious offense, and length of sentence. Twenty-eight percent of the respondents reported obtaining condoms from the vending machines and of those, 21 percent reported using the machines at least once a week. Forty percent of respondents used condoms for sex, 25 percent for self-masturbation, and 19 percent to store other substances such as tobacco. Of the 14 percent of respondents who reported they had participated in at least one sexual act while incarcerated, 59 percent reported that they used condoms during anal sex every time or often compared with 21 percent who reported never using a condom; and 30 percent indicated they used condoms during oral sex every time or often compared with 44 percent who said never. Eleven of the 13 senior officials interviewed agreed with the condom distribution program, one disagreed, and one was undecided. Of the 37 correctional officers interviewed, 43 percent agreed with the program and 43 percent disagreed. No incidents compromising prison security or safety were documented although minor acts of misuse (water balloons, water fights, and littering) were recorded. An incident occurred that involved an inmate throwing a used condom filled with shampoo at an officer. No incidents of hiding drugs were documented (Dolan et al., 2004).

Although distributing condoms is targeted primarily to consensual sex in correctional facilities, it may also protect some survivors of prison sexual assault from disease. Some inmates have been able to negotiate for the use of condoms especially when the assault results from threats or coercion. Stop Prisoner Rape, the leading U.S. prison rights advocacy group on this topic, provides self-help information to prisoners not only on how to prevent sexual assaults but also provides information on how to reduce the risk of contracting HIV. This advice includes ways to limit the assault to one assailant and only certain sexual acts, and how to negotiate with an assailant to use a condom (Donaldson, 1996). Often women are in no position to make or encourage their male partners to use condoms even outside of prison due to cultural and societal conditions (Reyes, 2001b). Negotiating for condom use in prison would likely present further obstacles.

Syringe Exchange, Bleach, and Other Disinfectants

Harm reduction is a pragmatic and sympathetic approach that recognizes many intravenous drug users cannot stop injecting drugs in the short term. The strategy is to help individuals to reduce the frequency with which they inject and to increase injection safety. Depending on factors like temperature and humidity HIV can survive in used needles for several days and hepatitis C for several weeks (WHO Europe, 2005). A syringe exchange program provides clean equipment to reduce the risk of transmitting HIV, HCV, and other infectious agents. In Europe, six countries have introduced syringe exchange programs into their correctional systems: Belarus, Germany, Kyrgyzstan, Republic of Moldova, Spain, and Switzerland (Lines et al., 2004). In 2001, Spain's general director of the Correctional System ordered all of the country's 68 prisons to provide drug users free access to sterile injection equipment (Stöver and Nelles, 2003). To date, syringe exchange programs are not permitted in U.S. correctional facilities (Hammett et al., 1999). Arguments against prison-based exchange programs are that they will increase and condone drug use and produce unintentional needle pricks, and syringes can be used as weapons. To date, evaluations of syringe exchange programs have not supported these fears: no documented increase in either overall drug use or intravenous drug use, syringes have not been used as weapons, and there have been no new or increased cases of HIV, HCV, or HBV. Syringe disposal has been safe and the programs acceptable to prisoners and staff members (Menoyo et al., 2000; Dolan et al., 2003; Stöver and Nelles, 2003; Lines et al., 2004). WHO Europe recommends that all prison systems "move quickly" to introduce syringe exchange programs equivalent to those in the community, especially where the local prevalence of HIV or hepatitis is high or if intravenous drug use is known to occur in the prison (WHO Europe, 2005).

In 1991, 16 of 52 prison systems surveyed in Europe made bleach available to prisoners for sterilizing injection equipment. Since then, the number has grown and no system has reversed the policy. Bleach is now available in Australian and Canadian prisons (Jürgens, 2004; Canadian HIV/AIDS Legal Network, 2004/2005a). Still there is controversy about using bleach and other disinfectants to sterilize injection equipment in prison. It is effective only when done with strict adherence to timely procedures and may give a false sense of security with respect to the safety of sharing injection equipment (Jürgens, 2004; WHO Europe, 2005). A qualitative study of 20 recently incarcerated male IDUs found that inmates agreed bleach distribution was not an adequate harm-reduction tool (Small et al., 2005). They reported that it was not used consistently and when employed was performed too quickly to be effective. In addition, the bleach supply was inconsistent and often diluted. WHO Europe recommends that bleach or other disinfectants should be made available to inmates along with information and training on their use in prison systems where syringe exchange programs are not feasible or desirable (WHO Europe, 2005). A 1997 U.S. government survey asked correctional facilities if they were making bleach available to inmates "for any purpose." It assumed that if bleach was offered to inmates for cleaning and other allowed purposes, it could also be used for disinfecting injection equipment. Twenty percent of the prisons (10 of 51) and jails (8 of 41) that responded reported that bleach was available (Hammett et al., 1999).

At present there appears to be a small risk of transmitting HIV when women have sex with other women through oral sex or contact with objects (e.g., dildos) carrying HIV-infected vaginal secretions. If used properly, bleach could be used to disinfect these objects (Reyes, 2001b).

Looking Ahead

Because incarcerated individuals are nearly completely dependent on the powers that confine them, those authorities are legally and ethically responsible for their health and safety. Failure to meet that responsibility allows millions to be exposed to disease, injury, and premature death. Prisoners engage in sex and all too often are subject to rape. They use drugs and are forced by others to use drugs. Most correctional systems do not have sufficient resources to make prisons safe. That would include having and properly training enough staff members to monitor all inmates around the clock. Facilities would have to be renovated to remove blind spaces and prisoners would be housed in single-occupant cells. Everyone who enters and all prisoners would be consistently and thoroughly searched for contraband. There would have to be sufficient resources to provide preventive and comprehensive health services including vaccination for diseases like HBV, mental health, and drug treatment programs. Given that high-risk sex and intravenous drug use continue in prisons and that complete elimination of these behaviors in the near future seems unrealistic, a prudent public health approach would be to afford prisoners the opportunity to protect themselves through proven harm-reduction measures like safe injection equipment and condoms. Education on disease risk and preventive measures beyond abstinence would also be far-sighted (Council of Europe, 1993). Such measures could put into practice a practical self-help approach and thereby offer inmates the opportunity—indeed the human right—not to contract disease. Even if not offered to the outside community, self-help programs in prisons seem to be a prudent strategy in prisons where resources are limited.

Substantial planning and cooperation among stakeholders is needed to successfully introduce self-help measures into prison systems. In places where there is resistance, it may work to start with pilot programs like evaluations; and recognize that perhaps not all settings are appropriate for every harm-reduction modality. For example, a syringe exchange program may not be suitable in a prison population with a high prevalence of serious mental illness. Nevertheless, the obligation remains for states to move quickly toward ensuring that prisoners are provided effective means of protecting themselves from the risk of deadly disease. Recent estimates put the number of incarcerated persons in the United States at more than 13 million, and millions more are in prison elsewhere around the globe. The vast majority of them will be released. Preserving and promoting their health and safety is prudent public health policy for the inmates in state care and for the general society.

References

Baillargeon, J., Black, S. A., Leach, C. T., Jenson, H., Pulvino, J., Bradshaw, P., and Murray, O. 2004. The infectious disease profile of Texas prison inmates. *Preventive Medicine* 38:607–12.

Beyrer, C., Jittiwutikarn, J., Teokul, W., Razak, M.H., Suriyanon, V., Srirak, N., Vongchuk, T., Tovanabutra, S., Sripaipan, T., and Celentano, D.D. 2003. Drug use, increasing incarceration rates, and prison associated HIV risks in Thailand. *AIDS and Behavior* 7 (2):153–61.

Beyrer, C., Zambrano, J., Mair, J. S., Golden, D., and Fornaci, P. 2005. *From the inside out: Talking to incarcerated women about health care.* Washington, D.C.: D.C. Prisoners' Legal Services Project (November 2005).

Canadian HIV/AIDS Legal Network. 2004/2005a. *HIV/AIDS in prisons.* 3rd ed. no. 5: *Prevention: Bleach.* www.aidslaw.ca/Maincontent/infosheets.htm#isohaap.

Canadian HIV/AIDS Legal Network. 2004/2005b. *HIV/AIDS in prisons.* 3rd ed. no. 4: *Prevention: Condoms.* www.aidslaw.ca/Maincontent/infosheets.htm#isohaap.

Centers for Disease Control and Prevention (CDC). 1992. Transmission of multidrug-resistant tuberculosis among immunocompromised persons in a correctional system, New York, 1991. *Morbidity and Mortality Weekly Report* 41 (28):507–9.

Centers for Disease Control and Prevention (CDC). 2001. Hepatitis B outbreak in a state correctional facility, 2000. *Morbidity and Mortality Weekly Report* 50 (25):529–32.

Centers for Disease Control and Prevention (CDC). 2002a (September). *Hepatitis C virus and HIV coinfection.* www.cdc.gov/idu/hepatitis/hepc_and_hiv_co.pdf.

Centers for Disease Control and Prevention (CDC). 2002b (September). *Viral hepatitis and injection drug users.* www.cdc.gov/idu/hepatitis/viral_hep_drug_use.pdf.

Centers for Disease Control and Prevention (CDC). 2004. Transmission of hepatitis B virus in correctional facilities, Georgia, January 1999-June 2002. *Morbidity and Mortality Weekly Report* 53 (30):678–81.

Centers for Disease Control and Prevention (CDC). 2005. Controlling tuberculosis in the United States: recommendations from the American Thoracic Society, CDC, and the Infectious Diseases Society of America. *Morbidity and Mortality Weekly Report* 54 (RR-12):1–82.

Centers for Disease Control and Prevention, National Center for HIV, STD and TB Prevention. (CDCa). How does HIV cause AIDS? *Frequently Asked Questions on HIV and AIDS.* www.cdc.gov/hiv/resources/qa/hivaids.htm (accessed October 20, 2006).

Centers for Disease Control and Prevention, National Center for HIV, STD and TB Prevention. (CDCb). How Is HIV passed from one person to another? *Frequently Asked Questions on HIV and AIDS.* www.cdc.gov/hiv/pubs/faq/faq16.htm (accessed October 20, 2006).

Centers for Disease Control and Prevention, National Center for HIV, STD and TB Prevention. (CDCc). Is there a connection between HIV and other sexually transmitted diseases? *Frequently Asked Questions on HIV and AIDS.* www.cdc.gov/hiv/pubs/faq/faq24.htm (accessed October 20, 2006).

Centers for Disease Control and Prevention, National Center for HIV, STD and TB Prevention. (CDCd). Why is injecting drugs a risk for HIV? *Frequently Asked Questions on HIV and AIDS.* www.cdc.gov/hiv/pubs/faq/faq25.htm (accessed October 20, 2006).

Centers for Disease Control and Prevention, National Center for HIV, STD and TB Prevention. (CDCe). 2005. *TB and HIV Coinfection.* www.cdc.gov/nchstp/tb/pubs/TB_HIVcoinfection/default.htm.

Centers for Disease Control and Prevention, National Center for HIV, STD and TB Prevention. (CDCf). November 1999. *The deadly intersection between TB and HIV.* www.cdc.gov/hiv/resources/factsheets/hivtb.pdf.

Champion, J. K., Taylor, A., Hutchinson, S., Cameron, S., McMenamin, J., Mitchell, A., and Goldberg, D. 2003. Incidence of hepatitis C virus infection and associated risk factors among Scottish prison inmates: a cohort study. *American Journal of Epidemiology* 159:514–19.

Choopanya, K., Vanichseni, S., Des Jarlais, D. C., Plangsringarm, K., Sonchai, W., Carballo, M., Friedmann, P., and Friedman, S. R. 1991. Risk factors and HIV seropositivity among injecting drug users in Bangkok. *AIDS* 5:1509–13.

Convention against Torture and Other Cruel, Inhuman or Degrading Treatment or Punishment. G.A. res. 39/46 of 10 December 1984, entered into force 26 June 1987 www.ohchr.org/english/law/index.htm.

Cornell Law School, Legal Information Institute. *International Law.* www.law.cornell.edu/wex/index.php/International_law.

Council of Europe, Explanatory Memorandum to Recommendation. 1993 (6) on Prison and criminological aspects of the control of transmissible diseases including AIDS and related health problems in prison, adopted by the Committee of Ministers 10 October 1993. http://cm.coe.int/stat/e/Public/1993/ExpRep(93)6.htm.

Dolan, K., Lowe, D., and Shearer, J. 2004. Evaluation of the condom distribution program in New South Wales Prisons, Australia. *Journal of Law, Medicine and Ethics* 32 (1):124–28.

Dolan, K., Rutter, S., and Wodak, A. D. 2003. Prison-based syringe exchange programmes: a review of international research and development. *Addiction* 98: 153–58.

Dolan, K. A., and Wodak, A. 1999. HIV transmission in a prison system in an Australian state. *Medical Journal of Australia* 171:14–17.

Donaldson, S. 1996. Hooking up: protective pairing for punks. *Stop Prisoner Rape.* www.spr.org/en/ps_hookingup.asp (accessed December 1, 2005).

Durose, M. R., and Langan, P. A. 2004 (December). *Felony Sentences in State Courts, 2002.* U.S. Department of Justice, Bureau of Justice Statistics, Bulletin NCJ 206916.

Fischer, B. 1995. Drugs, communities, and "harm reduction" in Germany: the new relevance of "public health" principles in local responses. *Journal of Public Health Policy* 1995:16 (4):389–411.

General Comment No. 06 (1982) of the Human Rights Committee concerning the right to life (art. 6) of the International Covenant on Civil and Political Rights. www.unhchr.ch/tbs/doc.nsf/(Symbol)/84ab9690ccd81f c7c12563ed0046fae3 ?Opendocument.

General Comment No. 14 (2000) of the Committee on Economic, Social and Cultural Rights concerning the right to the highest attainable standard of health (art. 12) of the International Covenant on Economic, Social and Cultural Rights. www .unhchr.ch/tbs/doc.nsf/(Symbol)/40d009901358b0e2c1256915005090be? Opendocument.

Gibbs v. Martin, No. 01-74480, 2003 WL 21909780 (E.D.Mich. July 28, 2003).

Gostin, L. O., and Z. Lazzarini. 1997. Prevention of HIV/AIDS among injection drug users: the theory and science of public health and criminal justice approaches to disease prevention. *Emory Law Journal* 46:587.

Grob, G. N. 2004. Deinstitutionalization of the mentally ill: policy triumph or tragedy? *New Jersey Medicine* 101 (12):19–30.

Hammett, T. M., Harmon, P., and Maruschak, L. M. 1999 (July). *1996–1997 Update: HIV/AIDS, STDs, and TB in Correctional Facilities.* Washington, D.C.: U.S. Department of Justice, National Institute of Justice, NCJ 176344.

Heilpern, D. M. 1998. *Fear or favour: Sexual assault of young prisoners.* Lismore, NSW, Australia: Southern Cross University Press.

Hellard, M. E., Hocking, J. S., and Crofts, N. 2004. The prevalence and the risk behaviours associated with the transmission of hepatitis C virus in Australian correctional facilities. *Epidemiology and Infection* 132:409–15.

Hensley, C. 2001. Consensual homosexual activity in male prisons. *Corrections Compendium* 26(1): 104.

Hiller, M. L., Webster, J. M., Leukefeld, C., Narevic, E., and Staton, M. 2005. Prisoners with substance abuse and mental health problems: use of health and health services. *American Journal of Drug and Alcohol Abuse* 1:1–20.

International Covenant on Civil and Political Rights, G.A. res. 2200A (XXI) of 16 December 1966, entered into force 23 March 1976. www.ohchr.org/english/law/ index.htm.

International Covenant on Economic, Social and Cultural Rights, G.A. res. 2200A

(XXI) of 16 December 1966, entered into force 3 January 1976. www.ohchr.org/english/law/index.htm.

Jones, T. F., Craig, A. S., Valway, S. E., Woodley, C. L., and Schaffner, W. 1999. Transmission of tuberculosis in a jail. *Annals of Internal Medicine* 131(8):557–63.

Jürgens, R. 2004 (September). Is the world finally waking up to HIV/AIDS in prisons? A report from the XV International AIDS Conference. *Infectious Diseases in Corrections Report* 7 (9):1–5. www.idcronline.org/archives/sept04/article.html (accessed November 28, 2005).

Jürgens, R., and Bijl, M. 2001a. High-risk behaviour in penal institutions. In *HIV in prisons: A reader with particular relevance to the newly independent states*, ed. Paola Bollino, 21–29. Copenhagen, Denmark: WHO Regional Office for Europe. http://nicic.org/Library/020671.

Jürgens, R., and Bijl, M. 2001b. HIV prevention in penal institutions. In *HIV in prisons: A reader with particular relevance to the newly independent states*, ed. Paola Bollino, 49–64. Copenhagen, Denmark: WHO Regional Office for Europe. http://nicic.org/Library/020671.

Kang, S. Y., Deren, S., Andia, J., Colon, H. M., Robles, R., and Oliver-Velez, D. 2005. HIV transmission behaviors in jail/prison among Puerto Rican drug injectors in New York and Puerto Rico. *AIDS and Behavior* 9(3):377–86.

Karberg, J. C., and James, D. J. 2005 (July). *Substance Dependence, Abuse, and Treatment of Jail Inmates, 2002.* U.S. Department of Justice, Bureau of Justice Statistics, Special Report, NCJ 209588.

Koscheski, M., Hensley, C., Wright, J., and Tewksbury, R. 2002. Consensual sexual behavior. In *Prison Sex: Practice and Policy*, ed. Christopher Hensley, 111–31. Boulder, CO: Lynne Rienner Publishers.

Koulierakis, G., Gnardellis, C., Agrafiotis, D., and Power, K. G. 2000. HIV risk behaviour correlates among injecting drug users in Greek prisons. *Addiction* 95 (8):1207–16.

Krebs, C. P., and Simmons, M. 2002. Intraprison HIV transmission: an assessment of whether it occurs, how it occurs, and who is at risk. *AIDS Education and Prevention* 14 (Suppl. B):53–64.

Kunselman, J., Tewksbury, R., Dumond, R. W., and Dumond D. A. 2002. Nonconsensual sexual behavior. In *Prison sex: Practice and policy*, ed. Christopher Hensley, 27–47. Boulder, CO: Lynne Rienner Publishers.

Lines, R., Jürgens, R., Betteridge, G., Stöver, H., Laticevschi, D., and Nelles, J. 2004. *Prison needle exchange: lessons from a comprehensive review of international evidence and experience.* Toronto, Ontario: Canadian HIV/AIDS Legal Network. www.aidslaw.ca/Maincontent/issues/prisons/pnep/toc.htm.

Macalino, G. E., Vlahov, D., Sanford-Colby, S., Patel, S., Sabin, K., Salas, C., and Rich, J. D. 2004. Prevalence and incidence of HIV, hepatitis B virus, and hepatitis C virus infections among males in Rhode Island prisons. *American Journal of Public Health* 94 (7):1218–23.

Mair, J. S., Frattaroli, S., and Teret, S. P. 2003. New hope for victims of prison sexual assault. *Journal of Law, Medicine and Ethics* 31:602–6.

Mariner, J. 2001. *No escape: Male rape in U.S. prisons.* New York: Human Rights Watch. http://hrw.org/reports/2001/prison/report.html.

Marlatt, G. A. 1996. Harm reduction: come as you are. *Addictive Behaviors* 21 (6):779–88.

May, J. P., and Williams, E. L., Jr. 2002. Acceptability of condom availability in a U.S. jail. *AIDS Education and Prevention* 14 (Suppl. B):85–91.

Menoyo, C., Zulaica, D., and Parras, F. 2000. Needle exchange programs in prisons in Spain. *Canadian HIV/AIDS Policy and Law Review* 5(4):20–21. www.aidslaw.ca/Maincontent/otherdocs/Newsletter/vol5no42000/issue.htm.

Mumola, C. J. 1999 (January). *Substance abuse and treatment, state and federal prisoners, 1997.* U.S. Department of Justice, Bureau of Justice Statistics, Special Report NCJ 172871.

National Commission on Correctional Health Care. 2002 (March). *The health status of soon-to-be-released inmates: A report to congress,* vol. 1. pp. 15–28. Chicago, IL: National Commission on Correctional Health Care. www.ncchc.org/pubs/pubs_stbr.vol1.html.

Nerenberg, R. 2002 (January). Spotlight: condoms in correctional settings. *HIV Education Prison Project News* 5 (1). www.thebody.com/hepp/jan02/spotlight.html.

O'Sullivan, B. G., Levy, M. H., Dolan, K. A., Post, J. J., Barton, S. G., Dwyer, D. E., Kaldor, J. M., and Grulich, A. E. 2003. Hepatitis C transmission and HIV post-exposure prophylaxis after needle-and-syringe-sharing in Australian prisons. *Medical Journal of Australia* 178:546–49.

Penal Reform International. 2001. *Making standards work: An international handbook on good prison practice,* 2nd ed. Huntingdon, United Kingdom: Astron Printers. www.penalreform.org/english/MSW.pdf (accessed December 1, 2005).

Post, J. J., Dolan, K. A., Whybin, L. R., Carter I.W.J., Haber, P. S., and Lloyd, A.R. 2001. Acute hepatitis C virus infection in an Australian prison inmate: tattooing as a possible transmission route. *Medical Journal of Australia* 174:183–84.

Prison Rape Elimination Act, 42 USCS § 15601 et seq.

Reuter, P., and Caulkins, J. P. 1995. Redefining the goals of the National Drug Policy: recommendations from a working group. *American Journal of Public Health* 85 (8):1059–63.

Reyes, H. 2001a. Health and human rights in prisons. In *HIV in prisons: A reader with particular relevance to the newly independent states,* ed. Paola Bollino, 9–20. Copenhagen, Denmark: WHO Regional Office for Europe. http://nicic.org/Library/020671 (accessed December 1, 2005).

Reyes, H. 2001b. Women in prison and HIV. In: *HIV in prisons: A reader with particular relevance to the newly independent states,* ed. Paola Bollino, 193–217. Copenhagen, Denmark: WHO Regional Office for Europe. http://nicic.org/Library/020671.

Small, W., Kain, S., Laliberte, N., Schechter, M. T., O'Shaughnessy, M. V., and Spittal, P. M. 2005. Incarceration, addiction and harm reduction: inmates experience injecting drugs in prisons. *Substance Use and Misuse* 40:831–43.

Srikameswaran, A. 2005. Iran tackles AIDS head on: 2 young doctors lead establishment of clinics. *Pittsburgh Post-Gazette.* March 13. www.post-gazette.com/pg/05072/470052.stm (accessed December 1, 2005).

Stephan, J. J. 2001(August). *Census of jails, 1999.* U.S. Department of Justice, Bureau of Justice Statistics, NCJ 186633.

Stern, V. 2001. Problems in prisons worldwide, with a particular focus on Russia. *Annals New York Academy of Sciences* 953:113–19.

Stöver, H., and Nelles, J. 2003. Ten years of experience with needle and syringe exchange programmes in European prisons. *International Journal of Drug Policy* 14:437–44.

Taylor, A., Goldberg, D., Emslie J, Wrench, J., Gruer, L., Cameron, S., Black, J., Davis, B., McGregor, J., Follett, E., Harvey, J., Basson, J, and McGavigan, J. 1995. *British Medical Journal* 310:289–92.

Tewksbury, R. 1989. Measures of sexual behavior in an Ohio prison. *Sociology and Social Research* 74 (1):34–39.

White House. 2005 (February). *National drug control strategy: Update.* Washington, D.C.: Office of National Drug Control Policy. www.whitehousedrugpolicy.gov/publications/policy/ndcs05/ndcs05.pdf.

Universal Declaration of Human Rights, G.A. res. 217A(III) of 10 December 1948. www.ohchr.org/english/law/index.htm.

Weinbaum, C., Lyerla, R., and Margolis, H. S. 2003. Prevention and control of infections with hepatitis viruses in correctional settings. *Morbidity and Mortality Weekly Report* 52 (RR-1):1–35.

World Health Organization (WHO). 2005 (March). *WHO model list of essential medicines.* www.who.int/medicines/publications/essentialmedicines/en/.

World Health Organization, Regional Office for Europe. 2001. *HIV in prisons: A reader with particular relevance to the newly independent states,* ed. Paola Bollino. Copenhagen, Denmark: WHO Regional Office for Europe. http://nicic.org/Library/020671.

World Health Organization, Regional Office for Europe. 2005 (May). *Status paper on prisons, drugs and harm reduction.* Copenhagen, Denmark: WHO Regional Office for Europe. www.euro.who.int/document/e85877.pdf.

Zamani, S., Kihara, M., Guoya, M. M., Vazirian, M., Ono-Kihara, M., Razzaghi, E. M., and Ichikawa, S. 2005. Prevalence of and factors associated with HIV-1 infection among drug users visiting treatment centers in Tehran, Iran. *AIDS* 19:709–16.

PART II

Methods

6

Using Molecular Tools to Track Epidemics and Investigate Human Rights and Disease Interactions

Chris Beyrer, M.D., M.P.H.

"From a public health perspective, the advent of molecular epidemiology, which allows tracking of pathogens based on unique genetic sequences or antigenic properties, has revolutionized how epidemiologists investigate and evaluate epidemics and assess endemic diseases" (Robertson and Nicholson, 2005). The development of genetics-based analytic assays and the multiple applications of these methods have changed science and medicine, botany, microbiology, and evolutionary theory—almost every field of inquiry in which they have been applied. The results of the human genome project, the complete sequencing of the human genetic code, are one spectacular example of the potential power of genetic tools for scientific endeavor. And the extraordinary impact of these technologies has not been limited to science. Genetic analyses have revolutionized the law as potently as they have affected medicine. DNA evidence, properly used, has a definitive precision that has led to the conviction of some criminals and to the freedom of other men and women falsely convicted, in some cases after years or decades of incarceration. The technologies have given forensic investigations arguably their most powerful tool—one that can transcend the time limits of other kinds of data. DNA evidence linked the charred bones buried in Yekaterinburg in 1918 with a living relative, Prince Philip of England, and confirmed the remains as those of the Romanovs. And DNA findings, brought together with archaeology and linguistics, have allowed us to answer seemingly unanswerable questions about human origins, our earliest migrations out of Africa, and the peopling of the continents by genetically modern yet Stone Age humans (Cavalli-Sforza, 2000).

Molecular tools have transformed the study of infectious diseases and have expanded exponentially the scientific speed, accuracy, and sensitivity of testing for microbial pathogens, including viruses, bacteria, fungi, and parasites. Among the first diseases for which these tools have been used is one of mankind's oldest foes: *Mycobacterium tuberculosis*, the causal agent of tuberculosis (TB). As an example of the utility of these tools, genotyping of TB bacteria from patients has allowed for the tracking of TB strains as they move through chains of infection in families and communities (Daley, 2005). Because TB can spread through respiratory droplets, exposure in geographic settings plays an important role in the spread of the disease. The spread of TB has been extensively documented in households, in workplaces, in institutional and hospital settings such as nursing homes, in schools, jails, and prisons, and in more informal settings, including bars, crack houses, and church choirs (Daley, 2005). Molecular methods have lent enormous precision to these kinds of study. In epidemiological investigations of a 1996–97 tuberculosis outbreak in central Los Angeles, genetic typing of TB strains showed that family and household transmission was rare, but that homelessness, and clustering at three specific gathering spots for other homeless persons within the city, was the key link for the majority of cases (Barnes, Yang, and Preston-Martin, 1997). Genetic tools can tell us, in like manner, if persons in a prison setting acquired TB before incarceration or while in custody, and whether ongoing spread of TB is occurring in an institution, a key question for disease control (Mohle-Boetani, 2002). Because TB is so common in most of the developing world and relatively uncommon in developed countries, a large proportion of TB cases in the United States and Western Europe are among foreign-born immigrants, workers, and residents. Molecular evaluations of disease spread in these contexts have allowed for targeted control programs, and enforced TB screening and treatment for immigration to a variety of states.

These examples of genetic tools for TB can also suggest the potential harm to civil liberties and human rights from the misuse of the technologies, which could include restrictions on legal immigration, and discrimination based on TB status or presumed TB status for foreign-born individuals from high-prevalence countries of origin. Used properly, molecular tools can tell us where a microbe likely originated, and through what chains of transmission it has moved. It is surely no coincidence that DNA mapping of microbes is often referred to in the medical literature as DNA fingerprinting—for genetic markers are like fingerprints—and can be used, albeit with far greater accuracy, to identify microbial culprits from TB to HIV.

A review of the recent literature suggests a great range of uses for these tools. Molecular methods have been used to study the genetic origins and transmission patterns of hepatitis B viruses (HBV) in an increasingly multicultural Spain (Echevarria, Avellon, and Magnius, 2005). A recent Spanish study looked at indigenous Spaniards and immigrants from Africa, Asia, and Eastern Europe. Genetic analysis revealed that viruses among persons born in China remained distinct, while viruses of West African origin were emerging among native Spanish patients, suggesting that HBV immunization for all residents of Spain may be required for epidemic control and also marking distinct social mixing patterns for those at risk for this potent liver pathogen.

There is perhaps no more striking example of the recent advances in molecular biology than the swift identification and rapid full-length sequencing of the severe acute respiratory syndrome (SARS) agent, now referred to as the SARS Corona virus, SARS-CoV. This virus was identified and its genome fully sequenced within 3 months of the first SARS patient samples becoming available to science (Shih, S. R., et al., 2005). Rapid development of a polymerase chain reaction (PCR) assay followed. And this assay allowed for rapid understanding of the relationship between cases, and between outbreaks, revealing, for example, that the SARS outbreak in Taiwan came from not one, but two introductions of the virus to the island (Shih, M. C., et al., 2005). Similar approaches have been applied to influenza outbreaks in Taiwan, to the spread of hepatitis C virus among a network of injection drug users in Australia (Aitken et al., 2004), and to HIV epidemics in a range of settings, populations, studies, and contexts.

The Molecular Epidemiology of HIV-1 and Heroin Trafficking

Are there potential applications of these powerful new tools for human rights efforts? And, if so, what would a molecular epidemiology of human rights look like? One example comes from work using the genetic variability of the HIV-1 virus to investigate heroin-trafficking routes out of the narcotics-based dictatorship of Burma.

HIV is a genetically diverse pathogen with high rates of genetic change. The virus has at least two predominant species: HIV-1, the principal global cause of AIDS epidemics, and HIV-2, which has been found principally in West Africa and India. Within HIV-1 there are multiple subtypes, commonly named subtype or clade (from the Greek Klados, for type) A, B, C, D, and so forth. High rates of mutation in the viral genome allow for diversification within each subtype, and indeed, within each HIV-infected individual over time. This inherent instability is part of the viruses' biologic strategy for evading the human immune system, and also allows for mutations leading to resistance to AIDS drugs—a daunting issue for patients and clinicians. To further complicate the picture, we now know that HIV-1 subtypes not only mutate within patients, but also can recombine across subtypes to generate new forms that are recombined offspring of two parents. A recombined virus with genetic material from an A clade and a B clade parent would be referred to as an A/B recombinant. The ability of HIV to generate these new recombinant forms sharply increases the genetic diversity of the virus. When one of these recombinant forms spreads within a population (the usual test is at least three unlinked cases with the same genetic structure), it is designated a circulating recombinant form, or a CRF. Those found in only one or two individuals are termed unique recombinant forms, URFs. In parts of East Africa, including Kenya and Tanzania, up to a third of new infections in 2004 were due to URFs—a daunting level of viral variation (McCutchan, 2005). This kind of genetic diversity is an enormous challenge to attempts to control HIV spread—most notably for the development of an HIV vaccine, which will likely need to control multiple forms of the virus to be effective. But it is also useful for adding new levels of precision to epidemiological investigations—and, it could be argued, for investigations in which the sources of HIV infection or its route of spread may have human rights and/or political implications. Like many powerful tools, it can be used (and, of course, misused) in a wide array of investigative approaches.

In 1990 Burma held its first free and fair elections since the military seizure of power in 1962 by General Ne Win. The military was defeated in the election, but refused to hand over power, jailed most of the newly elected leadership, and closed the country. Over the next two years, Burma rapidly became the world's largest producer of opium and exporter of heroin (Beyrer, 1998). By 1996, severe outbreaks of HIV among injection drug users (IDUs) were reported in China's Yunnan Province and India's Manipur State, which share long forested borders with northern and western Burma, respectively (Beyrer et al., 2000). Based in northern Thailand during this period as field director for the Johns Hopkins-Chiang Mai University collaborative Preparation for AIDS Vaccine Evaluations (PAVE) Project, I saw that Burmese heroin was flooding Thailand as well. It was soon clear that Burma's heroin exports could be a prime driver of the emerging regional epidemic of HIV—but how to investigate this, given the secretive nature of the ruling junta and the difficulty of generating evidence linking Burmese heroin to HIV outbreaks in India, China, Thailand, and farther afield?

This investigative effort began with basic "shoe leather epidemiology" for formulating hypotheses. With local colleagues, we visited affected zones along known or purported drug routes out of Burma, including investigative trips to northeast India, inside Burma proper, to southwest China, eastern Laos, and northern Vietnam, meeting with rights activists, physicians dealing with HIV/AIDS, drug users, police and security officials, and others. This effort led to the identification of four principal overland heroin-trafficking routes out of Burma, all associated with recent uptake of heroin use among local youth, swift transitions to injection, and explosive spread of HIV. In most settings, in particular, in India and China, drug users themselves were the most reliable and well-informed sources for sources and routes of Burmese heroin trafficking. Next, we secured *LandSat* satellite images of the opium poppy cultivation zones in Burma from U.S. intelligence service colleagues. Bringing poppy cultivation satellite images and heroin routes together was revelatory: we could now trace heroin to its sources and identify the specific mountain passes, roads, truck routes, and border points on overland heroin routes across South and Southeast Asia. As shown in Figure 6.1, with few exceptions, the satel-

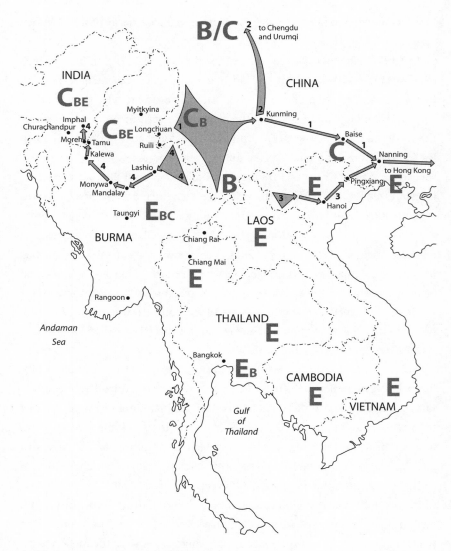

Figure 6.1. Overland heroin-trafficking routes and spread of HIV subtypes in South and Southeast Asia, 2000

lite images confirmed what local users and nongovernmental organization (NGO) staff members had reported: there were a limited number of routes, principally four, for the majority of heroin exports—and HIV epidemics were already well established along each route by the end of the 1990s. I then realized that if heroin were moving out of Burma, and HIV was following in its wake, molecular subtyping of HIV strains in the trafficking zones might be the "smoking gun" to connect Burmese heroin to HIV/AIDS spread in the region. Partnering with the virologist Xiao-Fang Yu at Johns Hopkins, and regional investigators in Thailand, Burma, and India, we began an effort to collect all that was known about HIV subtypes in the heroin-trafficking region, and, where possible, to do molecular subtyping of HIV isolates from IDUs in those areas along heroin routes where the molecular epidemiology of HIV-1 was unknown or unclear.

The molecular findings of HIV-1 fit remarkably well with what we now knew about heroin routes, indeed, all four primary routes were associated with specific viral subtypes and circulating recombinant forms (CRFs) (Beyrer et al., 2000). These HIV-1 molecular associations have since been confirmed and further refined by several other groups working in the region; and the association of HIV-1 spread and overland heroin trafficking is now recognized as a key mode of the introduction and spread of HIV into human populations (McCutchan et al., 2003; Takebe et al., 2003; Hammett et al., 2005).

From a political and human rights perspective, this work has had wide-reaching consequences, as these findings have been among the few "hard" facts tying Burma's narcotics-based economy under the generals to health and social consequences for the neighbor states. The elected leaders of Burma, including Daw Aung San Suu Kyi and her party leaders, have been briefed on these findings, as well as the U.S. Department of State, the U.S. Drug Enforcement Agency, the U.S. House of Representatives, the Centers for Disease Control and Prevention, and the Bush White House. In 1999–2000, I wrote talking points for then Secretary of State Albright on her visits to the region. Secretary Albright and Secretary Powell are both on record calling for the restoration of civilian rule in Burma and explicitly linking the ruling junta to the narcotics trade and to HIV/AIDS spread in Asia.

Trafficking Zones, Prevention Failures, and Human Rights

Although it is now confirmed that HIV can spread along overland heroin routes, this mechanism has been aided and abetted by the difficulty for many states to accept, support, and implement necessary HIV prevention measures for injection drug users. (Chapter 14 by Wolfe and Malinowska-Sempruch examines these failures in detail.) One of the clear and simple results of this work is that communities along or around heroin-trafficking routes (or by analogy, along cocaine-trafficking routes in the Americas) should be targeted for primary prevention of HIV spread. HIV prevention for drug users needs to be available wherever drugs are flowing. Instead, these areas, in general, have been dominated by legalistic, not public health approaches—by police, border patrol, and security forces—and have too often been virtually off limits to public health workers and others willing to work with drug users, particularly during the early, critical periods of viral dissemination (Beyrer, 2003). The result has been sharp limits on health care access and services for drug users, consistent reports of human rights limitations against drug users by security forces, and unimpeded spread of the HIV virus—a terrible synergy that has affected all too many communities in these regions. This has been true in Burma itself, and in the hills of northern Thailand, the states of northeast India, southwest and northwest China, in Laos, and in the western mountains of Vietnam (Beyrer, 2003).

An additional challenge in almost all of these areas is that the opium poppy, the source plant for opium and its derivative heroin, is grown in the highlands, and these hills and mountain tracts are peopled by ethnic minorities. The rice-growing majority peoples of the lowlands dominate all the modern states of Southeast Asia. And in all of these affected states, limitations on minority rights and ethnic tensions have colored responses to poppy cultivation, heroin trafficking, and HIV spread among injectors (Beyrer, 1998). In what is certainly one of the more painful outcomes of this complex scenario, HIV rates in China, India, Burma, and Thailand have been highest among ethnic minorities in these zones (Weiwel, 2005). For peoples like the Manipuris of India, the Wa of China and Burma, the Kachins of China and Burma, and the Akha of China, Burma, Thailand, and Laos, the brutal realities of life in these heroin zones have only been compounded by the spread of AIDS among their young people. And when police and the military and their U.N.

and First World allies appear to burn the fields and defoliate the crops in the name of poppy eradication, it is these subsistence farmers who lose their families' yearly cash crop in an afternoon. As the case study on the War on Drugs in Thailand demonstrates, state violence in these ethnic minority communities has not stopped at the burning of poppy fields.

How relevant are these approaches and findings for other regions? Related work is under way in another region facing an HIV explosion, and severe human rights violations—Central Asia and the States of the former Soviet Union. Here Afghanistan has emerged as the leading heroin-exporting state, with a 2003 crop estimated at 4,500 metric tons of opium, yielding an estimated 420–450 metric tons of heroin (U.N. Office on Drugs and Crime, 2003). The U.N. Office of Drug Control found 2003 to be the year Afghanistan overtook Burma as the world's leading heroin exporter. And as with Burma and its neighbors, it appears that heroin-trafficking routes out of Afghanistan are driving the emerging HIV epidemics in Central Asia. And again the affected communities have extremely limited prevention programs in the trafficking zones, and extensive human rights concerns for drug users. Human Rights Watch documented these interactions in their 2003 report on Kazakhstan, *Fanning the flames: How human rights abuses are fueling the AIDS epidemic in Kazakhstan* (pp. 22–24). A particular feature in this new epidemic zone has been the level of police and state security involvement in corruption and the narcotics industry. This kind of corruption allows for ongoing growth of the regional narcotics-based economy and undermines civil society—at a time when many of these states are struggling to emerge from decades of Soviet domination. These weak states have only nascent or highly threatened human rights movements, limited freedom of the press, weak or corrupt judiciaries, and public health systems at best in difficult transitions from Soviet times, and at worst, in collapse—all poor prognostic indicators for effective responses to HIV/AIDS epidemics.

A collaborative study investigating these interactions has just been completed in Tajikistan, on Afghanistan's northern border, where we have identified an emerging epidemic of HIV-1 associated with an Afghan heroin-trafficking route (Stachowiak et al., 2006). This collaboration included virologists at The Henry M. Jackson Foundation for the Advancement of Military Medicine laboratory for full-length HIV-1 subtyping; The Open Society Institute Tajikistan Office, whom we worked with to access drug users and shooting galleries;

AIDS Infoshare, a Russian AIDS service organization that trained our Tajik team in research methods, and voluntary counseling and testing; and the Tajik National Virological Institute. (To implement this project, we first had to assist the Tajik Government in creating their first Human Subjects Protections review committee, and in securing Tajikistan's first Federal Wide Assurance documents from the U.S. Office of Human Research Protections, a regulatory requirement for receiving U.S. federal research dollars.)

The data from this and related studies have been striking and suggest a distinct new pattern of HIV subtypes in Tajikistan and Uzbekistan, which differs sharply from Russia and the rest of the former Soviet Union. Across Russia, from St. Petersburg to Moscow and east across Siberia, the predominant virus found is subtype A of HIV-1 (Bobkov et al., 1998). This vast area has one major risk factor, needle sharing among injection drug users, and this one HIV variant, with strikingly low levels of genetic variation (Carr et al., 2005). Subtype A has been the predominant virus not only in Russia itself, but also in Ukraine, Belarus, and the Russian Far East (Carr et al., 2005). Central Asia has been an unknown, and Afghanistan, at the epicenter of the narcotics production driving these epidemics, remains an unknown.

What about Tajikistan? The Tajik epidemic turns out to be predominantly subtype A, but with roughly a half of infections due to a virus previously found largely in West Africa, a recombinant form known as CRF02_A/G for its clade A and G parentage (Carr et al., 2005). Neighboring Uzbekistan, like Tajikistan, sharing a long border with northern Afghanistan's heroin zones, had an almost identical picture. At present there is no simple explanation for the appearance of this West African variant of HIV-1 in Central Asia. But these findings do suggest a distinct Central Asian epidemic picture with Afghanistan playing a role in Central Asia similar to that played by Burma in Southeast Asia: and in both situations, molecular epidemiology can help clarify the regional relationships, define HIV epidemics, and underscore the key roles chaotic states like Burma and Afghanistan can play in regional health threats. Afghanistan itself is something of an unknown in terms of molecular epidemiology and urgently needs exploration. Given the Afghan poppy economy, poor human rights protections, and weak HIV prevention programs for drug users across this region, it will be critical to expand this work to other affected states in the coming years to prevent the ongoing concentrated epidemic in the region from becoming generalized.

Other Applications for Molecular Methods in Human Rights Work

Genetic analyses of HIV have been used in civil and criminal law cases where sexual abuse or knowing spread of HIV was suspected. In an infamous case of a dentist in Florida, HIV genetic sequences of virus isolated from a dentist and several of his patients were used as evidence to conclude that the provider had, in fact, spread HIV among his patients through use of unsterile and reused equipment (Ou et al., 1992). Such genetic linkages can also be used to link sexual partner pairs, including, for example, a rapist and his victim, should the victim become infected. This use of molecular methods has obvious implications in investigations of individual cases of sexual violence, but has been little used in investigations of population-level sexual crimes, such as those occurring in war. Are there potential applications of these tools for investigating war crimes? In June 2004 a working group was convened by the Council on Foreign Relations and UNAIDS to develop a policy for the U.N. Secretary General on HIV/AIDS and other infectious diseases as security concerns, including HIV spread among and by United Nations and regional peacekeeping forces (Garrett, 2005). This group proposed that molecular epidemiology be used as a tool to investigate HIV spread among peacekeeping forces in HIV epidemic zones, and HIV spread *by* peacekeeping forces in these zones. Here again, human rights violations (in this case use of civilian populations for sex by U.N. or other forces' troops) could potentially be tracked using novel epidemiological methods.

From an HIV epidemiological perspective, the global dispersion of HIV variants has been, and will likely continue to be affected by the movement of foreign troops in conflict zones. Nine African nations sent troops into the 1998–2002 war in Democratic Republic of Congo (DR Congo), the bloodiest conflict since World War II, and DR Congo had the most genetically diverse epidemic of HIV-1 yet described *before* the war. At this writing, investigations are underway to assess allegations of sexual exploitation by U.N. peacekeeping forces in the Bunia region of DR Congo. Here, too, a genetic approach to forensic investigations could be a powerful tool for prosecutors.

China has had at least two distinct outbreaks of HIV-1 infection (Piriyasilip et al., 2000). The first was, as we have described, among ethnic minority injection drug users along China's long mountainous border with Burma. This epidemic spread eastward into southern China, eventually leading to an epidemic encompassing most of Yunnan Province, and the neighboring provinces of Guangxi and Sichuan. This epidemic continued to spread north along a heroin-trafficking route to reach China far west—the Muslim majority province of Xinjiang, formerly East Turkestan, sharing borders with Kazakhstan and Tajikistan. The molecular epidemiology of this vast outbreak has been characterized by the predominance of two related viruses, both recombinant forms of HIV-1 and each with subtype B and subtype C parents. These viruses, called CRF07_B/C and CRF08_B/C, are thus far unique to these regions of China and to northern Burma, where they appear to have been generated among injectors, and have remained genetically stable for several years (McCutchan et al., 2003). More than 75 percent of all infections with these two strains are among IDUs in both Burma and China.

China's second HIV epidemic is much less well understood and involves different regions, populations, and modes of spread. This has been an outbreak among paid blood donors in the central Chinese provinces of Henan, Hebei, Anhui, and Shaanxi and described here in detail in the chapter by Wan Yan Hai and Li. Starting in the early 1990s, and continuing to at least 1996, for-profit agencies collected blood, mainly for plasma components, in rural districts of these provinces. To cut costs, blood collectors reused equipment, often repeatedly and without proper sterilization. Because too-frequent donation can lead to anemia, blood-collection agencies apparently reinfused red cell components in donors, often in pooled fashion, to allow for more frequent blood draws. In many impoverished villages, high proportions of young adult men and women were selling blood. This resulted in unprecedented rates of HIV-1 infection in some communities, where rates as high as 40 percent of all community adults have been reported (Beyrer, 2003). The scale and scope of this iatrogenic outbreak are still largely unknown, understudied, and politically sensitive in China. One estimate is that perhaps 500,000 adults in Henan province alone may have been infected with HIV through blood donation from 1990 to 1996 (Kaufman and Jing, 2002). China has passed strict new laws and guidelines to curtail the practices that led to this outbreak, but the extent to which these donor cases have led to wider spread is unknown. Perhaps even more troubling, the fate of the hundreds of thousands, if not millions, of infected units of blood and blood products also remains unknown.

The many human rights implications of this tragedy are ongoing—at this writing, no senior official in either the Provincial government of the affected provinces, nor in any of the companies who profited, have been charged or tried. Full epidemiological investigation of this epidemic has yet to be undertaken, and China continues to deny both the scale and scope of this outbreak.

Although Chinese authorities have continued to resist fully investigating this second outbreak, emerging data from molecular epidemiology shed light on the situation. Given the geographic, temporal, and causal relationships between these outbreaks (spread among drug users in Southwest China and among rural blood donors in Central China) a logical prediction would be that the viruses involved in each outbreak would differ. In the case of the Southwestern epidemic, as we have seen, two viral subtypes emerged and proved to be signature markers for the outbreak, both being B/C recombinants found only in affected parts of China and in Burma. A challenge for this comparison was that the authorities in those provinces affected by the blood products industry repeatedly refused to allow investigators to collect specimens from affected individuals and communities. If Chinese investigators had done so, their results were not available to the scientific community. But in 2004, the first HIV subtyping report did appear from Dr. David Ho and his collaborative group (Zhang et al., 2004). As expected, they reported that the HIV outbreak among paid donors was homogenous, and characterized by only one subtype of HIV; subtype B[prime], a variant found primarily in Thailand, and hence that the epidemic was, indeed, unlinked to the Southwestern outbreak of B/C recombinants among drug users (Zhang et al., 2004). Is this finding of interest beyond the world of HIV genetics research? Yes, because the molecular data are hard evidence that the blood donor outbreak is indeed a distinct entity from the drug use epidemic, and that those who would seek to muddle the question of origin and routes of spread can do so only by denying the evidence. This has direct bearing on the human rights arguments put forward by Wan Yan Hai and Li Xiao Rong in Chapter 3 and could be further hard evidence of epidemiological connections across the many provinces involved in China's blood-borne epidemic should larger molecular investigations be possible.

Looking Ahead

There are several challenges to furthering synthesis of epidemiology and human rights. Clearly, perpetrators will always resist documenting human rights violations on the part of state actors, and this is as true for genetic evidence as for other kinds of documentation. Increasing the kinds of evidence available and measuring the population-level effects of flawed policies can be potent tools for advocacy and can meet with resistance, hostility, and denial precisely because these kinds of data can be so compelling to policy makers. This has been the case with genetic evidence, in particular, because policy makers quickly grasp the power and precision of the evidence. Indeed, as genetics have been applied to criminal law, they have led at least one U.S. governor to suspend the death penalty in his state, Illinois, because so many persons serving sentences in his state were exonerated by DNA evidence (Davey, 2004).

A more subtle challenge has been the tradition in international health and relief work of the desire to maintain political neutrality. There is mounting evidence to suggest that apolitical stances in the face of human rights violations are both unethical and bad science. As science improves in power, and human rights begins to use molecular tools more widely, these tensions will likely increase. Political and rights-based analyses of disease outbreaks are demanded by the complexity of our time—and the technology now available will almost certainly begin to be used in this arena. It is therefore critically important that both the human rights and the public health communities understand and use these tools—others with less concern for human rights, but interest in the power of the new technologies, will undoubtedly want to employ them in a wide range of investigations as well.

References

Aitken, C. K., McCaw, R. F., Bowden, D. S., Tracy, S. L., Kelsall, J. G., Higgs, P. G., Kerger, M. J., Nguyen, H., and Crofts, J. N. 2004. Molecular epidemiology of hepatitis C virus in a social network of injection drug users. *Journal of Infectious Diseases* 190 (9):1586–95. Epub 2004 September 23.

Barnes, P. U., Yang, Z., and Preston-Martin, S. 1997. Patterns of tuberculosis transmission in central Los Angeles. *Journal of the American Medical Association* 278:1159–63.

Beyrer, C. 1998. Burma and Cambodia: Human rights, social disruption, and the spread of HIV/AIDS. *Health and Human Rights* 4:85–97.

Beyrer, C. 2003. HIV infection rates and heroin trafficking: Fearful symmetries. *Bulletin on Narcotics: The Science of Drug Use Epidemiology* 14 (2):400–417.

Beyrer, C., Razak, M. H., Lisam, K., Wei, L., Chen, J., and Yu, X. F. 2000. Overland heroin trafficking routes and HIV spread in South and Southeast Asia. *AIDS* 14:1–9.

Bobkov, A., Kazennova, E., Selimova, L., Bobkova, M., Khanina, T., Ladnaya, N., et al.

1998. A sudden epidemic of HIV type 1 among injecting drug users in the former Soviet Union: identification of subtype A, subtype B, and novel gagA/envB recombinants. *AIDS Research and Human Retroviruses* 14:669–76.

Carr, J. K., Saad, M., Nadai, I., Tishkova, F., Eyzaguirre, L., Strathdee, S. A., Stachowiak, J., Beyrer, C., Earhart, K., Birx, D., and Sanchez, J. L. 2005. Outbreak of a West Africa HIV-1 recombinant, CRF02_AG, in Central Asia Abstract MoOa0407. Third International AIDS Society Conference on HIV Pathogenesis and Treatment, 24–27 July 2005, Rio de Janiero.

Cavalli-Sforza, L. L. 2000. *Languages, genes, and peoples.* New York: North Point Press.

Daley, C. L. 2005. Molecular epidemiology: a tool for understanding control of tuberculosis transmission. *Clinical Chest Medicine* 26 (2):217–31.

Davey, M. 2004. Illinois governor in the middle of new death penalty debate. *New York Times.* March 15. Available at: www.nytimes.com.

Echevarria, J. M., Avellon, A., and Magnius, L. O. 2005. Molecular epidemiology of hepatitis B virus in Spain: Identification of viral genotypes and prediction of antigenic subtypes by limited sequencing. *Journal of Medical Virology* 76 (2):176–84.

Garrett, L. 2005. *HIV and national security: What are the links?* Special Report. New York: Council on Foreign Relations.

Hammett, T. M., Johnston, P., and Kling, R. 2005. Correlates of HIV status among injecting drug users in a border region of southern China and northern Vietnam. *Journal of Acquired Immune Deficiency Syndromes* 38 (2):228–36.

Human Rights Watch. 2003. *Fanning the flames: How human rights abuses are fueling the AIDS epidemic in Kazakhstan.* New York: HRW.

Kaufman, J., and Jing, J. 2002. China and AIDS—the time to act is now. *Science* 296 (5577):2339–40.

McCutchan, F. E. 2005. Molecular epidemiology of HIV. Plenary Presentation. Paper presented at Third International Conference on HIV Pathogenesis and Treatment, July 2005, Rio De Janeiro.

McCutchan, F. M., Carr, J. K., Tovanabutra, S., Yu, X-F., Beyrer, C., and Birx, D. L. 2003. HIV-1 and drug trafficking: Viral strains illuminate networks and provide focus for interventions. In *Proceedings of the 5th Global Response Network, Barcelona,* Spain, pp.112–19.

Mohle-Boetani, J. C., Miguelino, V., and Dewsnup, D. 2002. Tuberculosis outbreak in a housing unit for HIV-infected patients in a correctional facility: transmission risk factors and effective outbreak control. *Clinical Infectious Diseases* 34:668–76.

Ou, C. Y., Ciesielski, C. A., Myers, G., Bandea, C. I., Luo, C. C., Korber, B. T., et al. 1992. Molecular epidemiology of HIV transmission in a dental practice. *Science* 256 (5060):1165–71.

Piriyasilip, S., McCutchan, F., Carr, J.K., Sanders-Buell, E., Liu, W., Chen, J., Wagner, R., Wolf, H., Shao, Y., Lai, S., Beyrer, C., and Yu, X-F. 2000. A recent outbreak of HIV-1 infection in southern China was initiated by two highly homogenous, geographically separated strains: circulating recombinant for AE and a novel BC recombinant. *Journal of Virology* 74 (23):11286–95.

Robertson, B. H., and Nicholson, J. K. 2005. New microbiology tools for public health and their implications. *Annual Review of Public Health* 26:281–302.

Shih, M. C., Peck, K., Chan, W. L., Chu, Y. P., Chen, J. C., Tsai, C. H., and Chang, J. G. 2005. SARS-CoV infection was from at least two origins in the Taiwan area. *Intervirology* 48 (2–3):124–32.

Shih, S. R., Chen, G. W., Yang, C. C., et al. 2005. Laboratory-based surveillance and molecular epidemiology of influenza virus in Taiwan. *Journal of Clinical Microbiology* 43 (4):1651–61.

Stachowiak, J. A., Tishkova, F., Strathdee, S. A., Stibich, M., Latypov, A., Mogilnii, V., and Beyrer, C. 2006. Marked ethnic differences in HIV prevalence and risk behaviors among IDU in Dushanbe, Tajikistan, 2004. *Drug and Alcohol Dependence* 82 (Suppl. 1): S7–S14.

Takebe, Y., Motomura, K., Tatsumi, M., Lwin, H. H., Zaw, M., and Kusagawa, S. 2003. High prevalence of diverse forms of HIV-1 intersubtype recombinants in Central Myanmar: geographical hot spot of extensive recombination. *AIDS* 17 (14):2077–87.

United Nations Office on Drugs and Crime. 2004. *Statistics*, Vol. 2 of *World Drug Report on Afghanistan.*

Wiewel, E. W., Go, V. F., Kawichai, S., Beyrer, C., Vongchak, T., Srirak, N., Jaroon, J., Suriyanon, V., Razak, M. H., and Celentano, D. D. 2005. Injection prevalence and risks among male ethnic minority drug users in northern Thailand. *AIDS CARE* 17:103–10.

Zhang, L., Chen, Z., Cao, Y., Yu, J., Li, G., Yu, W., Yin, N., Mei, S., Li, L., Balfe, P., He, T., Ba, L., Zhang, F., Lin, H. H., Yuen, M. F., Lai, C. L., and Ho, D. D. 2004. Molecular characterization of human immunodeficiency virus type 1 and hepatitis C virus in paid blood donors and injection drug users in China. *Journal of Virology* 78 (24):13591–99.

7

Documenting the Effects of Trafficking in Women

Cathy Zimmerman, M.Sc., and Charlotte Watts, Ph.D.

Tatiana lost her mother, father, and younger brother to an automobile accident when she was sixteen years old in Ukraine. When she was eighteen and living on her own, she lost her job. A friend introduced her to Sasha who promised her work as a nanny in the United Kingdom. On arrival in the United Kingdom, Sasha informed her and the two other girls with whom she traveled that they would be working as prostitutes. Tatiana sobbed and refused. Sasha threw her to the floor, slapped her and raped her. The following evening, when her "minder" was not looking, Tatiana fled the apartment in her nightgown on a cold December night. Nine months later, the rape resulted in a baby girl who required treatment for congenital syphilis. Living alone with her daughter, each night Tatiana slept with a knife under her pillow and the fear of being found by her trafficker. Awaiting her asylum decision, distressed and anxious, Tatiana contemplated suicide on numerous occasions. When referred to a psychiatrist specializing in care of refugees, Tatiana was advised that anxiety among refugees was common, and that all would be well when her asylum papers were approved—the sexual and physical violence she experienced and her present fears of being found by her trafficker were never addressed. Tatiana was subsequently refused asylum.

The trafficking of women and adolescents into forced labor, including forced sex work and other exploitative or slavery-like conditions, is increasingly recognized as one of the world's fastest-growing crimes and most significant human rights violations (U.N. High Commissioner for Human Rights, 2001; International Organization for Migration, 2003). Few corners of the world are free from this form of violence against women. Although trafficking and sexual slavery are by no means new to the world, the rapidly globalizing market has turned individual hardship into an unlimited resource that feeds an insatiable demand for exploitable labor.

Trafficking is a complex, diverse, and controversial phenomenon, which has made the search for a definition a "terminological minefield" (Skeldon, 2000). The most commonly accepted definition is found in the *United Nations Protocol to Prevent, Suppress, and Punish Trafficking in Persons, Especially Women and Children, Supplementing the United Nations Convention against Transnational Organized Crime* (generally known as the Palermo Protocol), which defines it as follows:

> The recruitment, transportation, transfer, harbouring or receipt of persons by means of threat or use of force or other forms of coercion, of abduction, of fraud, of deception, of the abuse of power, or of a position of vulnerability or of the giving or receiving of payments or benefits to achieve the consent of a person having control over another person, for the purpose of exploitation. Exploitation shall include, at minimum, the exploitation of prostitution of others or other forms of sexual exploitation, forced labor or services, slavery or practices similar to slavery, servitude or the removal of organs (United Nations, 2000).

Although the trafficking of women is commonly associated with sexual exploitation, women are regularly trafficked for other forms of forced labor, such as domestic servitude, forced marriage, factory or agricultural labor, construction, and street begging (Anderson, 1993; Derks, 1997; Wijers and Lap-Chew, 1999; International Organization for Migration, 2003; U.N. Economic and Social Council, 2004). While working in any of these sectors, it is not uncommon for women to be sexually abused and/or exploited. Women are trafficked and transported internationally, regionally, and within their national borders. Internal trafficking, although likely to account for a greater number of trafficked persons, receives significantly less attention than international trafficking (International Labor Organization, 2005).

The need for a response to the physical and psychological harm caused to individuals has been acknowledged in a number of international instruments, such as Article 6 of the Palermo Protocol, which states, "Each State Party shall consider implementing measures to provide for the physical, psychological and social recovery of victims of trafficking in persons . . . in particular, the provision of . . . (c) Medical, psychological and material assistance" (United Nations, 2000).

Despite the weak language ("shall consider"), this seminal document recognizes that governments should address the health consequences of trafficking. However, the subject of health has received relatively little attention and even less evidence-based inquiry, despite widespread acknowledgment that trafficking in women involves an extraordinary range of abuses that cause profound and enduring personal harm (Zimmerman et al., 2003).

In 2001 a team of researchers from the London School of Hygiene and Tropical Medicine began to study the health effect of trafficking on women and adolescents who were trafficked for sexual exploitation and domestic services. Having previously worked with survivors of other forms of violence, such as domestic violence, we understood that women's health is likely to be a belated area for research and action—frequently following legal interventions—despite the associated morbidity and mortality (Heise, 1994). And, like other forms of violence, while ultimately the aim is to eliminate abuse, the reality is that trafficking shows no signs of abating, and increasing numbers of women around the world urgently need informed and appropriate care.

Drawing on our experience conducting qualitative and quantitative multiple-country studies on trafficking and health in Europe, this chapter discusses the methodological and ethical issues associated with carrying out research on this subject. After presenting a brief overview of what is known about trafficking, trafficked persons, and traffickers, we outline some of the particular conceptual and practical complexities inherent in studying trafficking and health. We discuss the political and cultural sensitivities that are likely to affect research and policies on trafficking. We describe the pervading ethical and safety issues and their impact on various methodological stages and review key considerations in selecting study instruments to examine health. We then suggest a public health perspective on trafficking, and finally propose future directions for research in this challenging subject area.

What Is Trafficking, Who Are Trafficked Women, and Who Are Traffickers?

Statistics on the scale of trafficking have proven elusive and still remain somewhat of a Holy Grail (Laczko and Gramegna, 2003; Loff and Sanghera, 2003). Annual estimates have ranged from 800,000 to 900,000 persons trafficked across international borders (U.S. Department of State, 2003), to 2,450,000 trafficked into forced labor worldwide (International Labor Organization, 2005). Of those trafficked into forced labor, not surprisingly, women are said to make up the majority of the victims of economic exploitation (56%) and those exploited in commercial sex (98%).

In terms of regional numbers, again, accurate figures are hard to come by. It has been estimated that most trafficked persons are from Asia and the Pacific (Miko and Park, 2002; International Labor Organization, 2005), although women trafficked from the Commonwealth of Independent States or central and Eastern Europe often make the headlines (Specter, 1998; U.N. Economic and Social Council, 2004; Cowan, 2005). Although less information has been available on Africa, the Middle East, and Central and Latin America, trafficking undoubtedly abounds in these regions as well (U.S. Department of State, 2005).

The dynamics of trafficking are no easier to pinpoint than the statistics. Features of the crime—such as recruitment tactics, financial arrangements, trafficking networks, travel and visa documents, border crossings, and the types of exploitation and abuse—may vary by cultural and geographical setting, and can radically differ from trafficker to trafficker (Salt and Stein, 1997). For example, one underacknowledged type of exploitation is the trafficking of women and children (often elderly or disabled) from Cambodia to Thailand or Roma girls to Western Europe for street begging (Derks, 1997; International Organization for Migration, 1999; Feuk, 2003). The strategies used by traffickers are also mutable, with traffickers regularly changing their methods and routes to evade detection and gain the most profit. Annual profits from human trafficking were estimated to be U.S. $32 billion in 2005 and are now thought to account for more than drug and weapons trafficking combined (International Labor Organization, 2005).

Although the variation between trafficking experiences can be significant, one theme that seems to be symbolic of the entire process is that of "control." The trafficker has it and uses it; the woman loses it and suffers for this loss.

Who are trafficked women? While it is tempting to imagine a naïve, poverty-stricken, young, and uneducated virgin girl from the countryside, or the opposite, a savvy woman who knows what she is getting into, but believes the money will be worth it, in reality, there is no single portrait of a trafficked woman. It is more useful to look instead at the causes of trafficking and, from there, to consider who might be most vulnerable to one or more of these factors. Most literature describing trafficking discusses the "push" and "pull" factors that contribute to trafficking (Sanghera, 1997; Zimmerman, 2003). Push factors, such as gender inequity, social deprivation and poverty, or civil and political unrest are said to cause women to migrate, while images of good jobs, political freedoms, and media images of wealth pull women toward what they hope will be a better life.

Listening to women's accounts of their recruitment, it seems that there is a "facilitating" factor that becomes the lynchpin. Women explain that their trust in the person making the offer (e.g., relative, friend of the family, referral by someone who has gone and profited, etc.) tipped the balance in their decision to accept risks that they might otherwise have refused. (See Figure 7.1.)

The abuses that trafficked women experience and the ways in which women are affected by abuse are also difficult to characterize. Some women will suffer the most unspeakable violence and humiliation and may be less affected than another who is not as severely violated. It is not unusual, however, for women on either end of the continuum of abuse to feel that they are no longer the same person they once were. One Eastern European woman poignantly explained: *I feel as if they took my smile and I will never get it back* (Zimmerman et al., forthcoming).

Who are traffickers? Information from law enforcement experts suggests that, like victims of trafficking, there is no single description that accurately captures all traffickers (Graycar, 1999). In practice, the category "traffickers" can include both males and females who may be amateur or opportunistic operators (such as those who provide a one-off service, such as transport); small groups of organized criminals (e.g., based on family connections); and international trafficking networks (often involved in other criminal activities) (Graycar, 1999; Schloenhardt, 1999). In this category, it is also reasonable to include others who buy or sell or exploit women, such as brothel owners

Push & Pull Factors

Facilitating Factors

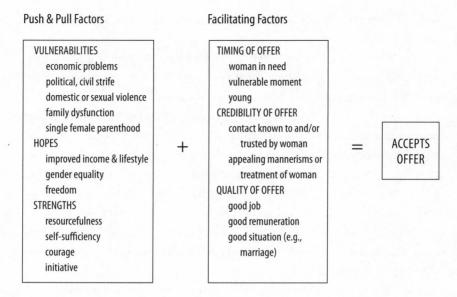

Figure 7.1. Recruitment equation

and employers of domestic workers. Importantly, in the case of trafficking for sexual exploitation, the demand is created almost wholly by men.

When trying to examine the dynamics and health aspects of trafficking, it is useful to recognize that traffickers of women are perpetrators of an extreme form of gender-based violence who use a range of strategies to obtain and maintain power over the women (see Chapter 16). The process employed to inculcate dependence and submission has also been likened to the stages of mental manipulation employed by totalitarian regimes (Tchomarova, 2001). First, the person is put in "extreme survival conditions" in which she is forced to face the possibility of death. The perpetrator makes the woman know that she no longer controls her safety—the perpetrator does. The second stage involves "physical exhaustion." Individuals are forced to work long hours with no free time and minimal rest, which gives perpetrators significant control, and, in the case of trafficking and labor exploitation, increased profits. Without time to recuperate, the individual is exhausted, unable to plan or contemplate self-defense strategies, and must simply focus on responding appropriately to commands and perceived immediate threats. The final elements to ensuring dependence are control and isolation.

Research on Trafficking and Women's Health

Migration Stages of the Trafficking Process: A Theoretical Model

For our study, we developed a conceptual framework, based on a migration model (Salt and Stein, 1997; Gushulak and MacPherson, 2000) which outlines the chronological developments and geographical movements that women may make to help conceptualize the range of health risks that trafficked women may face (Zimmerman, 2003). From this perspective, the trafficking process can be divided into five stages:

1. Predeparture stage
2. Travel and transit stage
3. Destination stage
4. Detention, deportation, and criminal evidence stage[1]
5. Integration and reintegration stage

(See Figure 7.2.) This model offers a good starting point for a study on health and trafficking because it proposes a way of looking at health and morbidity both singularly—according to each individual stage of the trafficking process—and cumulatively, as the sum of the different stages.

The *predeparture stage* is the period before an individual is recruited into the trafficking situation. This stage reflects a trafficked person's mental and physical health characteristics at departure, which in turn may affect her health and health-related behavior throughout the trafficking process, and ultimately, her strength and resilience later. Frequently, many of the factors that negatively influence health during the predeparture stage are also those that predispose individuals to being trafficked (e.g., gender inequity, poverty, unemployment, interpersonal violence, child abuse, sexual abuse, family dysfunction, environmental destruction, agricultural decline, civil unrest, and displacement). An example of pretrafficking vulnerability is the case of Angela (not her real name), who was the oldest child in her family when her mother began a new relationship. From the age of fourteen to eighteen, her mother's new partner sexually abused Angela. This only ended when she left home to seek work overseas (Dickson, 2004). Data from an assistance program in London show that 68 percent of women using their services reported having experienced violence before being exploited in the destination setting (Dickson, 2004).

DESTINATION STAGE

Risks and abuse affecting:
- Physical health
- Sexual health
- Mental health
- Substance abuse and misuse
- Social health (isolation, exclusion)
- Economic well-being
- Occupational and environmental health
- Access to health information and care

TRAVEL AND TRANSIT STAGE
- High-risk, arduous travel conditions
- Violence, sexual abuse, threats
- The "initial trauma"
- Debt-bondage, being bought and sold
- Confiscation of documents
- Absence of information and care

PREDEPARTURE STAGE
- Personal history
- Experience with home country health services and health education and promotion
- Epidemiological and socioeconomic conditions of the country

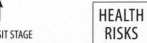

DETENTION, DEPORTATION, AND
CRIMINAL EVIDENCE
- Lack of attention to health by all law enforcement, immigration, and justice officials
- Lack of official health-related procedures
- Absence of victim-sensitive procedures
- Reprisals by trafficking agents resulting from contact with authorities
- Anxiety, trauma resulting from contact with authorities, evidence-giving or trial proceedings
- Unsafe, inhumane deportation and return procedures
- Retrafficking, retribution and trauma associated with deportation

INTEGRATION AND REINTEGRATION
- Personal security risks
- Risks associated with being a refugee, immigrant, or returnee
- Practical, social, economic, cultural, and linguistic barriers to care
- Isolation and exclusion
- Immediate and longer-term mental health consequences
- Retrafficking

Figure 7.2. Conceptual model: stages of the trafficking process

Women's backgrounds may also influence their later ability to protect their health or access health services. For example, trafficked persons often come from areas where health systems are underresourced and difficult to access, and women may be relatively uninformed about their sexual and reproductive health and methods to protect themselves from pregnancy or sexually transmitted infections. Even if the woman is informed and the opportunity to seek care arises at a later stage, she may be hesitant to seek help for legal, practical (e.g., travel logistics, finances, language), and cultural reasons.

The *travel and transit stage* begins at the time of recruitment when an individual agrees to go or is forced to depart with a trafficker (whether or not she is aware that she is being trafficked), and ends when the she arrives at the work destination. Because illegal activities (e.g., abduction, rape, forged papers, illegal border crossing) generally start at this stage and a trafficker's primary concern is to avoid detection rather than to protect the women who are being trafficked, the dangers to women may significantly increase at this time. For many women, the journey exposes them to hazardous modes of transportation, high-risk border crossings, arrest, threats and intimidation, and violence.

> S saw her companion drown when trying to swim against the fast running currents at night while the traffickers transported them from Poland to Germany (La Strada Ukraine, November 28–30 2002).

Psychologically, this stage is frequently when the "initial trauma" occurs, because it is often at this time that a woman first realizes that she has been misled and is in life-threatening danger (Zimmerman, 2003). She may suspect this from a trafficker's behavior ("I saw my fiancé meeting some young men who called him 'boss' . . . and he was promising to three foreign women to arrange for their trip to Italy, as well" [Zimmerman, 2003]), or may be beaten or raped to groom her for the work to come. As this period reflects the point at which women's hopes turn to nightmares, many women have trouble recalling or discussing details of events that occur at this time. Recall difficulty and discrepancies in autobiographical memories by traumatized persons have been demonstrated in many different settings (Herlihy et al., 2002). Unfortunately for the women, this is often the period about which law enforcement and immigration and asylum officials demand the greatest detail.

> Abortion was forbidden because of the faith. I was past my fifth month when the abortion was done. I didn't know I was pregnant. The abortion was done illegally in terrible unsanitary conditions. The operation was very difficult, so I was nearly dead. There was no anaesthetic. The doctor said he would inject soap water into the uterus and the foetus would go out (Elena was 13 when she was trafficked from Ukraine to the UAE). (Zimmerman, 2003)

The *destination stage* is the period when a woman is put to work most often in irregular, unregulated labor sectors, and subjected to the forms of violence and exploitation commonly associated with trafficking. Many of the abuses and health risks that occur during this stage are similar to those associated with other forms of violence against women (e.g., domestic violence), including physical abuse, sexual abuse, psychological abuse, social restrictions, and emotional manipulation. Other types of abuse—such as forced and coerced use of drugs and alcohol, economic exploitation, and hazardous working conditions—are more regularly linked to sex work or forms of labor exploitation (International Labor Organization, 2005). There are also abuses unique to trafficking, including debt bondage, confiscation of women's legal and identity documents, and forced legal insecurity. Broader risks include those associated with being a socially marginalized migrant in an unfamiliar location, bereft of any supportive social network.

It is rare that a trafficked person has an opportunity to seek adequate or any medical assistance or information during this phase. Many women acquire infections, injuries, or illnesses, and develop complications resulting from lack of treatment.

> Generally we try not to become involved with the welfare of people we send back. (Immigration Official). (Zimmerman, 2003)

The *detention, deportation, and criminal evidence stage* is when an individual is in the custody of police or immigration authorities, for alleged violation of criminal or immigration law, or is cooperating, voluntarily or under threat of prosecution or deportation, in legal proceedings against a trafficker, exploitative employer, or other abuser. In some locations, the conditions at detention facilities are extremely harsh and pose additional physical health risks (e.g., poor sanitary conditions, violence, poor food, heat, space, or light deprivation, and so on), leading to further deterioration. In other facilities, physical health and basic needs are adequately met. In most cases, however, negative effects on mental health are difficult to avoid when a woman is arrested, held in detention, obliged to give evidence, or testify in a criminal proceeding. Counseling or psychological support is rarely available during detention.

> My friend phoned and said that everyone is saying that I am a prostitute. My aunt said that they should ask me to dance on the table. I am horrified by myself and what my friends think of me (Zimmerman et al., forthcoming).

The *integration and reintegration stage* consists of a long-term and multi-faceted process that is not completed until the individual becomes an active member of the economic, cultural, civil, and political life of a country and perceives that she has reoriented and is accepted by her community (European Council on Refugees and Exiles, 1999). Although women may be freed from the trafficking situation, their health problems do not necessarily disappear, and it is not always a direct road to recovery. Indeed, it appears as if the health complications accumulated throughout the trafficking process may be compounded by the multiple challenges that emerge during this stage. Trafficked persons frequently face administrative, financial, or language challenges within government systems, and stressful emotions similar to those identified among immigrant and refugee populations, such as loneliness and alienation. According to support workers, the clients of shelter services experience anxiety, isolation, aggressive feelings or behaviors, self-stigmatization or perceived stigmatization by others, barriers communicating needs and accessing necessary resources, and they may develop negative coping behaviors (e.g., excessive smoking, drinking, or drug use) (Zimmerman et al., 2003; International Organization for Migration, 2004).

When thinking of health and trafficking, one may be tempted to attribute all manifestations of ill health to the period of labor exploitation alone. Yet, as this model shows, health risks and protective factors occur at each stage of the journey. An illustration of this is found in the study we are currently completing, which looks at, inter alia, the mental health status of women in service settings during the integration-reintegration stage (Zimmerman et al., forthcoming). For example, of two women who reported nearly identical symptom levels of anxiety and panic reactions, one explained that she had always had these feelings before leaving home, while the other said that she never felt any of these symptoms until after being abused and exploited.

This model also offers a framework to consider how different issues might fit into the overall picture of the trafficking process, and how they piece together to determine patterns of need. Additionally, the framework can be used to explore intervention options. Research questions on interventions might focus on a single stage, exploring, for example, "Under what conditions are presumptive protocols for sexually transmitted infections appropriate during the integration-reintegration stage?" Or, one could use the model to try to understand the impact of policy change across multiple stages: reviewing, for example, how international instruments, treaties, and national legislation and procedures hinder or foster access to support and medical care at different stages of the trafficking process.

Similarly, this model might be used to develop and investigate theories about factors that fuel the trafficking phenomenon, for example, delineating different causal influences at each stage of the process, examining, for example, different societal levels: personal, family, community, and political structures (Heise, 1998).

Methodological Complexities of Studying a Highly Vulnerable Group

In conducting any research on health and trafficking, investigators encounter a variety of methodological challenges (Laczko and Gozdziak, 2005). Some are related to the recent emergence of the subject, which means that there is limited baseline data or tested theories. Many are associated with the highly sensitive nature of the topic and the extreme vulnerability of the study population. For this reason, in studying women who have been trafficked, one must think beyond traditional methodological approaches and standard ethical guidance to ensure that any research does not put individuals or groups of individuals at risk of imminent or future harm, while still gaining high-quality data.

Features of Trafficking That Challenge Standard Methodologies

Renzetti and Lee define a sensitive research topic as "one that potentially poses for those involved a substantial threat, the emergence of which renders problematic for the researcher and/or the researched the collection, holding, and/or dissemination of research data" (Renzetti and Lee, 1993). There can be no doubt that trafficking of women fits this description. Trafficking is a subject that is laden with threats. To understand the implications of these threats, it is useful to delineate those features of trafficking that are (a) politically sensitive or (b) socially sensitive, and those that (c) raise legal issues or (d) create serious ethical and safety concerns. (See Figure 7.3.)

Social and cultural sensitivity have long been a matter for discussion within social science literature (Neuman, 1991; Seale, 1998), and in medicine the term "cultural competency" has begun to enter the common lexicon (American Medical Association, 1999). Sensitivity associated with race, religion, or

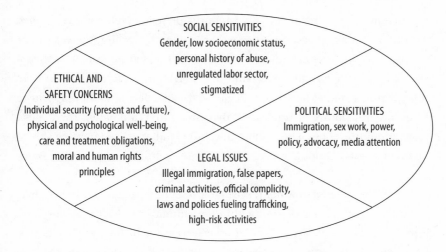

Figure 7.3. Features of trafficking that place additional demands on researchers

ethnicity is generally included under this heading (Huisman, 1997; Fortune, 2001). Because trafficking, especially international trafficking, can involve women from diverse backgrounds moving between different countries and cultures, addressing these social sensitivities can be an especially complex aspect of any study. Moreover, although trafficking occurs globally, its characteristics are frequently tied to cultural contexts.

For work on trafficking, the category of social and cultural sensitivity must be expanded to include less recognized characteristics that make trafficked women extraordinarily marginalized, including gender inequities; personal history of abuse, including sexual abuse; low socioeconomic status; membership of unregulated, underground sectors; and the strong potential for stigmatization.

Social marginalization for many trafficked women begins before they leave home and increases as they move through the trafficking process. Numerous women who are trafficked already fall within a marginalized population; they may be single parents, victims of domestic violence or child sexual abuse, orphans, or refugees. During the trafficking cycle, women move even further to the margins of society, working in unregulated sectors, doing degrading work, and in some cases, they are literally locked up and hidden from view. For example, women trafficked into domestic work can be entirely secluded, some being confined within the home for months or years. Isolation perpetrated by exploiters may be accomplished either by literally locking up women, or through various types of intimidation, such as threatening women with violence, harm to their family, arrest and/or deportation (Human Rights Watch, 2001; Zimmerman et al., 2003). Racial and social discrimination appear to be an integral feature of trafficking. By coming from a different race, social class, or culture, those who exploit, purchase, and abuse women are able to see them as merchandise, rather than as entirely human (Cox, 1999; Brennan, 2005).

Even once released, a woman may later be stigmatized by the experience, and tainted both to herself and within her community. For those who have been sexually abused, if married they may be rejected by their husbands, and if unmarried, they may be considered ineligible for marriage. It is not only sex that will cause a woman to be shunned; women have also been rejected because they failed to bring home the income that the family expected (Skrobanek et al., 1997).

Social sensitivities can make it difficult to access women in ways that do not put them at risk of harm, shame, or exposure leading to ostracism or social exile. These sensitivities can influence what women should be asked about their experiences, how it should be asked, and whether others close to the woman can be contacted or interviewed. Because so much of the information gathered has social implications, how findings are interpreted and presented is important to avoid fueling stereotypes, prejudices, and policy overreactions. If, for example, women are found to have high rates of sexually transmitted infections, government officials in some countries may use these findings to impose mandatory medical testing on women who have been trafficked. This has already happened in Nigeria, where women deported back to Lagos were forced to undergo medical tests, including HIV testing. No tests were required of men who returned, however (Pearson, 2002).

The relationship between these many factors that cause women's vulnerability, or contribute to the perpetuation of trafficking and the associated harm is an important area for future research for primary prevention.

Legal Issues

Legal issues associated with trafficking, such as immigration violations and vice crimes, weigh heavily on many aspects of research. The effects of laws and policies can affect women on an individual level, such as when they knowingly or unwittingly become involved in criminal activities (e.g., illegal border crossing, using forged papers, illegally selling sex or drugs), and can influence the treatment of trafficked women as a group, such as when they are profiled as illegal entrants and targeted by police or immigration officials and deported without recognition of their rights to protection.

Practically, because so many aspects of trafficking are illegal, women are usually reluctant to respond to questions. Frequently they are highly mobile and hidden, many taking care to avoid outsiders, especially anyone they believe might represent a local authority. Whether it is because the women are aware that they have done something illegal, because they believe that officials might be complicit with those exploiting them (as many are told this by traffickers), or because they are afraid of being unable to earn enough money to pay back their debts or return home financially better than they left, most women avoid anything that has to do with police, immigration officials, and others who may be perceived as "authorities"—which can often include researchers.

Sensitivity around legal dimensions of trafficking also emerges at the governmental level. Trafficking frequently involves officials that are complicit, such as consular representatives, border police, and local police (Asia Watch Women's Rights Project, 1993; Human Rights Watch Asia, 1995). In one study on gambling, arms, and human trafficking in Thailand, for example, a researcher was threatened with arrest and the research was "denigrated on the radio" when he exposed police corruption (Phongpaichit et al., 1998).

Legislation on areas related to trafficking—such as increasingly restrictive immigration laws (Morrison and Crosland, 2000), laws on "reflection delay" (a period of temporary legal residence during which a woman must decide if she wishes to cooperate with authorities), and expeditious removal and deportation procedures—can have an influence on the conduct of a study. Conversely, and importantly, well-founded research has the capacity to influence procedures and laws applied in cases of trafficking. For example, research demonstrating the negative effects of trauma on an individual's memory can contribute to how discrepancies in reports by asylum claimants are perceived (Herlihy et al., 2002).

Political Sensitivities

Politically sensitive research topics have been described as those that are, or have the potential to be, "controversial" (Sieber and Stanley, 1998). This sensitivity often relates to debates that take place in the larger political environment (governmental, policy, legal). Sensitive issues can have broad social implications (public attitudes, prejudices, stereotypes), or imply something about power, who holds it, and to what effect.

Trafficking is a politically loaded subject. Situating trafficking politically helps to gain insight into the etiology of trafficking and to consider potential interventions. First and foremost, trafficking in women is a form of violence against women in which exploitation for profit—the selling of women, their bodies, and their labor—is a fundamental feature. That this phenomenon has spread so quickly and that demand seems never to be sated is testimony to a global socioeconomic environment that undervalues women, the poor, and migrants. The exploitation of the disadvantaged, while rhetorically decried, seems to have become normative, and has benefited sex traffickers and certain labor sectors. A host of discriminatory economic and social conditions have increased women's need to seek income, safety and/or freedom, while simultaneously spurring the growth of a multibillion dollar sex industry and market for cheap labor.

On a policy level, trafficking involves two of today's most controversial issues: immigration and sex work (Anderson and O'Connell-Davidson, 2002). Immigration is an issue that holds great capital for politicians. Promising to remove so-called undeserving migrants, and rescuing the population from foreigners, can earn politicians political points. Trafficking of women offers governments a convenient and moral argument for cracking down on immigrants. To "save" vulnerable women, governments tighten restrictions on all migrants. As suggested above, experts on migration assert that sweeping initiatives to control labor migration do not help reduce trafficking and cause harm to voluntary migrants (Busza et al., 2004). Many argue that the evidence shows that restrictions only increase business and profits for traffickers and smugglers, and pushes them to resort to more dangerous routes and brutal methods, which ultimately cause further harm to the women they are claiming to protect (Morrison and Crosland, 2000; Davies, 2002; Gallagher, 2002). Further, there is a significant grey area between "trafficking" and "smuggling." Anderson and O'Connell-Davidson note that the ambiguities in "the trafficking/smuggling distinction represents a gaping hole in any safety net for those whose human rights are violated in the process of migration" (Anderson and O'Connell-Davidson, 2002). Researchers working on trafficking must understand the implications of the definitions they choose. For example, research on immigration and exploitation may include "trafficked persons" and "smuggled persons."

Equally charged are the conflicting positions (and animosity) between the factions in the "prostitution-sex worker" debate. When broaching the subject of sex work and prostitution, even women's organizations and human rights groups working toward the same humanitarian purposes (the well-being of women) can often hold seemingly irreconcilable and heartfelt positions. Sex work is viewed by one faction as a fundamental labor right that should be legalized (Bindman and Doezema, 1997; Ditmore, 2005), whereas the other declares prostitution to be immoral, and a severe form of violence against women that must be eliminated (Hughes and Roche, 1999). The latter view has influenced major donor agencies to attach strict anti-prostitution criteria to the funding they give to outreach programs for sex-workers (Ditmore, 2003; Amin, 2004; Busza et al., 2004; Henry Kaiser Family Foundation, 2005). Researchers working on the health of women in trafficking situations may be accused of studying "slaves" rather than trying to "free" them.

In any research on health and trafficking, neither of these subjects can be ignored, because both sides of either debate have the potential to lay claim to the protection of women's health. Anderson and O'Connell-Davidson, in their report looking at the demand side of trafficking, summarize the effect of restrictions in either realm: "In the current global economic and political climate, prioritizing the control of illegal immigration or the suppression of prostitution is not necessarily consistent with the goal of protecting migrants from abuse and exploitation by traffickers and other third parties, and may indeed cause or encourage human rights violations" (Anderson and O'Connell-Davidson, 2002, p. 63). In either the immigration or the sex work debate, there is a risk that by highlighting the vulnerability and "innocence" of victims of trafficking, people who are smuggled, or voluntary migrants and sex workers, may be thus labeled "guilty."

The choice of terms in trafficking is important, and researchers should be aware of the politics of language. Notable examples are the terms prostitution, sex work, and forced prostitution, which each have political connotations that can place a researcher/author in one camp or another (i.e., "prostitution" is more often used by individuals whose aim is to eliminate it; "sex work" is more often used by those who do not take a position or who support the rights of women in sex work). Similarly, terminology for migrants must be chosen carefully to accurately describe each person's status, and to avoid stigmatizing individuals (e.g., illegal versus undocumented or irregular migrant). "Trafficking" is politically laden. It is criticized for undermining the rights of migrant sex workers and giving governments license to raid sex worker venues and deport women (Murphy and Ringheim, 2002). Researchers need to be mindful and understand the political connotations of the terms they select, even before a study begins.

Journalists and filmmakers who have shown an interest in trafficking simultaneously call attention to the problem, while, in some cases, they inadvertently further ignite the politics of the subject. This means that extra caution must be taken with findings that can easily be exaggerated and spun out of control.

As the number of persons trafficked continues to grow, it becomes increasingly apparent that trafficking does not occur in a vacuum, but in modern social, cultural, and economic environments that, to varying degrees, ignore, tolerate, or condone it (Amnesty International, 2001). The politics surrounding the subject cannot be avoided, because they ultimately will affect research, prevention, protection, and care.

Ethical and Safety Concerns

Dimensions of the topic of trafficking that are of ethical and safety concern include those that are related to personal security and may affect the physical and psychological well-being of study participants or members of the research team. Ethical dimensions can also be viewed as those that adhere to moral and human rights standards.

As health studies have increasingly begun to focus on society's most marginalized individuals, traditional ethical guidelines for research, such as the CIOMS *International Ethical Guidelines for Biomedical Research Involving Human Subjects,* now seem somewhat limited in scope, because they are unable to anticipate many of the risks involved in investigating highly vulnerable groups (Council for International Organizations of Medical Sciences, 1993). Current rights-based documents written to protect trafficked persons, on the other hand, are often too broad in scope to offer specific guidance for the research context (U.N. High Commissioner for Human Rights, 2002).

In conducting research on trafficking, the basic ethical standards to protect participants, such as do no harm, informed consent, and confidentiality, require reevaluation and added scrutiny. The potential for harm, not only to the participants but also to others associated with them (e.g., family, friends) or to the research team, can be so great, and can emerge from so many different directions that researchers have an ethical obligation to go beyond "doing no harm." They must not rely solely on responsive techniques (e.g., providing referral information), but should develop and implement dynamic protective strategies (e.g., on-site psychological support). Moreover, in the case of trafficked women, because the individuals involved are already in situations of harm, and in general at risk of greater harm, the underlying ethic should aim not simply to do no further harm, but to improve the situation for individuals in the study and for the group as a whole. In particular for health research, avenues leading to improved individual and population well-being should be built into the methodology.

As part of our research on trafficking, we worked with the World Health Organization (WHO) to develop guidelines on how to conduct research that involves women who have been trafficked. As described in detail in the resulting *WHO Ethical and Safety Recommendations for Interviewing Trafficked Women*, we propose ten principles for conducting research (Box 7.1), and describe in practice the range of issues that need to be considered when conducting research in this area (Zimmerman and Watts, 2003).

As discussed further below, a key consideration is the importance of collaborating with experienced service providers or support groups who work in the community being studied, and who can provide care or assistance. Local groups are able to competently advise on security issues, understand safe means of accessing and speaking with individuals, and respond to many of women's needs. From a research perspective, researchers who work with these service providers are more likely to be trusted by the women who are being asked to provide highly personal, often shameful, and sometimes dangerous details. For example, collaborating with a local nongovernmental organization (NGO) that offers psychological counseling may mean that interviews will be conducted by someone who is trusted by the woman, and who will

---

Box 7.1. Guiding principles for the ethical and safe conduct of interviews with women who have been trafficked

1. Do no harm.
2. Know your subject and assess the risks.
3. Prepare referral information; do not make promises that you cannot fulfill.
4. Adequately select and prepare interpreters and coworkers.
5. Ensure anonymity and confidentiality.
6. Get informed consent.
7. Listen to and respect each woman's assessment of her situation and risks to her safety.
8. Do not retraumatize a woman.
9. Be prepared for emergency intervention.
10. Put information collected to good use.

---

know how to ask sensitive questions and how to respond to emotional reactions. Not only is this an ethical approach, it is the one most likely to garner truthful and detailed responses.

For all members of a research team, it is helpful to keep in mind that fear is a defining element of the trafficking experience and the subsequent integration/reintegration period. In most cases, women who have been trafficked have an overwhelming, irrepressible feeling that they are not safe—even after they are out of the exploitative situation. Every attempt must be made to quell a woman's insecurity—both real and perceived. Standard considerations for privacy (i.e., a closed door) may not be enough. An overabundance of care for the physical setting and for the atmosphere of the encounter must be taken, because what an interviewer might believe is a private and safe environment may not be perceived this way by the woman. Researchers should explore with each woman what she needs to feel confident and to speak freely, in particular, if she is still under threat from traffickers. A change in the tone of women's responses during an interview, for example, may indicate that the woman no longer feels safe.

A second characteristic emotion felt by most women who have been trafficked is shame. For a researcher who is not sensitive to a woman's sense of humiliation, disclosure will be a problem. Equally, if an interviewer feels uncomfortable or embarrassed by a woman's report, this will negatively affect the interview and, more important, the woman's psychological state. Support workers assisting trafficked women explain the importance of being nonjudgmental, empathetic, and reassuring the woman that she is not to blame for what happened to her.

Ethical considerations may also be broader, less tangible, as in the application of concepts, such as gender. Campbell and Dienemann propose that by ignoring gender, the researcher risks adopting a "male perspective as normative," yet overemphasizing gender may condemn women to victimhood, overlooking their coping skills and resourcefulness (Campbell and Dienemann, 2001).

In the case of trafficking, one of the more common conceptual problems has been the neglect of the "demand" side of the equation. Although difficult to investigate, leaving out those who create the demand for trafficked labor promotes the impression that women are victims of a neutral and intangible marketplace and its consumers, and may relieve governments of their responsibility to eliminate these exploitative markets.

Carrying out research on sensitive topics places additional responsibilities on researchers, both in terms of the process of doing research, and the obligation to effectively and responsibly disseminate findings. In the public arena, ethically sensitive topics can have profound political, social, or policy implications. Study results must therefore be presented in ways that foster progressive policy discussions and avoid inflaming public discrimination, generating bias, or encouraging stereotypes (World Health Organization, 2001).

Ethical challenges can affect different stages of a study, from conceptualization of the subject, to the conduct of the interview, to the dissemination and reception of the findings. If unrecognized or unaddressed, these complications and dangers can render study results meaningless, or, worse, can leave individuals or groups exposed to harm. The potential for physical and psychological injury is not simply hyperbole, but a possibility associated with research on a subject involving illegal activities and tremendous profits, severe violence, such high-stakes politics, all centering on an extraordinarily vulnerable study population.

Research Tools: Do Suitable Instrument Exist to Measure the Physical and Mental Health of Women Who Have Been Chronically at Risk, Abused, and Traumatized?

An issue emerging from our current research on the self-reported health status of trafficked women in service settings is the degree to which standard research instruments that have been developed to document different aspects of health functioning and/or ill health or the impact of single traumatic events apply when trying to document women's physical and mental health needs (Zimmerman et al., forthcoming). Women who have been trafficked are, for the most part, individuals who have been exposed to extreme physical risks, sexual abuse, and/or psychological trauma sustained over an extended period. However, existing health survey tools are often designed to look at physical health in a general population, examine a specific health issue, or explore the aftermath of one traumatic episode (e.g., earthquake, rape). Moreover, from our search for tools to suit our study population, it appeared as if, to date, there are few tools designed to take a gendered approach to assessing the health of women who have been chronically or repeatedly violated physically, sexually, and psychologically, or to chronicle how their health status changes over time. For example, in our study, in which we were interviewing women who had recently emerged from a trafficking situation, questions from the Short Form Health Survey (SF) 36, a commonly used tool to assess health status, were not useful to understanding our population's health concerns. Questions such as: "During the past week, to what extent has your physical health or emotional problems interfered with your normal social activities with family friends, neighbors, or groups?"(Ware and Sherbourne, 1992) were mainly irrelevant to highly traumatized women residing in a shelter or single-resident secure housing.

Common indices for assessing physical health are generally based on the concept of "functioning," such as surveys based on the International Classification of Functioning, Disability and Health (ICF), and aimed to gather data on limitations in functional activities (seeing, hearing, communication, walking, and using stairs) and in activities of daily living (ADLs). For women who are either still in a trafficking setting or have recently emerged and are in a care setting, many of these questions are likely to be either irrelevant or uninformative (unless trying to compare them against the general population, or examining women who have been out of the trafficking situation for a longer time and have returned to their "normalized" lifestyle). These instruments may not reflect the nature of the harm, nor the specific health needs.

For mental health, epidemiological instruments for studying individuals who have been exposed to a single circumscribed event or war-related trauma (e.g., soldiers or refugees) are numerous (Derogatis et al., 1974; Mandoki-

Arata et al., 1991; El-Bassel et al., 1997). However, few of these instruments are specifically designed to take account of the features inherent in the type of gender-based abuse that aims to maintain a chronic state of fear and anxiety, and which usually does this in a highly intimate and personal way. The gender dimensions of trafficking in women underlie the type of abuses inflicted, the way they are carried out, and women's perceptions of and responses to them.

In our study we were also interested in looking at how women's health status, in particular, mental health, changed over time. We therefore designed an instrument that was modified to be implemented over three periods: within seven days after arrival at a service setting, and then two weeks and three months after the first interview to explore women's needs at a crisis intervention point, once their immediate needs have been met, and several months later, after they have had time to think about their future.

When exploring mental health, it is also important to be attentive to issues such as stigma, guilt, and shame. To approach these subjects, women in our study, were asked, for example: "Do you think being trafficked has changed the way you feel about yourself/the way others feel about you?" Qualitative questions such as these helped illuminate the impact of the experience on women's identity and self-perception, which were issues that were not brought up in the quantitative section. Many women in our study responded as L did: "It's changed dramatically. I cannot live as I lived before," or as P did: "I feel like I am not like any other human being—like I am useless; I feel ashamed" (Zimmerman et al., forthcoming).

Public Health Implications

The difficulty obtaining reliable information on trafficking makes it hard to assess how, in the broader sense, trafficking in women might be affecting public health. Although identifying specific implications of trafficking in women is problematic, trafficked women can be considered a subset of other marginalized populations, in particular, irregular migrants and sex workers—populations for whom the public health dimensions are better understood. The public health impact of human trafficking is likely to reflect many of the dimensions of irregular migration. The relationship between migration, epidemiological patterns, migrants' social context, and infectious diseases is well recognized (Dodson, 1998; Skeldon and Hsu, 2000; Caballero et al., 2002; Lurie, 2004; Physicians for Human Rights, 2004). Mobile populations may act as a primary source of change in regional prevalence rates, as individuals move between disparate epidemiological environments (Gushulak and MacPherson, 2004). Yet, to date, for trafficking in women a lack of specific data on whether they contribute to infectious disease prevalence in this same way remains. It thus is unclear, for example, in which contexts women might be contributing to certain epidemics (e.g., HIV), and in which contexts women instead become ill because they have been trafficked into populations where certain infectious diseases are epidemic or endemic. We can only infer women's risks and roles based on data from other migrant populations.

In terms of awareness of public health information, access to services, and responsiveness to treatment, trafficked women are situated at the extreme end of what might be termed a "vulnerability continuum." Women and girls who have been trafficked into sex work, or those who are subjected to sexual violence in other labor sectors (e.g., domestic servitude, factory or agricultural labor), rarely have control over their movement, the type of sexual encounter that takes place, or access to health information or services. For example, early data from our recent study indicate that 80 percent of the women interviewed reported having "never" been free to do what they wanted or go where they wanted, and nearly 70 percent said that they had never had a sexual health check while trafficked (Zimmerman et al., forthcoming). It is reasonable to speculate that trafficked persons will be even less able to access services than undocumented migrants or unbonded sex workers, both of whom already face significant barriers. This hidden and restricted existence has numerous implications for public health, and these require further examination. For example, trafficked persons are likely to be excluded from vaccination programs, disease surveillance, and outreach and awareness campaigns.

Even after escaping the trafficking situation, women may continue to have difficulty using medical services of any kind—because of financial constraints, stigma, or concerns over breaches of confidentiality—and they may continue to be excluded from public health programs, including maternal and child health campaigns. Like others who suffer from chronic trauma, without mental health support, a certain portion of women who are trafficked will struggle to participate in the economic sector, to care for their families, or to care for themselves. As such, it is worth contemplating the generational effects that might be associated with trafficking, as well.

The magnitude of the international pandemic cannot be overstated, and for numerous trafficked women HIV becomes an awful medical reality. Vulnerability to HIV/AIDS has been clearly associated with gender inequality and the types of human rights violations associated with trafficking in women, indicating that it should be part of any HIV/AIDS program (U.N. Development Program et al., 2005). Defining HIV as the central health concern of trafficking in women is misleading, however, and inappropriate for many reasons.

First, being trafficked, even into commercial sex, does not universally result in HIV infection. Although in some countries the number of trafficked women testing positive for HIV might be quite high (Beyrer, 2001), in other locations, assistance centers have thus far encountered relatively low rates of infection (Zimmerman et al., forthcoming). Trafficking assistance centers in Western and Eastern Europe, for example, report low numbers of women testing positive (London School of Hygiene and Tropical Medicine, 2005).

Second, research on health and trafficking should start from the premise that a trafficked woman's health status is complex and her chief concerns may not be the same as those of service providers or the medical establishments. Women in assistance programs usually have numerous health complications to address—many of which are more urgent than HIV testing. In addition to infections and injuries acquired during trafficking, women may present with pre-existing medical problems that have worsened over time; they may be pregnant; have severe headaches, dental pain, and likely require crisis counseling for profound anxiety and psychological distress (Zimmerman et al., 2003; Tudorache, 2004). In other words, a trafficked woman's health is more than the sum of her reproductive parts.

Third, and not least, to focus on HIV as the dominant issue in health and trafficking in women not so subtly implicates the women as "vectors" of disease. In fact, trafficked women are better viewed as the victims of those who use (abuse) their sexual services. An HIV focus may unwittingly create prejudices and stigmatize women who are trafficked. In many circumstances it is more justifiable to identify men who regularly purchase sex from trafficked women as the "high-risk" group that promotes infection transmission. Future research that highlights HIV should take care to put this subject in perspective.

Methodological Steps to Good-Quality Information

How can a researcher gather good-quality data on a population accompanied by so many political and social sensitivities, personal vulnerabilities, and practical hindrances, while upholding the highest ethical standards? As it turns out, overcoming barriers, avoiding political pitfalls, and acquiring good-quality data depend on prioritizing women's well-being. Following the guidance offered in the *WHO Ethical and Safety Recommendations* and placing women's safety first generally results in the most effective research techniques for each methodological stage of a study, including: (1) prestudy preparation; (2) selecting and accessing a study sample; (3) conducting fieldwork; (4) interpreting data; and (5) disseminating findings. In practice, prioritizing individual safety often translates to working with groups that are on the ground providing direct services to women who have been trafficked.

In the planning phase, it can be helpful to think about other marginalized groups that pose similar research challenges and sensitivities. Figure 7.4, which situates trafficked women at the center of spheres representing other similarly vulnerable populations, was drafted for the first study on health and trafficking (Zimmerman, 2003). Thinking about and reviewing available literature on migrant women, exploited women laborers, sex workers, and women experiencing sexual abuse and domestic violence, and victims of torture helped us anticipate many methodological challenges. Not surprisingly, gender underpins each of these categories.

During the preparation activities for a study on trafficking in women, a researcher should become informed about trafficking in general, and about the specific trafficking situation (i.e., for each woman) that will be investigated. This means learning about the broader international or theoretical picture and about the local context, the main actors, the government's public position and its actual stance, and the unwritten rules (e.g., realities about contacting women, how authorities view and treat them, etc.). Knowing the local context is vital, as trafficking from Vietnam to Cambodia is not the same as trafficking from Lithuania to the United Kingdom, Mali to the Ivory Coast, or from Mexico to the United States. In some locations, such as Cambodia, trafficking into prostitution is visible and, an unspoken, yet recognized part of the local fabric. By contrast Lithuanian women trafficked to the United Kingdom are hidden and menaced.

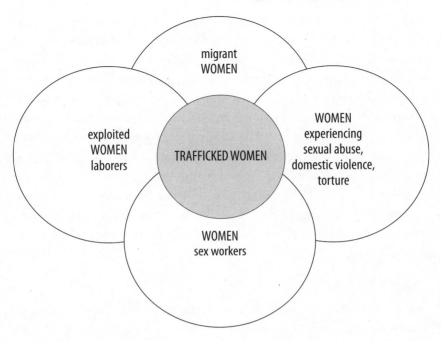

Figure 7.4. Spheres of marginalization and vulnerability

Selecting and accessing women is the stage that requires some of the most serious thought and planning. Gaining access is ordinarily not a simple matter of approaching a woman with a form that explains the purpose for the study, outlines any possible side effects, and requests her signature approving her participation. Selecting and recruiting women for a study on trafficking has significant implications for both the researcher and the women. This is why it is beneficial to collaborate with groups who are familiar with the local scene and understand which women can be approached, know how to contact a woman, ask for an interview, and can detect when situations become in any way detrimental to the woman or the researcher, and know how to react.

The same is true for the fieldwork. Organizations who have worked with trafficked women have the knowledge to help develop interview questions that are relevant and meaningful and to avoid poorly phrased questions. They are able to compose introductions and closing statements that address key issues in ways that will be understood and well received. Perhaps most important, working with service providers ensures that resources and experienced personnel are available to respond to women's needs. Trained service personnel are also likely to collect the most reliable data because they communicate in nonjudgmental and emphatic ways and are trusted by the women to maintain confidentiality. Whether collaborating with a service group or not, it is important that at the conclusion of an interview women are not left feeling "used" and alone, but understand that support is available to them even after the encounter, either directly with the organization conducting the interview or through referral information provided by the interviewer.

Interpreting data is when all the good work can come together into meaningful findings, or may fall apart if data are not correctly understood within the cultural and local context, and placed within the prevailing social and political climate.

Looking Ahead

The inequities of poverty, unemployment, the societal subordination of women, and the corruption and lax law enforcement that underpin the trafficking problem are not going away any time soon. For these same reasons, the work of being an investigator in this context is sometimes dangerous and almost always emotionally demanding. Trafficking is a complex problem that requires sensitive and well-planned investigation. Quantitative and qualitative research on trafficking in women is fundamentally about investigating extraordinarily vulnerable and marginalized members of society. This is an important area of research, but as discussed above, it is an area that requires caution both during the research and with the findings. Additional resources, energy, and a commitment to effective collaboration are needed to ensure that any research involving women who have been trafficked is conducted in an ethically sound manner that prioritizes women's safety and well-being.

Though the process of documenting the health impacts of trafficking is young, there are some near-term needs we can point to and evidence-based information that is urgently required to inform the development of prevention efforts and support services. Needed is better information on the following: the specific and broader health service requirements of women who have been trafficked; how health care providers can effectively respond while women are in a trafficking situation and once they have left; the micro and macro level factors that fuel the trafficking process; potential individual and governmental intervention options; and a systematic examination of strategies to work across sectors and across international boundaries. We must expand the sample size of future research projects and conduct rigorous studies in Asia, Africa, Latin America, and the Middle East where populations are difficult to access and law enforcement is often ineffective. Our initial work relied heavily on women's self-reporting in structured qualitative interviews, and our second study gathered quantitative data on health effects based on women's perceptions. A next step is to collect quantitative data based on medical histories, physical examinations, laboratory testing, psychological testing, and the results of treatment. Long-term follow-up of subjects is extraordinarily difficult, but much needed.

In addition, extremely little work has been carried out on those who create the demand for exploited labor (Anderson and O'Connell-Davidson, 2001, 2002). Those who purchase the sexual services of trafficked women and girls and those who exploit their labor in factories, farms, or domestic services are rarely a subject of systematic investigation. Although this is an area that poses profound challenges for research, because of the causal role demand plays in trafficking, it is one in which dedicated inquiry can have influential consequences. Moreover, as previously noted, ignoring those who foster the demand for trafficked labor is to create the impression that women are laborers in an invisible marketplace. This has the potential of relieving governments of their responsibility to deal with the abuses committed by those who knowingly consume exploited labor.

The physical and psychological harm caused to an individual woman's health is one of the primary reasons why trafficking is denounced as a serious human rights violation. Health should therefore be considered central to any discussion about trafficking, and should not be sidelined by the health community. Although health and trafficking in women is not an uncomplicated field of study, because the subject is so emotive and highly political, accurate and specific evidence-based information is all the more valuable. Findings grounded in well-designed studies can foster effective interventions that are instituted at a structural level, and improve targeted assistance for individual women, who can sometimes get lost or stereotyped amid the rhetoric and politics.

Notes

1. This stage is of particular relevance for international trafficking, where women are frequently detained or asked to participate in a criminal proceeding. Criminal proceedings also occur in cases of internal trafficking, but it is much less common.

References

American Medical Association (AMA). 1999. *Cultural Competence Compendium.* Chicago: AMA.

Amin, A. 2004. *Risk, morality, and blame: a critical analysis of government and U.S. donor responses to HIV infections among sex workers in India.* Takoma Park, MD: Center for Health and Gender Equity.

Amnesty International. 2001. *Broken bodies, shattered minds: Torture and ill-treatment of women.* London: Amnesty International.

Anderson, B. 1993. *Britain's secret slaves.* London: Anti-Slavery International and Kalyann.

Anderson, B., and O'Connell-Davidson, J. 2001. The demand side of trafficking. A multi-country pilot study. Part 2. (draft) www.childtrafficking.com/ (accessed November 18, 2005).

Anderson, B., and O'Connell-Davidson, J. 2002. *Trafficking: A demand led problem?* Part I: *Review of evidence and debates.* Stockholm: Save the Children.

Asia Watch-Women's Rights Project. 1993. A modern form of slavery. *Trafficking of Burmese women and girls into brothels in Thailand.* New York: Human Rights Watch.

Beyrer, C. 2001. Shan women and girls in the sex industry in Southeast Asia: Political causes and human rights implications. *Social Science and Medicine* 53:543–50.

Bindman, J., and Doezema, J. 1997. *Redefining prostitution as sex work on the international agenda.* London: Anti-Slavery International and the Network of Sex Work Projects.

Brennan, D. 2005. Methodological challenges in research with trafficked persons: Tales from the field. In *Data and research on human trafficking: A global survey,* ed. F. Laczko and E. Gozdziak. Geneva: International Organization for Migration.

Busza, J., Castle, S., et al. 2004. Trafficking and health. *British Medical Journal* 328:1369–71.

Caballero, M., Dreser, A., et al. 2002. Migration, gender and HIV/AIDS in Central America and Mexico. Cuernavaca, Mexico: Center for Health Systems Research, National Institute for Public Health.

Campbell, J. C., and Dienemann, D. D. 2001. Ethical issues in research on violence against women. In *Sourcebook on violence against women,* ed. C. M. Renzetti, J. L. Edleson, and R. K. Bergen. Thousand Oaks, CA: Sage Publications.

Council for International Organizations of Medical Sciences (CIOMS). 1993. *International ethical guidelines for biomedical research involving human subjects,* ed. Z. Bankowski. Geneva: CIOMS.

Cowan, R. 2005. Migrant women forced into cheap sex trade. *The Guardian.* London. http://www.guardian.co.uk

Cox, R. 1999. The role of ethnicity in shaping the domestic employment sector in Britain. *Gender, migration and domestic service,* ed. J. H. Momsen. London: Routledge.

Davies, J. 2002. *The role of migration policy in creating and sustaining trafficking harm.* Sussex: Migration Research Centre, University of Sussex.

Derks, A. 1997. *Trafficking of Cambodian women and children to Thailand.* Phnom Penh: International Organization for Migration / Center for Advanced Study.

Derogatis, L., Lipman, R., et al. 1974. The Hopkins symptom checklist (HSCL): A self-report symptom inventory. *Behavioral Science* 19 (1):1–15.

Dickson, S. 2004. *When women are trafficked: Quantifying the gendered experience of trafficking in the UK.* London: Poppy Project, Eaves Housing.

Ditmore, M. 2003. Morality in new policies addressing trafficking and sex work. Paper presented at "Women working to make a difference" Institute for Women's Policy Research.

Ditmore, M. 2005. Sex work and law enforcement. *Research for Sex Work* (8):1–17.

Dodson, B. 1998. Women on the move: Gender and cross-border migration to South Africa. Migration Policy Series No. 9. Cape Town: South African Migration Project.

El-Bassel, N., Schilling, R.F., et al. 1997. Sex trading and psychological distress among women recruited from the streets of Harlem. *American Journal of Public Health* 87 (1):66–70.

European Council on Refugees and Exiles (ECRE). 1999. *Good practice guide on the integration of refugees in the European Union.* Geneva: ECRE.

Feuk, R. 2003. ODIHR CPRSI assessment trip to Albania on trafficking in children from Roma and Egyptian communities. Vienna, Austria: Organization for Security and Co-operation in Europe (OSCE) Office for Democratic Institutions and Human Rights.

Fortune, M. 2001. Religious issues and violence against women. In *Sourcebook on violence against women,* ed. C. M. Renzetti, J. L. Edleson, and R. K. Bergen. Thousand Oaks, CA: Sage Publications.

Gallagher, A. 2002. Trafficking, smuggling and human rights: tricks and treaties. *Forced Migration Review* 12:25–28.

Graycar, A. 1999. *Trafficking in human beings.* Paper presented at the International Conference on Migration, Culture and Crime, Israel, July 5–8.

Gushulak, B., and MacPherson, D. W. 2004. Globalization of infectious diseases: The impact of migration. *Clinical Infectious Disease* 11 (3):171–74.

Gushulak, B. D., and MacPherson, D. 2000. Health issues associated with the smuggling and trafficking of migrants. *Journal of Immigrant Health* 2:67–78.

Heise, L. 1994. Violence against women: The hidden health burden. World Bank Discussion Papers 255. Washington, DC: World Bank.

Heise, L. 1998. Violence against women: An integrated ecological framework. *Violence against Women* 4:262–90.

Henry Kaiser Family Foundation. (February 8, 2005). Bush administration to require U.S. AIDS groups take pledge opposing commercial sex work to gain funding. Menlo Park, CA: The Henry Kaiser Family Foundation: kaisernetwork.org.

Herlihy, J., Scragg, P., et al. 2002. Discrepancies in autobiographical memories: Implications for the assessment of asylum seekers: Repeated interviews study. *British Medical Journal* 324 (9 February):324–27.

Hughes, D., and Roche, C. 1999. Making the harm visible. Amherst, MA: The Coalition against Trafficking in Women.

Huisman, K. A. 1997. Studying violence against women of color. In *Researching sexual violence against women. Methodological and personal perspectives,* ed. M. D. Schwartz. Thousand Oaks, CA: Sage Publications.

Human Rights Watch. 2001. *Hidden in the home.* New York: Human Rights Watch.

Human Rights Watch Asia. 1995. *Rape for profit: Trafficking of Nepali girls and women to India's brothels.* New York: Human Rights Watch.

International Labor Organization (ILO). 2005. *A global alliance against forced labor.* Geneva: ILO.

International Organization for Migration (IOM). 1999. *Paths of exploitation. Studies on the trafficking of women and children between Cambodia, Thailand and Vietnam.* Geneva: IOM.

International Organization for Migration (IOM). 2003. World migration, 2003. *Managing migration. Challenges and responses for people on the move.* Geneva: IOM.

International Organization for Migration (IOM). 2004. Psychosocial support to groups of victims of human trafficking in transit situations. *Psychosocial Notebook* 4 (February):1–115.

Laczko, F., and Gozdziak, E. E. 2005. *Data and research on human trafficking: A global survey.* Geneva: IOM.

Laczko, F., and Gramegna, M. 2003. Developing better indicators of human trafficking. *Brown Journal of World Affairs* 10 (1):179–94.

La Strada Ukraine. 2002. Final workshop: Responding to the health needs of trafficked women, 28–30 November, London.

Loff, B., and Sanghera, J. 2003. Distortions and difficulties in data for trafficking. *The Lancet* 363:9408.

London School of Hygiene and Tropical Medicine. 2005. Meeting report for multi-country study on health of trafficked women in service settings, 13–15 November (draft). London: London School of Hygiene and Tropical Medicine.

Lurie, M. N. 2004. Migration, sexuality, and the spread of HIV/AIDS in rural South Africa. Migration Policy Series, No. 31. Cape Town: Southern African Migration Project.

Mandoki-Arata, C., Saunders, B. E., et al. 1991. Concurrent validity of a crime-related post traumatic stress disorder scale for women within the symptom checklist-90-revised. *Violence and Victims* 6 (3):191–99.

Miko, F. T., and Park, G. J.-H. 2002. Trafficking in women and children: The U.S. and international response. Washington, DC: Congressional Research Service/The Library of Congress-CRS Report for Congress.

Morrison, J., and Crosland, B. 2000. The trafficking and smuggling of refugees: The end game in European Policy? Geneva: U.N. High Commission for Refugees.

Murphy, E., and Ringheim, K. 2002. An interview with Jo Doezema, of the Network of Sex Work Projects: Does attention to trafficking adversely affect sex workers'

rights?. *Reproductive Health and Rights—Reaching the Hardly Reached.* http://path
.org/publications/pub.php?id=505.

Neuman, W. L. 1991. *Social research methods: Qualitative and quantitative approaches.*
New York: Simon & Schuster.

Pearson, E. 2002. *Human traffic, human rights: Redefining victim protection.* London:
Anti-Slavery International.

Phongpaichit, P., Piriyarangsan, S., et al. 1998. *Guns, girls, gambling, ganja. Thailand's illegal economy and public policy.* Bangkok: Silkworm Books.

Physicians for Human Rights, USA. 2004. No status: Migration, trafficking and exploitation of women in Thailand. Health and HIV/AIDS risks for Burmese and hill
tribe women and girls. Boston: Physicians for Human Rights.

Renzetti, C. M., and Lee, R. M., eds. 1993. Overview and introduction. *Researching
sensitive topics.* Newbury Park, CA: Sage Publications.

Salt, J., and Stein, J. 1997. Migration as a business: The case of trafficking. *International Migration* 35 (4):467–91.

Sanghera, J. 1997. In the belly of the beast: Sex trade, prostitution and globalization. *Moving the whore stigma: Report on the Asia and Pacific regional consultation on
prostitution.* Global Alliance against Traffick in Women/Foundation for Women,
17–18 February.

Schloenhardt, A. 1999. The business of migration: organized crime and illegal
migration in Australia and the Asia Pacific Region. *Adelaide Law Review* 21 (1):
96–97.

Seale, C. 1998. *Researching society and culture.* Thousand Oaks, CA: Sage Publications.

Sieber, J. E., and Stanley, L. J. 1998. Ethical and professional dimensions of socially
sensitive research. *American Psychologist* 43:49–55.

Skeldon, R. 2000. Trafficking: A perspective from Asia. *Perspectives on Trafficking of
Migrants* 38 (3-Special Issue 1/2000):7–28.

Skeldon, R., and Hsu, L. 2000. *Population mobility and HIV vulnerability in South East
Asia: An assessment and analysis.* Bangkok: U.N. Development Programme.

Skrobanek, S., Boonpakdi, N., et al. 1997. *The traffic in Women: Human realities of the
international sex trade.* Bangkok: Foundation for Women.

Specter, M. 1998. Contraband women—a special report. Traffickers' new cargo: Na-
ive slavic women. *New York Times.*

Tchomarova, M. 2001. Trafficking in women: Personal, psychological and social
problems in (non)-united Europe. *Trafficking in women.* Sofia, Bulgaria: Animus
Association Foundation, Strada.

Tudorache, D. 2004. General consideration on the psychological aspects of the trafficking phenomenon. *Psychosocial support to groups of victims of human trafficking
in transit situations,* ed. G. Schinina. Geneva: International Organization for Migration. *Psychosocial Notebook,* vol. 4, February.

U.S. Department of State. 2003. Trafficking in Persons Report. Washington, D.C.:
U.S. Department of State.

United Nations. 2000. United Nations Protocol to Prevent, Suppress, and Punish
Trafficking in persons, especially women and children, supplementing the United

Nations Convention against Transnational Organized Crime. G.A. res. 55/25, annex II, 55 U.N. GAOR Supp. (No. 49) at 60, U.N. Doc. A/45/49 (Vol. I).

United Nations Development Program, Office of the United Nations High Commissioner for Refugees, et al. 2005. High-level meeting on HIV/AIDS. Follow-up to the outcome of the twenty-sixth special session: Implementation of the Declaration of Commitment on HIV/AIDS. Geneva: United Nations. A/59/CRP.3.

United Nations Economic and Social Council. 2004. Integration of the human rights of women and the gender perspective. Report of the Special Rapporteur on trafficking in persons, especially women and children. GE.04-16928 (E) 040205. Geneva: United Nations Economic and Social Council.

United Nations High Commissioner for Human Rights. 2001. Traffic in women and girls Commission on Human Rights. Resolution 2001/48.

United Nations High Commissioner for Human Rights. 2002. Principles and Guidelines on Human Rights and Trafficking. Geneva: United Nations High Commissioner for Human Rights.

U.S. Department of State. June 2005. Trafficking in persons report. Washington, DC: U.S. Department of State.

Ware, J. J., and Sherbourne, C. D. 1992. The MOS 36 Item Short Form Health Survey (SF-36). Conceptual framework and item selection. *Medical Care* 30:473–83.

Wijers, M., and Lap-Chew, L. 1999. *Trafficking in women, forced labor and slavery-like practices in marriage, domestic labor and prostitution.* Utrecht: Foundation against Trafficking in Women, Global Alliance against Traffic in Women.

World Health Organization (WHO). 2001. *Putting women first: Ethical and safety recommendations for research on domestic violence against women.* Geneva: World Health Organization Department of Gender and Women's Health (WHO/FCH/GWH/01.1).

Zimmerman, C. 2003. Trafficking in women: a qualitative study to conceptualise and map health risks. Doctoral thesis draft. Health Policy Unit. London: London School of Hygiene and Tropical Medicine.

Zimmerman, C., Hossain, M., et al. Forthcoming. *The physical and mental health status of trafficked women in seven service settings in Europe.* London: London School of Hygiene and Tropical Medicine/European Commission.

Zimmerman, C., and Watts, C. 2003. *WHO ethical and safety recommendations for interviewing trafficked women.* London: London School of Hygiene and Tropical Medicine/World Health Organization.

Zimmerman, C., Yun, K., et al. 2003. *The health risks and consequences of trafficking in women and adolescents. Findings from a European study.* London: London School of Hygiene and Tropical Medicine, European Commission.

8

Documenting Sexual Violence among Internally Displaced Women

Sierra Leone

Chen Reis, J.D., M.P.H.

At the request of the U.N. Mission in Sierra Leone, in early 2001, Physicians for Human Rights (PHR) conducted a population-based assessment of the prevalence and effects of sexual violence and other human rights abuses perpetrated against internally displaced persons (IDPs) in Sierra Leone. At the time of our study, Sierra Leone had been embroiled in a devastating ten-year-long civil war. The international press and various nongovernmental relief organizations had reported on widespread violence and human rights violations against the civilian population, but there had been no rigorous population-based investigation to document prevalence and downstream health effects. In highlighting horrific individual cases, the press reports pointed to a deliberate policy on the part of combatants designed to intimidate and brutalize noncombatants. By the time PHR went to Sierra Leone, we were aware of an extraordinary pattern of brutal human rights abuses, such as summary killings, sexual violence against women and girls, abductions, amputations, and the forced conscription of children soldiers. We also were aware that our work in Sierra Leone had context and use beyond the conflict in West Africa and Sierra Leone. Throughout the 1990s, world attention had been focused on the use of rape and sexual violence against women and girls as part of the ethnic cleansing campaigns in the breakup of the former Yugoslavia and in the Rwandan genocide.

PHR is a nongovernmental organization (NGO) based in the United States, and its findings and recommendations from the work in Sierra Leone may be found in the report *War-Related Sexual Violence in Sierra Leone: A Population-Based Assessment* and elsewhere (www.phrusa.org/publications/sl_report .html; Amowitz et al., 2002). This chapter focuses on PHR's study methodologies and how they may be adapted to other settings of civil conflict. Its purpose is to focus on how researchers obtain valid and reliable population data in the challenging context of civil conflict with a special emphasis on how to assess the health effects of human rights violations perpetrated against girls and women. For the purposes of this chapter and PHR's study approach, human rights abuses include the array of violence that occurs during civil strife, as well as the negligent and complicit behavior of government that permits it to occur, and societal conditions that subordinate women and further permit violence and abuse. PHR is a pioneer in the use of a study methodology we call "triangulation research," which incorporates collecting qualitative and quantitative data with the relating of true human stories amassed in the data-collection process, to provide a complete and compelling picture of rights violations and their effects on populations. This chapter focuses on how we did this in Sierra Leone.

Context

Slightly smaller than the U.S. state of South Carolina, the West African country of Sierra Leone gained independence from the United Kingdom in April 1961 (Figure 8.1). The population is estimated at approximately 6 million, of which 60 percent are Muslim, 30 percent follow indigenous beliefs, and 10 percent are Christian. Sierra Leone's climate is largely tropical with a hot and humid rainy season that lasts from May to December and a dry winter season from December to April. Sierra Leone, one of the poorest nations in the world, is caught in a vicious circle of economic and political disarray. The central government is weak, and corruption and malfeasance are rampant.

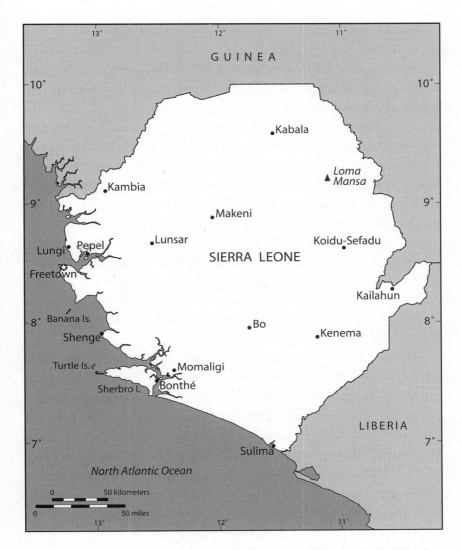

Figure 8.1. Sierra Leone. After map from the University of Texas at Austin Libraries, Perry-Castañeda Library Map Collection (available at www.lib.utexas.edu/maps/ cia05/sierra_leone_sm05.gif)

Political instability, inadequate infrastructure, and crime inhibit the inflow of foreign capital.

Sierra Leone's public health system also is extremely weak. In 1999 only 34 percent of the population had access to safe drinking water and only 11 percent had adequate sanitation (U.N. Children's Fund [UNICEF], 1999). The risk of acquiring bacterial and protozoan waterborne agents that cause diarrhea, as well as hepatitis A and typhoid fever, is high and widespread across the country. There also is malaria and yellow fever, as well as schistosomiasis and Lassa fever. Sierra Leone may have the highest infant (316/1000) and child (182/1000) mortality rates and the lowest life expectancy at birth (estimates vary between 38 and 44 years) in the world (www.cia.gov; UNICEF, 1999). The capacity to track the health of the population with epidemiological research is as poor as the overall health delivery system, so these figures are gross estimates. The ten-year civil war exacerbated the already bleak situation for tracking the health of Sierra Leoneans, similar to that discussed by Beyrer et al., as a result of the civil conflict in the Democratic Republic of Congo.

Though Sierra Leone has significant mineral resources, including diamonds, its people are some of the poorest in the world. The per capita income is estimated at about 600 U.S. dollars a year. Explosive population growth is certainly a factor. The average birth rate is estimated to be 5.72 children per woman. The population is young and growing fast, but there is almost no viable economic infrastructure to provide jobs to handle the influx of young, new workers. About two-thirds of the working age population is engaged in subsistence agriculture. While there are no accurate numbers for the unemployment rate, it is estimated that more than two-thirds of the population lives in poverty. Meanwhile the gap between poor and rich is staggering. According to one 1999 estimate, 0.5 percent of the nation's wealth is in the hands of the lowest 10 percent of the population, while the highest 10 percent controls 43.6 percent of the wealth. Even for people who are able to obtain an education, economic opportunities are extremely limited. Currently many of Sierra Leone's limited economic activities are degrading the environment through overharvesting timber and fish, extensive cattle grazing, and slash-and-burn agriculture that takes a toll on the land. The country's bauxite and rutile mines shut down during the civil war and have not reopened because political instability and inferior infrastructure are major impediments to foreign investment. Diamond mining is the major source of hard currency and illicit trade in diamonds has fueled the civil conflict.

Violence and political instability in Sierra Leone have been part of a wider regional problem in West Africa that includes Cote d'Ivoire, Guinea, and Liberia. Rebel groups are fluid across poorly controlled borders. They have a history of taking over geographic areas and then engaging in insurgencies and crime, smuggling, looting, arms trafficking, and violence, all with little regard to recognized international boundaries. Violence in one West African nation has frequently spilled over into another and cross-border infiltration has not been limited to armed rebel groups. In an attempt to control the violence, instability, and human rights catastrophe, since 1999 the United Nations has maintained more than 4,000 peacekeepers in Sierra Leone. This has not been the only time when international peacekeepers have had to step in to control violence in West Africa (Box 8.1).

Mass displacement also was a defining characteristic of the Sierra Leone crisis. More than 3,000 communities were destroyed (U.N. Office for the Coordination of Humanitarian Affairs [UNOCHA], 2000), and nearly half the country's population had to flee their homes. Many were displaced more than once. Approximately 400,000 people fled Sierra Leone into neighboring Guinea and Liberia (UNOCHA, 2001). By early 2002, the humanitarian community reported more than 400,000 cases of IDPs, which likely represented a fraction of the total (Pratt, 2001). More than half of the IDPs were estimated to be women and girls (UNOCHA, 2001).

In July 1999 the Lome Peace Accord was signed in hopes of ending the civil war that had killed an estimated 50,000 people, displaced an estimated 1 million, and made many thousands victims of mutilations and sexual violence. One militia in the Sierra Leonean conflict, the Revolutionary United Front (RUF), is often cited as the perpetrator of most of the cases of murder, rape, and mutilation in Sierra Leone (USCR, 2001). In addition to the sexual violence, which was the focus of PHR's research, the rebels cut off limbs and murdered people as popular methods of torture and intimidation. The Lome Peace Accord came in the form of a power-sharing arrangement between President Ahmad Tejan Kabbah, first elected in 1996, and rebel leaders who were granted cabinet posts.

In this context, a team of PHR researchers went to Sierra Leone with a goal of producing a reliable, scientific population-based assessment with

Box 8.1. Human rights timeline: Sierra Leone

1961	Sierra Leone gains independence from the United Kingdom.
1991	Civil war erupts in Sierra Leone when the Revolutionary United Front (RUF) attempts armed overthrow of the government. Over a ten-year period, tens of thousands will die and more than 2 million (about one-third of the population) will be displaced.
1996	Parliamentary and presidential elections are held; Dr. Ahmad Tejan Kabbah declared winner.
1997	A military coup negates a brokered peace agreement called the Abidjan Accord; the army and RUF form a ruling military junta. President Kabbah and his government go into exile.
1998	In February, ECOMOG forces, regional peacekeeping forces of the Economic Community of West African States, drive the RUF out of Freetown and reinstate President Kabbah. In June, the U.N. Security Council establishes an unarmed U.N. Observer Mission in Sierra Leone (UNOMSIL), which, under the protection of ECOMOG, documents and reports ongoing atrocities and human rights abuses against civilians. Fighting continues and rebel groups take control of half the country. UNOMSIL personnel are evacuated.
1999	On July 7, the government and rebels sign the Lome Peace Accord, providing for power sharing between President Ahmad Tejan Kabbah and rebel leaders who received cabinet posts. On August 20, the United Nations authorizes an increase in military observers to 210. In October, the United Nations terminates UNOMSIL and establishes UNAMSIL, a new and much larger mission. Médecins sans Frontières conducts health survey and estimates 14 percent of Freetown residents witnessed rape and war-related sexual assault.
1999–2000	Physicians for Human Rights (PHR) begins to plan research; the goal is to document the incidence and effects of conflict-related sexual violence against girls and women.
2000	Adoption of the Truth and Reconciliation Commission Act, which includes paying "special attention to the subject of sexual abuses."
2001	PHR conducts its population-based assessment of the prevalence and effects of sexual violence and other human rights abuses perpetrated against internally displaced persons in Sierra Leone.
2002	The war is declared over. The agreement establishing the Special Court for Sierra Leone is signed. PHR publishes a report of its research findings and releases findings in Sierra Leone. PHR meets with the Special Court and Truth and Reconciliation Commission to ensure that appropriate procedures, processes, and staff are in place to support and protect victims and witnesses, and it advocates for additional resources to assist survivors.

an emphasis on documenting the health effects of persistent human rights abuses. PHR and the international community were aware of the importance of documenting the nature and extent of the human rights abuses as an essential part of informing regional policy decisions, guiding humanitarian relief efforts, planning treatment and prevention programs for the survivors, and holding perpetrators accountable for their actions (Iacopino et al., 2001; PHR, 2001).

Planning the Research

Sexual violence has been common in armed conflicts throughout human history and across civilizations (PHR, 2002). Until recently the international community paid relatively little attention to documenting rigorously the effects on health of sexual violence during conflicts on populations, so that the relative paucity of information about its prevalence made it difficult to identify strategies for preventing sexual violence in crisis settings or addressing its consequences (Swiss and Giller, 1993). During the 1990s the view of the world community changed, in part, because of widespread media reports of rape and sexual violence being used as a tool in the civil conflict in the former Yugoslavia. It is likely that the historical lack of documentation about rape and sexual violence as a deliberate strategy in conflict has been due to the subordinate position of women in societies and the social stigma associated with rape and sexual violence. PHR knew it had to take these factors into account in planning its research work in Sierra Leone, a society in which most women live in a subordinate status to men.

In addition to the population sampling and data-collection methods described below, PHR knew it would need to record the stories of survivors. These anecdotes would give a human face to the trauma that the women experienced. The stories we heard were horrendous and shocking. One was from Isata,[1] a Sierra Leonean teenager who told us she had been brutally raped in front of her family. Before the assault, she was a virgin. Isata's attackers said to her parents, "Come and see how we use your children." This suggested that rape was used as a means to intimidate and brutalize the noncombatant population. Isata said, "They undressed five of us, laid us down, used us in front of my family and took us away with them. . . . When I escaped I couldn't walk— the pain. I was bleeding from my vagina. . . . Since I got back I have been so sick. I never used to get sick like this . . . I would like to go back to school but I can't concentrate anymore. I can't do anything." Here also was an indication of health effects (PHR, 2002).

In formulating the research plan, PHR realized that traditional research techniques, including even those used by traditional human rights investigators, would have to be adapted to the context of women's subordination and the social stigma associated with sexual violence in a society like that of Sierra Leone. Confidentiality arrangements would have to provide for the anonymity and protection of respondents. Further, the qualitative assessments used by human rights researchers usually involve nonprobability sampling for gathering testimonies. This can produce inaccuracies due to inherent bias, in particular, that the individuals interviewed are self-selected so as to identify themselves to receive assistance and may be those who have experienced the worst cases of abuse.

To avoid these biases, PHR employed the quantitative methods used in much public health research, in particular, the population-based survey to establish prevalence. As mentioned already, we also knew that presenting quantitative findings alone could appear to dehumanize events and thereby reduce their impact. Additionally, a structured survey questionnaire could not capture the full range of experiences that individual women may have had. Therefore, PHR developed a research strategy to link the qualitative (focused interviews) and quantitative methodologies with stories obtained in an open-ended interview. This research strategy enabled PHR to present our findings in a way that could be reliably generalized to a larger population, which we knew to be important for informing policies and programs, while retaining the multifaceted and compelling human face that is often better empathized with by leaders, journalists, and the general public.

Defining the Research Question

The first step to conducting a study is to identify and define the research question. This will determine the focus for the investigation and determine what methodologies should be employed. One key research objective for the Sierra Leone study was to determine the prevalence of war related sexual violence. PHR decided to use a population-based survey where parameters such as averages, rates, and proportions are compiled. We wanted to obtain the prevalence of experiences within the at-risk population rather than just the experiences of individuals (Coggon et al., 1997; Schoenbach and Rosamond, 2000).

Sampling Technique

At the time Physicians for Human Rights conducted this study, registered IDPs were living in a total of 21 camps or locales in seven districts and the western area of Sierra Leone. To obtain a representative sample of IDPs, we selected camps and/or locales on the basis of IDP arrival time and place of residence before displacement. Four districts were excluded because of safety and accessibility, or because the number of IDPs was small. The remaining four districts from which camps and locales were sampled housed 91 percent of the registered IDP population in Sierra Leone.

To have confidence that the sample included in the study was representative of the population to which the findings are generalized, we needed to estimate the expected prevalence of war-related sexual assaults. Using a previous survey-based estimate by Médecins sans Frontières (MSF) of 14 percent of Freetown residents witnessing rape in 1999, which was the best available data at the time (de Jong et al., 2000), we assumed a prevalence of war-related sexual assault between 10 and 20 percent. We then calculated it would be necessary to reach approximately 1,000 households to obtain a sample size sufficient to obtain reliable estimates of the prevalence of assaults. Households were then selected in each camp and/or locale in proportion to the distribution of IDPs in that location. A total of 1,048 households were selected from three camps and one town (Mile 91 Township). We obtained detailed existing maps of our sites from other NGOs, including those involved in camp management and water and sanitation, and in one case, we used a detailed map of each dwelling in the location that had been developed a few months before our study to help aid workers working with MSF to trace the spread of an infectious disease through the community. All study participants were selected using systematic random sampling or a combination of systematic random sampling and cluster sampling (Patton, 1990). Using the detailed map of a site showing the dwelling units (our sampling frame) and the number of interviews to be done in that location, we determined the sampling frequency. Each researcher was assigned a sector and instructed to approach every "*n*th" dwelling in their cluster starting with a randomly selected dwelling. In one location it was not possible to use this technique. The camp had been in existence since the start of the conflict and had grown haphazardly throughout the conflict, so that each influx of IDPs required establishing dwellings where space was available. In some cases, additions were built onto existing structures that were housing other families. Because of this, no accurate map of the dwellings in the camp existed and the camp was too large for us to map by alternative methods in the time we had available. We used cluster sampling at this location. The camp was divided into several administrative sections that were approximately equal in size. We determined from camp management and a review of the population registers that there was no significant difference between these sections in terms of place of origin or date of arrival of inhabitants and we randomly selected two sections (or clusters) in which to conduct the research. Within each of these clusters, we used systematic random sampling.

Developing the Study Instruments

PHR's survey contained 49 questions pertaining to demographics (age, sex, marital status, socioeconomic status, etc.), physical and mental health perception, experiences of war-related human rights abuses among household members, experiences of war-related sexual assault, assistance needs, opinions regarding punishment and justice for perpetrators, and attitudes on women's human rights and roles in society. The survey also assessed the lifetime prevalence of non-war-related sexual assault to highlight the importance of recognizing that sexual violence is not only a war-time phenomenon. The survey is available on PHR's website: www.phrusa.org/research/sierra _leone/pdf_files/08_appendixA.pdf.

To assess the prevalence of human rights abuses, we asked all women and girl respondents whether they or their household members had been beaten, shot, killed, tortured, seriously injured, sexually assaulted, raped, abducted, had amputations, or been subjected to forced labor by combatants during the 10 years since the start of the civil war. Respondents also were asked if their homes were burned and/or their property was looted. For each abuse, participants were asked to specify the sex of the abused person, the type of abuse, who they thought committed the violation, and the consequences of the abuse. Finally, all participants were asked about non-war-related sexual assault experiences in their lifetime committed by noncombatants, such as family members, friends, or civilian strangers, including age at assault, type of sexual assault, and identity of the perpetrators.

To assess the prevalence of war-related sexual assault experiences during the prior 10 years of war, we asked respondents when the incident occurred, where it took place, the type or nature of sexual abuse, the identity of the perpetrator, the number of attackers, the duration of the assault, and the consequences of the sexual assault. In addition, these women were asked their opinions regarding the punishment of perpetrators, and whether they were willing to give their name to the proposed Special Court or the Truth and Reconciliation Commission.

The survey concluded with open-ended questions for those respondents who reported war-related sexual violence to provide more details about their experiences and additional information about their health, their future, and other concerns. All participants were also encouraged to provide additional comments at the end of the interview.

The questionnaire was written in English, the official language of Sierra Leone, then translated into Krio, the nation's lingua franca, and then back-translated into English by someone not otherwise associated with the study. The questionnaire was developed by a team, which included Sierra Leonean women who conducted research in this area and who had experience providing treatment services to survivors of sexual assault in Sierra Leone. It was reviewed by seven regional human rights and sexual violence experts for content validity and was submitted to an ethics review. To ensure that the questions were clear and appropriate, the survey instrument was pilot tested among 12 IDP women in Freetown. Furthermore, input was sought from the locally recruited researchers, and their suggestions for clarity and cultural appropriateness of questions were incorporated.

Training the Field Research Team

Twenty-one Sierra Leonean women trained and supervised by the PHR/United Nations Mission in Sierra Leone (UNAMSIL) field team conducted the survey interviews. The five-member team had extensive experience in research, psychological counseling with survivors of sexual assault and torture, sexual assault aid programs for Sierra Leonean refugees and IDPs, and human rights issues.

Field researchers learned to administer the survey in Krio in which they all were fluent and then collaborated with the Sierra Leonean members of the team on a translation from the Krio into the two other main languages in Sierra Leone (Mende and Temne). Members of the PHR/UNAMSIL team checked these translations for accuracy. Researchers underwent nine days of classroom teaching and role-play, followed by several days of field observation and ongoing supervision throughout the duration of the study.

All interviews were conducted over a four-week period in 2001. After the interview, the completed questionnaires were reviewed for completeness and for correctness of recording by the researchers themselves, and then they were reviewed by the field supervisors at the end of each day to identify any concerns.

Accounting for Research Ethical Considerations

Given the sensitive nature of the study's subject matter, PHR was especially careful to ensure that the study was conducted in an ethical and sensitive manner. In addition to subjecting the research instrument and plan to ethics review, we made every effort, at each stage of the study, to ensure that the women understood they had a right to participate or not in the study and that they would not be harmed by speaking to us. Before conducting the study in a specific location, we made sure that we could refer women, with their consent, to medical or psychosocial services, if they were identified as needing these during conduct of the study. We did not conduct the study where these services were not available.

Because of the disturbing nature of what our interviewers would be hearing during the study, we checked in with them on a regular basis to ensure that they were able to continue. One of the supervisors on the team was a social worker with extensive experience working on gender-based violence including in the region. She was available to speak with interviewers negatively affected by what they heard.

Characterizing the Respondents

The first step in organizing and reporting data in this kind of research effort is to characterize the respondents that participated in the study and to calculate the response rate. Of the 1,048 households sampled, 991 female heads of household participated in the study (95% response rate). Seven women were ineligible, 41 were not available at the time of sampling, and nine were opposed to the survey, refused to participate, or requested that the interview be stopped.

The average age of the women and girls interviewed was 34 (range, 14–80 years). The majority were poorly educated, Muslim, married, and from either the Temne or Mende tribes; they most commonly reported their occupation as farmers, petty traders, and businesswomen. Nearly one quarter of the women were either separated or widowed due to war, had been displaced more than four times since 1990, and had, on average, lived in the surveyed sites for 18 months. Fifty-seven percent of the women reported that they had been displaced between one and six years, and 41 percent had been displaced between six and 10 years.

More than ninety percent of the women perceived their general health and mental health as fair or poor. Two hundred eighty women (28%) reported suicidal tendencies and 34 had attempted suicide (3%). In responding to the question of what would most help their state of mind, 960 (97%) indicated humanitarian assistance would help the most; 956 (96%) said medical assistance; 937 (94%) wanted income-generation projects; 879 (89%) sought religious counseling and support; 832 (84%) wanted skills training; and 714 (72%) desired mental health counseling.

Analyzing and Reporting the Results

The 991 household representatives reported on the experiences of 9,166 household members, which included themselves and those who lived with them before their displacement. Of the 9,166 household members, 55 percent were women and 44 percent were men. Overall, respondents reported a total of 1,157 incidents of specific forms of war-related human rights abuses. The most common were abduction, beatings, killings, sexual assault, kidnapping for less than 24 hours, forced labor, gunshot wounds, and amputations. Extrapolating the number of war-related sexual assaults reported by participants in our sample to the total female IDP population, PHR estimated that approximately 50,000 to 64,000 Sierra Leonean IDP women might have suffered wartime sexual violence.

Ninety-four of the 991 respondents (9%) reported one or more war-related sexual assault experiences. Study participants also reported war-related sexual assault among 396 (8%) female and six (0.1%) male household members. The prevalence of war-related sexual assault among female household members may be as high as 11 percent (554/5,001) if 158 women are included who did not report sexual assault per se, but did report abduction and pregnancy, vaginal bleeding, pain, swelling, uterine pain, vaginal discharge, or sexually transmitted disease—all possibly the consequence of sexual assault. Respondents reported that 36 female household members became pregnant as a consequence of their assault. In addition, 22 women reported being pregnant at the time of the attack with an average reported gestation of three months. Eighty-nine percent (89%) of women reporting sexual violence were raped; 33 percent were gang raped, and abduction and forced nudity were also reported. Some women were forced into marriage and some became pregnant as a result of the rapes. The most common consequences of the sexual assault as reported by the women interviewed included bodily injury and/or physical disability, sexually transmitted disease, and reproductive complications, including miscarriage.

More than half (60%) of the abuses lasted less than one week. Respondents reported that the majority of the abuses among household members occurred in the last three years of the conflict. Most of these occurred between 1997 and 1999, more than half while in their home villages, and nearly a quarter while fleeing.

For all abuses reported, the RUF was identified as the perpetrator in 1,490 instances (40%). Fifty-three percent of respondents who reported being sexually assaulted also reported "face-to-face" contact specifically with RUF forces, compared with fewer than 6 percent for any other combatant group.

Nearly two-thirds of the respondents subjected to war-related sexual assault indicated they reported the incident(s) to another person. The most common reasons given for not reporting the assault were: "feelings of shame or social stigma," fear of being stigmatized and/or rejected, and not trusting anyone to tell. More than half the women reported seeking help after the attack, and most informed a health care clinician (physician, nurse, or health care worker) of the attack. However, 20 percent of those seeking help in a medical setting indicated that they did not tell anyone about what had happened to them. On average, these women sought help five months after the assault(s) occurred. Hospitals, traditional healers, and health centers were the most common places women turned to for help following the assault. Women generally reported that what helped them the most after an assault was trying to forget about the incident, receiving support from family, counseling from a health care clinician, and receiving care from a traditional healer.

Understanding and Reporting Women's Concerns about the Future and about Their Health

Sexual violence can have serious physical and mental health consequences. In response to queries about future health concerns as a result of the sexual assault they experienced, most women expressed concern about having contracted a sexually transmitted disease or AIDS. Women also described experiencing diffuse abdominal and pelvic pains and worried that these were symptoms of diseases. Some, however, were afraid of the stigma associated with seeking help for rape-related health problems as stated by one respondent: "I don't want to have AIDS. I am afraid to go to the hospital. I don't want people to know if it is true that I have AIDS. I don't know whether I have AIDS or not." At the time, treatment for HIV/AIDS was not available in the country.

Other women expressed a desire for medical treatment, but spoke of their lack of access to medical assistance at the IDP camps. Many of the respondents, both those who reported experiencing sexual violence and those who had not, spoke in general terms of suffering physical and mental ailments, but expressed no hope of receiving the medical care they needed.

Assessing Attitudes about Women's Rights, Their Roles, and Justice

Research participants and attitudes, and their understanding of their own experiences, are critical components of any investigation that involves human subjects. At PHR we were aware that Sierra Leone is a traditional society with regard to women's roles and were therefore concerned to make certain their voices would be heard. To understand the societal context of any effort to address violence against women including the proposed justice mechanisms, we asked women to indicate whether they agreed or disagreed with a number of statements about women's rights and their roles in society. We also asked them to indicate whether they agreed or disagreed with a number of statements about justice. Ninety-four percent of the respondents agreed that women and girls should have the same access to education as men and boys. More than 80 percent agreed that women should be able to express themselves freely, that there should be legal protection for the rights of women, and that women and girls need to receive more education about their reproductive health. This was belied, however, by more than 80 percent agreeing with the statement that a good wife obeys her husband even if she disagrees with him. Most women felt that family problems should only be discussed within the family, that women have the right to control the number and spacing of their children, that more should be done to protect women and girls from having sex when they do not wish to, and that women and girls need more education about their right to refuse sex. More than 60 percent of the women, however, expressed the view that a man has the right to beat his wife if she disobeys and that it is a wife's duty/obligation to have sex with her husband even if she does not want to.

Regarding justice, the survey revealed that only 42 percent of those who responded to this question thought their perpetrators should be punished. Most commonly, women who wanted to grant immunity felt that this was in the "spirit of reconciliation." Other reasons included fear of reprisal; lack of confidence in the system to render punishment for these crimes; and the desire to forget about the incident(s). Many women believed their attacker's commander was aware of the assault. While no direct evidence of command responsibility was provided to PHR, several women blamed rebel leadership. A 30-year-old woman from the North who was abducted, raped, and beaten by RUF stated, "I just know that the leader of the fighters is the fault because if he stopped them, they would never do it—because he supported it—that's why." Fewer women believed that punishment of perpetrators would prevent sexual assault from happening to others, and even fewer (about one-fourth) were willing to give their names to the proposed Special Court and/or the Truth and Reconciliation Commission once these bodies were established.

Because of the long-standing civil war and the destruction that accompanied it, many Sierra Leoneans have no experience of a functioning judiciary—this may have been a factor in some responses. Some of the women indicated to PHR that their experiences were so horrific that they did not believe justice was possible. Some victims revealed that their attackers made explicit threats and that they still feared them. Their fear highlights the need for justice mechanisms to adequately protect those willing to provide information or testify, and for people to be able to rely on such protection. Many women who spoke to PHR did not seek justice or revenge, but rather peace and reconciliation, Mary J., a teenager, explained her reasons for not wanting to seek punishment for her persecutors:

> My parents died during the war—they were killed by rebels. I was there and saw it. They captured me and took me with them to the bush. I was a virgin. Two men used me, they ruined me. I escaped when we came near Freetown . . . [and have had] so many problems since. I became ill, stomach aches. . . . Finally I was taken to the hospital. I wanted to die. In the hospital, they told me they had to do emergency surgery. My people did not have any money. . . . If they catch them and try to do to them what they did to me, it won't even come near the hell I've been through. So they should just leave them. If they try to punish them, the punishment that I have gotten is more than theirs. I wanted to die during that time. If the emergency operation had not been performed, I would have died. . . . If I ask for punishment for them, it will never amount to what I went through, so the best thing is just to leave them so that we can have peace in Sierra Leone.[2]

The complexity of the relationship between victim and perpetrator that has on occasion developed in the bush may also complicate efforts to obtain justice for survivors of sexual violence. It has been reported that some women and girls who were abducted chose to remain with their captors. There are many possible explanations for this. The PHR survey revealed that some who became pregnant as a result of rape consider themselves married to their captors and believed they had no choice but to remain with their "husbands." Other possible factors contributing to abductees voluntarily remaining with their captors include: identification with the abductor; drug addiction; the more desirable food options reportedly available in the bush; fear of being rejected by their families and communities if they were to go home; and the fact that many abductees, particularly those who were captured as young girls, are now settled in a new way of life.[3]

Incorporating the Legal Context in Field Research

The United Nations called Physicians for Human Rights to Sierra Leone because acts of sexual violence, killing, and torture are crimes against humanity and war crimes as defined by international legal standards (Askin, 1997).[4] Rape and other forms of sexual violence, including reproductive crimes, are now regarded as means of inflicting terror and destruction on the civilian population and the armed forces protecting them. Several judgments rendered by the International Criminal Tribunal for Yugoslav (ICTY) and the International Criminal Tribunal for Rwanda (ICTR) tribunals have recognized various forms of sexual violence as instruments of genocide, means of torture, crimes against humanity, and war crimes, regardless of the nature of the conflict as international or internal.[5] Sexual violence, including rape and sexual slavery, is specifically included in the Statute of the Special Court for Sierra Leone.[6]

The legal instruments that constitute international humanitarian law, or the law of war, set out protections that apply in times of conflict. These overlap and supplement the protections offered by human rights law. In the case of an internal conflict, such as the one in Sierra Leone, the codified protections are less complete. Nonetheless, rape, extrajudicial killing, and torture are clearly prohibited under any circumstance. The origin of these standards is codified in Article 3 common to all four of the 1949 Geneva Conventions, which afford protections to civilians, prisoners of war, and others rendered *hors de combat* in internal armed conflicts.[7] The 1977 Additional Protocol I, which regulates international armed conflicts, and Additional Protocol II, which regulates noninternational armed conflict, expand on these protections.[8] Sierra Leone is a party to all four of the 1949 Geneva Conventions[9] and both additional protocols.[10]

Common Article 3, which applies to all parties in internal conflicts such as Sierra Leone's, prohibits "violence to life and person, in particular murder of all kinds, mutilation, cruel treatment and torture" and "outrages upon personal dignity, in particular humiliating and degrading treatment." Additional Protocol II, also regulating internal armed conflicts, expands on this and explicitly forbids "violence to the life, health and physical or mental well-being of persons, in particular murder as well as cruel treatment such as torture, mutilation" and "outrages upon personal dignity, in particular humiliating and degrading treatment, rape, enforced prostitution and any form of indecent assault."[11] The jurisprudence of the ICTY and ICTR has clarified that serious violations of these provisions constitute war crimes. As such, the acts of rape, killing, and torture documented in this report, which were committed with a nexus to the armed conflict, are war crimes.

In addition, Sierra Leone has signed or ratified several international human rights treaties that prohibit the abuses committed against civilians documented in the PHR report. These include the International Covenant on Civil and Political Rights,[12] the Convention against Torture and Other Cruel, Inhuman or Degrading Treatment or Punishment,[13] and the Convention on the Rights of the Child. Sierra Leone is also a party to the Convention on the Elimination of All Forms of Discrimination against Women.[14]

The Special Court for Sierra Leone

At the request of the Government of Sierra Leone, the United Nations proposed establishing an international court for prosecution of those responsible for the commission of atrocities during the war. U.N. Security Council Resolution 1315, adopted on August 14, 2000, requested negotiations for creation of a court to prosecute "crimes against humanity, war crimes and other serious violations of international humanitarian law,"[15] and to try those "persons who bear the greatest responsibility"[16] for these crimes.

Following negotiations, it was determined that the Court for Sierra Leone would differ from the ICTY and ICTR in several ways. The Sierra Leonean Court is based on a treaty or agreement between the United Nations and Sierra Leone. As such, unlike the ICTY and ICTR, it cannot assert primacy over national courts of other states, nor can it order accused individuals located in another state to surrender.

The staff for the Special Court, including the judges and prosecutors, is composed of both Sierra Leoneans and internationals.[17] The Court's subject matter jurisdiction includes acts in violation of international humanitarian law as well as certain crimes under Sierra Leonean law.[18]

The Statute of the Special Court for Sierra Leone explicitly includes gender-based violence in its definition of several categories of crimes that the Court has the power to adjudicate. The statute lists "rape, sexual slavery, enforced prostitution, forced pregnancy and any other form of sexual violence" as crimes against humanity,[19] prosecutable when "committed . . . as part of a widespread or systematic attack against any civilian population."[20]

The Court also expressly includes "rape, enforced prostitution and any form of indecent assault"[21] as violations of humanitarian law as enshrined in Common Article 3 and Additional Protocol II.[22] The Court has the power to try certain offenses under the laws of Sierra Leone. Some of these may be used to prosecute gender-based violence against girls under the age of fourteen.[23]

The Truth and Reconciliation Commission

The Lome Peace Agreement of July 7, 1999, provided for the establishment of a Truth and Reconciliation Commission (TRC) in Sierra Leone to "address impunity, break the cycle of violence, provide a forum for both the victims and perpetrators of human rights violations to tell their story [and] get a clear picture of the past in order to facilitate genuine healing and reconciliation"[24] by addressing human rights violations committed from the start of the conflict. Enacted in 2000, the Truth and Reconciliation Commission Act[25] provides more detail about the TRC. As part of its mandate to "work to restore the human dignity of victims and promote reconciliation,"[26] the TRC is supposed to pay "special attention to the subject of sexual abuses."[27]

PHR met with key staff members of and provided information to both the Special Court and the TRC and urged both bodies to be especially sensitive to gender-related crimes, including sexual violence, in particular, to ensure that appropriate procedures, processes, and staff are in place to support and protect victims and witnesses, learning from experiences with other international tribunals. PHR also urged that these bodies ensure, to the extent possible, that those who come forward should be protected when they return to their communities as well.

PHR published the findings in the form of a book-length report, which included copies of the survey instruments used (PHR, 2002). This report was distributed widely, including in Sierra Leone, and posted in full on its website. An article reporting the findings was simultaneously published in the *Journal of the American Medical Association*. Publication in general medical journals is an important step in establishing methodologies for research on health and human rights as valid and in establishing human rights as a relevant concern for a medical and scientific audience. In addition to the dissemination of the findings through distribution of publications, team members spoke to international and local media and conducted high-level advocacy with staff members at U.N. headquarters and officials of donor governments, including the United States and the United Kingdom.

It was also important for us to ensure that Sierra Leoneans had an opportunity to learn about the findings and use them. We returned to Sierra Leone to formally release the study. While there, we met with local NGOs to brief them about the findings and strategize with them about how they could use the findings in their own work; we also did extensive work with local media, including a televised press conference and several radio shows. We met with key international NGO and U.N. staff members to share our findings. We were also able to hold an open town meeting in one of the locations where we conducted the study. In this forum we presented the findings, and community members were able to ask questions, discuss responses, and relate experiences. We received positive feedback on this forum, in particular. Some people told us that they were grateful that we took the time to come back and tell them what we found, because others who did research in their communities simply asked questions and left. Unfortunately, such reporting back to affected communities is not standard practice of many researchers.

Looking Ahead

PHR's study in Sierra Leone documented the widespread use of sexual violence against women and girls and their public health effects during the civil war in Sierra Leone. The violence against women was part of an overall pattern of rights abuses against the civilian population, which also included abductions, beatings, torture, gunshot wounds, amputations, killings, "capturing" persons for less than 24 hours, and forced labor. Burning of homes and looting property also was common. The RUF was responsible for perhaps 40 percent of the violations, but they were not the only rights violators. Overall, a substantial segment of the population was affected. PHR found that 94 percent of household members surveyed experienced one or more human rights violations during the ten-year-long civil conflict, with most abuses occurring between 1997 and 1999 when the civil war raged most violently (Pratt, 2001). The adverse physical and psychological consequences of sexual violence are described in other studies (Schafran, 1996; Resnick et al., 1997). The prevalence of sexual assault, including war related or non-war related, among IDP women in this study suggests a serious health burden for individual and community members that cannot be addressed adequately by services that currently exist in Sierra Leone (Coker and Richter, 1998).

Further study is needed to document health consequences. One of the lessons PHR learned in conducting this type of research is that the societal context affects how this kind of research must be designed. Despite efforts to ensure privacy for respondents, PHR believes there is a high likelihood that the prevalence of war-related sexual violence in this study was underestimated because of intentional nondisclosure of sexual violence and the perceived lack of privacy in some of the interviews. All research on prevalence and consequences of violence against women should consider the reasons why women fail to disclose experiencing violence, such as fear of retribution by an assailant, being stigmatized and rejected, being blamed for the assault, and experiencing the psychological consequences of disclosure (Koss, 1993). Although PHR's interviewers were careful to explain that there would be no material or other gain by participating in the survey, we must also consider that the number of abuses reported in the study may have been overestimated, if those interviewed judged it in their material, political, or psychological interest to exaggerate claims of abuse. In other words, there are possible incentives for concealing and exaggerating historical accounts. It is, however, PHR's view that in this context the greatest likelihood is for the concealment and hence under-reporting of these painful and stigmatizing events.

Health care and public health professionals have a unique role to play in investigating and documenting wartime sexual violence and in the treatment of survivors. Collecting and presenting sound evidence may contribute to efforts to hold perpetrators accountable, restore the rule of law, and limit future violations. Furthermore, increasing knowledge about sexual violence in war will facilitate the development of strategies that allow the recovery of survivors of sexual violence and their families and communities. A better understanding of the underlying factors and characteristics of war-related sexual violence might contribute to the development of measures to better protect potential victims and deter perpetrators (Swiss and Giller, 1993). Documentation is also a key part of the development of international jurisprudence and of strengthening the interpretation and implementation of existing international legal standards. Survivors of human rights abuses, including sexual violence, deserve no less.

There are important methodological, ethical, and safety considerations to doing research on sensitive issues and in emergency settings. Violence including violence against women is now recognized as an important public health issue. As part of ongoing work on improving research on violence, there are efforts to identify the best methods for measurement of violence against women and to address challenges and gaps in this work (U.N. Division for the Advancement of Women [UNDAW], 2005). Despite this, such research is still often complicated or even obstructed by political considerations and discomfort with the issue of sexual violence. Furthermore, there are still those who consider violence against women a "social issue" rather than one that is relevant to health professionals or who deny that it is a commonplace occurrence. Ironically, it is these very notions that proper documentation of the prevalence and impact of sexual violence can dispel. Until these attitudes are addressed, therefore, it is unlikely that we will be able effectively to prevent and respond to violence against women in conflict settings.

Acknowledgments

The material in this chapter is based on work done by Physicians for Human Rights with the support of the UNAMSIL, and portions have been published previously in Amowitz et al., 2002, and Physicians for Human Rights, 2002.

Notes

1. Not her real name.

2. Interview with Physicians for Human Rights, March 2000, Freetown, Sierra Leone.

3. Conversations between PHR and Corinne Dufka, Human Rights Watch (January 2001), and between PHR and NGO representatives providing services to returned abductees (March 2000).

4. Rome Statute of the International Criminal Court, U.N. Doc. A/CONF.183/9 (1998) entered into force July 1, 2002, www.un.org/law/icc/statute/romefra.htm.

5. See especially *Prosecutor v. Jean-Paul Akayesu*, ICTR-96-4-T, September 2, 1998; *Prosecutor v. Anto Furundzija*, Judgment, IT-95-17/1-T, December 10, 1998; *Prosecutor v. Zejnil Delalic et al.*, IT-96-21-T, November 16, 1998; *Prosecutor v. Kunarac et al.*, IT-96-23-T and IT-96-23/1-T, February 22, 2001. www.un.org/icty/foca/trialc2/judgement/index.htm.

6. Statute of the Special Court for Sierra Leone, articles 2 and 3. www.sierra-leone.org/specialcourtstatute.html.

7. See, for example, Geneva Convention (IV) Relative to the Protection of Civilian Persons in Time of War, August 12, 1949, 75 UNTS (1950) 287–417.

8. 1977 Geneva Protocol II Additional to the Geneva Conventions of 1949, and Relating to the Protection of Victims of Non-International Armed Conflicts, June 8, 1977, 1125 UNTS (1979) 609–99 [hereinafter Additional Protocol II]. Protocol Additional to the Geneva Conventions of August 12, 1949, and relating to the Protection of Victims of International Armed Conflicts June 8, 1977, 1125 U.N.T.S. (1979) 3–434?, entered into force December 7, 1978 [hereinafter Additional Protocol I].

9. Succession: June 10, 1965.

10. Ratified October 21, 1986.

11. Additional Protocol II, Article 4(2).

12. Acceded August 23, 1996.

13. Signed March 18, 1985; ratified March 1, 2001.

14. Signed September 21, 1988; ratified November 11, 1988. (Sierra Leone's initial, second, and third periodic reports were due 1989, 1993, and 1997, respectively.)

15. SCOR Res. 1315, adopted on August 14, 2000 available at www.un.org/Docs/scres/2000/sc2000.htm.

16. Agreement on the Special Court for Sierra Leone.

17. Ibid., articles 2 and 3.

18. Statute of the Special Court for Sierra Leone, article 1. www.sierra-leone .org/specialcourtstatute.html>.

19. Article 2 (g).

20. Article 2 *chapeau.*

21. Article 3 (e).

22. Article 3 *chapeau.*

23. Article 5.

24. Lome Peace Agreement.

25. The Truth and Reconciliation Commission Act 2000, www.sierra-leone.org/trcact2000.html.

26. Ibid. Part III, article 6 (2)(b).

27. Ibid.

References

Amowitz, L. L., Reis, C., Hare-Lyons, K., Vann, B., Mansaray, B., Akinsulure-Smith, A., Taylor, L., and Iacopino, V. 2002. A letter from Sierra Leone: Prevalence of war-related sexual violence and other human rights abuses among internally displaced persons in Sierra Leone. *JAMA* 287 (4):513–21.

Askin, K. D. 1997. *War crimes against women: Prosecution in international war crimes tribunals.* The Hague: M. Nijhoff Publishers.

Central Intelligence Agency (CIA). 2005. *The world factbook.* https://www.cia.gov/cia/publications/factbook/index.html (accessed November 18, 2005).

Coggon, D., Rose, G., and Barker, D. J. P. 1997. *Epidemiology for the uninitiated.* 4th ed. Available at http://bmj.bmjjournals.com/epidem/.

Coker, A. L., and Richter, D. L. 1998. Violence against women in Sierra Leone: Frequency and correlates of intimate partner violence and forced sexual intercourse. *African Journal of Reproductive Health* 2:61–72.

de Jong, K, Mulham, M., et al. 2000. Doctors without Borders/Médecins sans Frontières special report, assessing trauma in Sierra Leone. Psychosocial questionnaire: Freetown survey outcomes. January 11. http://www.doctorswithoutborders.org/publications/reports/2000/sierraleone_01-2000.cfm

Iacopino, V., Frank, M. W., et al. 2001. A population-based assessment of human rights abuses against ethnic Albanian refugees from Kosovo. *American Journal of Public Health* 91:2013–18.

Koss, M. P. 1993. Detecting the scope of rape: A review of prevalence research methods. *Journal of Interpersonal Violence* 8:198–222.

Patton, M. O. 1990. *Qualitative evaluation and research methods,* 2nd ed., 169–283. Newbury, CA: Sage Publications.

Physicians for Human Rights (PHR). 2001. *Endless brutality: War crimes in Chechnya.* Cambridge, MA: Physicians for Human Rights. http://www.phrusa.org/publications/chechnya.html

Physicians for Human Rights (PHR). 2002. The prevalence of sexual violence and other human rights abuses among internally displaced persons in Sierra Leone: A population-based assessment. Boston: Physicians for Human Rights. January. Available online at: www.phrusa.org/research/sierra_leone/report.html (accessed November 18, 2005).

Pratt, D. 2001. Sierra Leone: Danger and opportunity in a regional conflict. Report to Canada's Minister of Foreign Affairs.

Resnick, H. S, Acierno, R., et al. 1997. Health impact of interpersonal violence: 2, medical and mental health outcomes. *Behavioral Medicine* 23:65–78.

Schafran, L. H. 1996. Topics for our times: rape is a major public health issue. *American Journal of Public Health* 86:15–17.

Schoenbach, V. J., and Rosamond, W. D. 2000. Understanding the fundamentals of epidemiology: An evolving text. Available at: www.epidemiolog.net/evolving/TableOfContents.htm (accessed November 18, 2005).

Swiss, S., and Giller, J. E. 1993. Rape as a crime of war: A medical perspective. *JAMA* 70:612–15.

United Nations Children's Fund (UNICEF). 1999. State of the World's Children 2000. Statistical tables, 81–113. U.N. Sales No. E.00.XX.1.

United Nations Division for the Advancement of Women (UNDAW). 2005. Violence against women: a statistical overview, challenges and gaps in data collection and methodology and approaches for overcoming them. Report of expert group meeting, 2005, Geneva, Switzerland. www.un.org/womenwatch/daw/egm/vaw-stat-2005/docs/final-report-vaw-stats.pdf (accessed November 18, 2005).

United Nations Office for the Coordination of Humanitarian Affairs (UNOCHA). 2000. *Consolidated inter-agency appeal for Sierra Leone,* 117. /www.reliefweb.int/appeals/2002/files/sle02.pdf (accessed November 18, 2005).

United Nations Office for the Coordination for Humanitarian Affairs (UNOCHA). February 2001. *Humanitarian situation report.* http://ochaonline.un.org/ (accessed November 18, 2005).

U.S. Committee for Refugees (USCR). 2001. Special report: Sierra Leone. www.refugees.org/news/crisis/sierraleone/sierraleone.htm (accessed November 18, 2005).

9

The Crime of Genocide

Darfur

Jennifer Leaning, M.D., S.M.H.

The 1948 Convention on the Prevention and Punishment of the Crime of Genocide characterizes genocide as a crime under international law that signatory nations must prevent and punish.[1] Under the statute, genocide must be charged against an individual and established in a court of law. It requires establishing the act itself (*actus reus*) and the intent of that act (*mens rea*). Yet the statute also confers in its title and in Article 3 the unequivocal and separate obligation on states that have signed and ratified the Convention to undertake to prevent the crime of genocide wherever it is found. Prevention implies intervening before something has happened, or before at least a process has been completed. To act in the real world in real time, however, is to act outside a courtroom, in a political arena where information is fragmentary and debate follows few rules of logic or procedure.

So how does one act to prevent a possible crime from taking place when it has not yet been judged in a court of law to be a crime? Is it ever possible to attach the label genocide to a set of events that are in the process of unfolding? Without proving intent in a court of law according to criminal rules of evidence, how can one establish that genocide, as defined in the convention, has taken place? Can one ever call anything genocide before the killings are over, the malignant government or the predatory authorities deposed, the memo of intent found in the files or the pockets of the offenders, the paper trail established, the witnesses deposed, and the legal process completed?

Finding a useful answer to these questions is becoming urgent to many scholars and policy analysts who have tracked events in the ugly ethnic and communal wars of the past fifteen years in the Balkans, the Great Lakes region, and now Darfur. Attention has turned to the methods of public health assessment and epidemiology, applied to population-based data on morbidity and mortality in crises, as a possible approach to strengthening our assessment of ongoing genocidal processes. The discussion that follows describes these methods, in particular, as they support the functions of early warning and pattern identification, and shows how they have been applied most recently in the case of Darfur.

The evidentiary base for this discussion is derived from many sources but principally from the work of Physicians for Human Rights in the Chad-Darfur region over the past 16 months (Leaning, 2004; Physicians for Human Rights, 2004).

Preventing a Crime When Intent and Action Are Clear

Arguing from domestic criminal law, intervening to prevent a crime appears relatively straightforward. Attempted murder exists as an accepted charge in domestic criminal law in virtually all countries. The crime of murder is sufficiently understood in its preparatory, escalating, and consequential modes that domestic police systems are permitted to intervene and restrict a potential perpetrator's capacity to carry out and complete a possible murder. In the subsequent court proceeding, the evidence is amassed and a decision is reached as to whether the charge was valid and whether the alleged perpetrator is to be found guilty or innocent.

The problem of defining intent and identifying the act exists in the prosecution of domestic crimes. The ordinary crime of murder, however, is sufficiently familiar that we are permitted within the law to intervene against a person who is holding a large knife against the throat of another who is screaming for help. It is evident, on the basis of precedent and common sense, that there is a high likelihood that harm may befall the person against whose throat the knife may about to be applied; and it is presumed reasonable for the authorities or even a courageous passer-by to intervene to stop the process. We infer, based on known patterns of previous knife murders, that what we are observing in this instance may indeed be the initial act of another knife murder and we assume intent based on our knowing that this pattern of behavior is highly unlikely to arise from any other than the intent to kill.

Preventing the Crime of Genocide

With regard to the Genocide Convention, however, these bastions of common sense reasoning and legal precedent are insufficient to provide that presumptive envelope, familiar in domestic criminal law, within which action to prevent is legally allowed to take place before establishing the definitive facts of the case. In mentioning the three main factors responsible for this insufficiency, the focus of the discussion will be on the third—the problem of prediction based on early warning and pattern identification.

The first factor is the opacity of the convention itself. The document does not address the steps required to apply the convention to an actual circumstance. It is silent on what information is relevant, says nothing about how to gather or interpret the kind of data that are available while a conflict or organized assault is taking place, and provides no guidance as to how intent might be determined or what information might be relevant in assessing intent. The need to establish intent, however, is central to the application of the Convention. Its entire force rests on the opening language of Article II, whereby all the acts specified as genocidal must be undertaken "with the intent to destroy, in whole or in part, a national, ethnical, racial or religious group, as such."

The second factor is the deep reluctance on the part of the international community to intervene for any reason against the sovereignty of a nation state. The discussion has been enriched in the past decade by several reports from the U.N. secretary general (on protection of civilians on war and on the stance to take toward prevention of armed conflict) (U.N. Doc, 1999, 2001). These reports, submitted for discussion and subsequently adopted by the U.N. General Assembly, have established a set of norms and expectations that now infuse international debate over the plight of civilians in Darfur, in Chechnya, in eastern Congo, and other people trapped in civil wars or oppressive circumstances. A comprehensive document, developed by the International Commission on Intervention and State Sovereignty and warmly received by the international community on the occasion of its release in 2001, reviewed the history, law, and policy behind the concept of "the responsibility to protect" (International Development Research Centre, 2001). It presented proposals for constructing a limited menu of rationales that might support a range of responses on the part of the international community, extending to a discussion of what might warrant international military intervention in a given set of circumstances. Yet as the examples of Rwanda, Chechnya, and now Darfur attest, the interests of great nations continue to maintain the threshold for intervention at a high level, despite the growing normative acknowledgment that there does exist in theory an international responsibility to protect civilian populations from sweeping assault by rapacious authorities.

The third factor is that the predictive parameters of historical genocide are not well understood. Much uncertainty exists among scholars, politicians, and international lawyers regarding when to say a genocidal process is unfolding—whether in the midst of an international war, a civil war, the suppression of a rebellion, or an oppressive state campaign against internal minorities or stigmatized groups (Staub, 1989). Historical turning points, where contemporaries should have known or should have acted, are hotly contested.

The controversy about turning points should be distinguished from the powerful growing consensus among genocide scholars that the overall features of a society veering toward genocide are clear (Gillately and Kiernan, 2003). When viewed through the long lens of history, the factors that in retrospect are seen to have contributed to genocide include: social tensions around ethnic or communal identities; a history of exclusion from the state or nationalist project; a sudden shift in the balance of power relationships between or among opposing groups; an event that serves as a flash point, often further manipulated by irresponsible leaders; and an inability or unwillingness of the state to contain escalations in violence against the despised subgroup. To carry out killings on a genocidal scale also appears to require significant bureaucratic capacity, sustained as in the case of Germany and Rwanda by population registries and a culture of respect for systems and hierarchy. Prolonged and brutal wars, waged by weakening regimes and poorly disciplined armies, can also turn into genocide, especially when communal tensions among civilians on all sides are whipped into frenzy by malevolent leaders.

The key problem with this scholarly consensus on contributory factors, however, is that from a policy standpoint the presence of these factors in any given instance does not predict whether a genocide may be about to take place. Many societies struggle for years to surmount these divisive and bitter factors in their midst or engage in bloody, protracted wars—and yet they do not descend into genocide. Our historical understanding of genocide is simply not complete enough to provide definitive guidance in a particular set of circumstances as to whether and when the international community should act to prevent the crime of genocide.

Yet genocide scholarship identifies a crucial space for contemporaneous investigation and analysis. The two major lines of genocide analysis—what makes a society plunge into genocide and what prevents another from doing so—affirm that there exists an historical moment in social crises, war, or violent oppression when events are taking shape, when there might be opportunity for decision, change, or intervention. The past is not comprehensively determining and the future is unpredictable. The investigative and analytic task is to discern, in the midst of events and in real time, whether a shift is occurring that marks a turn toward genocide.

Early Warning

Those who seek to intervene early in the genocidal process need methods that support the notion of early warning. As developed in public health and disaster response, *early warning* is the term used to describe the process of identifying early indicators of impending epidemic disease or famine (FEWS-NET). Adapted by human rights investigators, early warning indicators have been sought to alert the international community to deteriorating trends in social tensions or civil oppression (Leaning, 2002). Genocide scholars and historians have taught us that genocide is also a process, arising from an enabling context and an intensifying pace of targeted attacks against members of an identifiable group (Fein, 2001). Efforts have been made to develop a framework for political early warning, based on structural characteristics of a society and then "accelerators" or "triggers" that take an at-risk situation into a genocidal trajectory (Harff, 2002). To provide early warning information to policy makers about an unfolding genocide would require methods that could furnish irrefutable and robust information about the acts themselves and their effect on the targeted group as well as indicators of intent that would be difficult to dispute or dismiss.

Assessment and Analysis of Patterns

In late 2003 and early 2004, humanitarian organizations in Sudan began to report increasing attacks on Black African civilians in Darfur by forces of the Government of Sudan (GOS) and Janjaweed militia. Linked to these reports were communications about the bureaucratic impediments imposed by the GOS, thwarting relief workers in their attempts to import and deliver supplies and their efforts to travel throughout the region to reach populations fleeing attack. (See Figure 9.1.)

Denied visas to enter Sudan and reach the population in Darfur that was under direct attack, human rights investigators began to explore methods of gathering data from the 200,000 refugees who had moved into eastern Chad, along the western border of Darfur. In the past 18 months, these refugees have provided information, through surveys, interviews, and focus groups, to several human rights groups, including Amnesty International, the Coalition for International Justice, and Physicians for Human Rights (PHR).

In its first investigation in the summer of 2004 along the Chad-Sudan border (PHR, 2004), PHR gathered refugee testimony that presented a consistent picture of the village attacks in Darfur that prompted a mass population flight. The refugees recounted similar features of the village attack, in terms of timing, weapons, transport, targets[2] for killing and infliction of rape; similar tactics used in the destruction of villages, in terms of items destroyed, looted, pillaged, and contaminated; similar methods in abolishing evidence of land use and demolishing all infrastructure and stores; the same techniques of hot pursuit, for hours and days afterward; and widespread systematic rape of individuals and groups of women and girls. To PHR investigators, it became evident that the refugee testimony provided sufficient consistency and detail to warrant the effort to gather systematic data regarding overall patterns of attack, with a particular focus on the issue of deliberate assaults on livelihoods. Two subsequent investigations with this purpose were undertaken by PHR in 2005.

The process of gathering data to test for patterns is central to the methods of public health and epidemiology. Using standard sampling methodologies

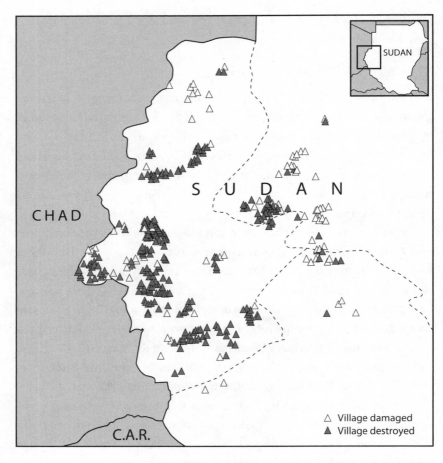

Figure 9.1. Sudan (Darfur)-Chad border region confirmed damaged and destroyed villages. After map from the University of Texas at Austin Libraries, Perry-Castañeda Library Map Collection (available at www.lib.utexas.edu/maps/africa/darfur_villages_0802_2004.jpg)

within a given population, investigators develop an instrument that seeks information on a given set of effects that are presumed to have taken place, along with descriptive information regarding social, economic, and demographic attributes of the target population. Based on the strength of the statistical sampling methods, the individual responses to the survey instrument and focus groups can be grouped into categories, which can then be assessed for possible patterns of effect. This information, when related to other information from other sources and from understanding of context and plausible causal pathways, allowed investigators to aggregate data, discern patterns, and advance notions of interpretation (Berkman and Kawachi, 2000).

These methods are always more difficult to use when data are fragmentary, populations are moving, or conditions are insecure. Yet with practiced modification, this methodological approach to population sampling has been used to good purpose in many humanitarian situations, where the effects of interest are nutritional status or crude mortality among the recipient population of interest. Several important studies from relief agencies using these techniques have been reported out of Darfur in the past year (Centers for Disease Control and Prevention [CDC], 2004; Depoortere et al., 2004; World Health Organization [WHO], 2004; Grandesso et al., 2005).

No standard instrument or set of sampling methodologies has been developed for a population-based assessment of morbidity and mortality that might shed light on whether a genocide is underway. Adapting the humanitarian public health approach to sampling and instrument design for such purposes introduces significant obstacles, because the populations at risk may be sequestered, in flight, or inaccessible and general insecurity may impede the gathering of information. The main challenge, however, is how to generalize from small samples. Humanitarian program assessment looks at relief impact in camps and villages over a past period of a few weeks or a few months. Assessments of widespread morbidity and mortality, at a scale that might furnish evidence of genocide, require gathering data that could speak to the experience of an entire population with deaths, births, migration, illness, injuries, assaults, and rapes from all causes over a longer time frame.

Denominators

The basic task in estimating morbidity and mortality in war is obtaining reliable counts for denominators (the numbers of people living in a given place) and numerators (the numbers of people from within that denominator sample who have been killed or physically harmed by the conflict) (Checchi and Roberts, 2005). These reliable counts can be based on actually counting everyone in the numerator and denominator or on statistically sound samples of the population at risk. In practice, even in stable and peaceful states, counts of total population (the national census) are reached by established sampling techniques, not by actually counting every single person who lives within the boundaries of that nation state. Internal or civil wars often take place in badly governed and poor countries that lack a recent reliable national census; the last one in Sudan was in 1983 and even that is seen as highly flawed, with marked undercounts in the more remote regions, like Darfur.

In the absence of a national census, the next option for obtaining the population denominator would be to design and implement almost a minicensus—a statistically sound sample of the population in the region of interest—in this case, all of Darfur. During conflict, however, a population-based sample is almost always unfeasible, because travel throughout the war zone becomes insecure and people are afraid to come forward to be counted. In Darfur, the war has introduced great insecurity and fear, much of the population has been in flight, the distances are vast, and the road network sparse, with large sections impassable in the rainy season. These factors combine to make a systematic sample of the entire population of Darfur almost impossible to accomplish in any useful time frame.

The remaining options for estimating population denominators become increasingly unreliable when the total population of interest is scattered widely and may have had highly variable but unknowably different experience. If in addition a significant but unknowable fraction of this scattered population cannot even be reached for assessment and sampling, because of insecurity, checkpoints, and bad transport conditions, then the denominators that are obtained through these incomplete sampling techniques are flawed in ways that cannot be compensated for in statistical models.

Add to these issues the problem of numbers. The larger the sample, the more valid it becomes, in terms of being representative of the underlying population. In the volatile context of Darfur, it is not safe for survey teams to stay for long even in areas that can be reached. So the numbers of people who are selected for sampling are quite small when compared with the large underlying population.

Because of these constraints, the construction of estimates of population denominators in Darfur is imperfect. Every study of morbidity and mortality that has been performed in Darfur in the past two and a half years is based on some combination of samples from populations within accessible internally displaced person (IDP) camps, in towns where IDPs are self-settled, and in accessible regions of the country where people are not in camps (Leaning and VanRooyen, 2005). Two main issues make it difficult to generalize from these samples. (1) In general, it is presumed that the populations who have been reached are in better shape than those who are living in areas inaccessible to the humanitarian community, and (2) it is entirely uncertain whether the experience of attack and flight reported by the populations who have been reached is similar to the war experience of those populations who remain inaccessible.

Numerators

To arrive at estimates of the number of people who have been killed or physically harmed from a conflict, one asks precise questions relating to these issues of every informant selected from within the sample denominator. Many studies conducted by humanitarian nongovernmental organizations (NGOs) in the field, however, are designed to elicit information about health conditions and nutritional status of target age groups. Obtaining reliable data about deaths, disappearances, forced flight, rapes, or injuries in a given family unit over a specified time frame requires many added questions, a more sophisticated interview process, and more complicated data analysis. These additions consume time and resources that hard-pressed humanitarian NGOs often cannot supply, in particular, if the information about deaths and conflict-related injury are not directly germane to their field operations.

Findings

Surveys and interviews conducted by several different human rights organizations, based on different methods of sampling and interviewing refugee populations in Chad, combine to form a composite picture of village attack and pursuit of survivors. These reports cannot be neatly summed in quantitative fashion but they provide independent portrayal and validation of events that taken together provide ample evidence of widespread infliction of atrocity and violations of basic human rights. The question here is whether the information provided is sufficient to raise the charge of genocide.

For the past two and a half years, in every attack on the Black African villages of Darfur, the government and Janjaweed forces have used a consistent and sweeping strategy that involves burning all dwellings, looting all personal possessions, destroying all food and seed supplies, stealing all livestock, poisoning or destroying all wells and irrigation systems, uprooting or burning fruit trees, and destroying all crops in the fields. Often the civic buildings in the larger towns, such as schools, are burned and looted. The inhabitants of these villages are all forced to flee through most immediate and violent means: surprise raids at dawn that find people in their homes undefended, outright killing of as many men as can be encountered, chasing women and raping whoever can be caught, and then chasing after the fleeing population using all means of transport (helicopter, land vehicles, horseback, on foot) to pursue scattered remnants for hours at a time, returning to the chase the next day and for several days thereafter.

This information reported independently by several human rights organizations was obtained on the basis of small samples taken from refugee populations only. Corroboration is provided by humanitarian agencies and analysts working with populations still in Darfur. Their formal findings from public health assessments include terse descriptions of current conditions and circumstances from recent past recall that are entirely consistent with the human rights reports. The narrative picture is more robustly rendered in first-hand accounts from foreign governmental officials and journalists. The reports are further reinforced by many photographs, films, and satellite images taken of the villages, both before and after attack, by a wide range of reporters, human rights investigators, and international commercial satellite sources.

The GOS has not denied these reports of physical destruction. It has chosen instead to dismiss or minimize reports of human death and rape, in an apparent effort to deflect what it considers the more serious allegations and the ones that are harder to prove. The GOS attributes the current situation in Darfur to an exacerbation of drought and communal strife in the context of a chronic conflict between Arab and African populations in the region. The government invokes the world's application of a familiar pattern—drought and disturbance in Africa. Yet the data from human rights investigations, humanitarian reports, and photographic imaging would suggest a different pattern, one that appears to be designed and directed by GOS forces to drive several million Black African inhabitants for removal from this region of the country—by death, rape, forced migration, and obliteration of livelihoods.

Establishing Acts as Genocide

To move from pattern identification to the charge of genocide requires establishing two independent lines of analysis: (1) that the acts framed in the pattern constitute genocidal acts in the terms of the convention and (2) that the pattern is so organized, coherent, and sustained that it could only have been accomplished through the intent and direction of the government.

In Article II, the Genocide Convention presents an exhaustive list of five separate and independent acts that would rise to the finding of genocide:

1. Killing members of a group;
2. Causing serious bodily or mental harm to members of a group;
3. Deliberately inflicting on a group conditions of life calculated to bring about its physical destruction in whole or in part;
4. Imposing measures intended to prevent births within a group;
5. Forcibly transferring children of a group to another.

No guidance is provided regarding the numbers or proportion of people within one of the four designated groups (identified by race, ethnicity, religion, or nationality) who must be so affected for any of these five categories to apply. From a practical standpoint, there is wisdom in this silence, because it is often impossible, even after the fact, to determine precisely how many people have been killed, raped, or otherwise seriously harmed. This silence, however, has continued to perplex those who attempt to apply the Genocide Convention to actual conflict settings, because the issue of numbers always intrudes. How many deaths, how many rapes does it take before one can raise concerns about a pattern, and a pattern suggestive of intent, and thus advance the charge of genocide?

Some advance in legal interpretation of the meaning of intent in the convention has been provided by the rulings in the two ad hoc criminal tribunals for Former Yugoslavia (ICTY) and Rwanda (ICTR). Systematic mass rape, as found in Rwanda, was determined by the ICTR to constitute genocide, in terms as defined under Article II (b), (d), and (e) (ICTR, 1998). The ICTR has also been helpful in narrowing the gap between legal definition and operational guidance when it comes to interpreting the meaning of "intent" in advance of the completed act. In Rwanda, examining the evidence after the fact and after the collapse and defeat of the genocidal Hutu regime, the ICTR determined that even in the absence of a definitely clear document or statement of intent, the overwhelming physical and testimonial evidence of sweeping attacks, rapes, and mass killings of Tutsi by Hutu could be advanced as sufficient indication of intent. In this important finding, the notion of pattern identification was advanced as a significant element in the argument establishing intent (ICTR, 1998). The pattern that the ICTR discerned from the evidence was gathered at the end of the genocidal process, not during it, and was gathered through a juridical process, rather than through population sampling techniques, yet the essential point of this ruling is that official intent could be inferred if evidence could be amassed to show a systematic pattern of planning, attack, and selective impact.

In Darfur, several analysts have attempted to estimate the numbers of people killed, based on extrapolation from small sample studies among internally displaced populations within Darfur or on extrapolations from data provided by refugees in Chad. The range is large (200,000 to 400,000 people killed) and the estimates lack statistical strength (Guha-Sapir and Degomme, 2005). For good reasons (known underreporting, small and biased samples), no one has even tried to develop a cumulative estimate of rapes, despite widespread indication in anecdotal reports that rape was inflicted on many Black African women, girls, and even young boys throughout this campaign (Amnesty International, 2004; Gingerich and Leaning, 2004; MSF Holland, 2005). Several million people have been driven from their homes and villages and now survive in difficult circumstances in IDP camps in Darfur, entirely dependent on international aid. An unknown number of displaced survivors of these attacks exist in desperate circumstances in more remote regions of Darfur, where access by the humanitarian aid workers is impeded by GOS and Janjaweed forces. On the basis of these findings and reports, ample evidence exists to suggest that these killings, rapes, and mass expulsions amount to genocide, under clauses IIa, IIb, and IId.

In addition, however, a particular feature of the war waged against the Black African Darfurians—the sweeping and systematic destruction of infrastructure and looting of all household wealth, including livestock—invokes consideration of II (c), "deliberately inflicting on a group conditions of life calculated to bring about its physical destruction in whole or in part." Considerable attention among human rights investigators, particularly PHR, has been directed at analysis of this clause and its application to the conflict in Darfur.

Assault on Livelihoods as Genocidal Action

War has often inflicted massive injury to the environment and inhabited countryside, in particular, when military strategies employ carpet bombing and laying of mines, as in World War II, or widespread use of defoliants and incendiary materials, as in Vietnam (Westing, 1980). Outrages against fragile ecosystems have begun to attract attention as violations of obscure sections of international humanitarian law, as in the burning of the oil fields and spillage of oil into the Persian Gulf during the Gulf war in 1990–91 (Omar et al., 2000). These attacks on the environment were not directed against the living conditions of specific groups as defined in the Genocide Convention, however, and for this reason at least could not be held up as possible instances of genocide as defined in Article II(c).

In Darfur, even in times of peace, the balance between resources and need was taut and precarious for these communities. Rains and disease determined the harvests, and in this harsh and dry terrain, war or conflict in any form would disrupt this ecological balance by extracting manpower, consuming resources, and distorting normal markets. The current war in Darfur has proved particularly damaging, not only by inflicting gross death and misery on the Black African population, but also by eradicating whole-scale their built, cultivated, and living environment.

It is suggested here that what the international community confronts in Darfur may be an early, well-documented instance of the kind of deliberate infliction of physical conditions of life that the framers of the convention envisioned. To pursue this line of argument, two major points need to be addressed successfully. The first point is whether the observed destruction of livelihoods meets the convention definition of physical conditions of life. The second point is whether the observed destruction of livelihoods is deliberate, in the terms of the convention. These are issues of law as well as of fact and in the remainder of this section these issues are explored in brief.

This clause in the convention has not been widely applied in human rights discussion of genocide nor is there much scholarly discussion of its meaning in the genocide literature.

The scant juridical precedent relating to this clause can be amplified by referring to the travaux preparatoires, the background documents and debate that supported the drafting process that produced the convention. Reference to similar materials behind the development of the Rome Statute for the International Criminal Court also supplies insight into the possible legal range and meaning of this clause. Several key elements emerge from this record (Schabas, 2002):

Physical Destruction: The framers of the Convention focused on the notion of the physical destruction of life itself. Actions aimed at destroyed cultural dimensions of life, for instance, did not meet their sense that in this clause they were considering sweeping systematic efforts to kill members of a group, doing so through means such as deprivation of food or water, forced marches, or other means of oppression that would clearly lead to the widespread loss of life of this particular population.

Calculation: The framers were seeking evidence that these actions were organized to lead to the outcome of widespread death, even if that outcome did not occur. Calculation could be found in the design of the acts, not in what consequences took place. If the design of the actions was to deprive a population of food to such an extent that, if carried out in full, everyone in that group would die, then even if the process did not run to full completion, the calculated attempt to impose these conditions would meet the meaning of this clause.

Deliberate: In terms of intent, two layers of context must be addressed. The first is that the entire Convention is read within the opening language of Article II, as noted earlier. The second layer is introduced into this clause (c) only, whereby it is said that these actions must be undertaken "deliberately." Here, based on the *travaux preparatoires* and commentaries, the interpretation of "deliberately" is that the deaths caused by infliction of these conditions would arise from conscious intended omission of necessary life supports. (Deaths from negligence or inattention would not meet this standard.) In the view of the framers of the Convention, actions such as those taken by the Turkish government to forcibly deprive Armenian populations of food on forced marches, and actions undertaken against the Indian populations in Guatemala, whereby all means of livelihood were stripped away from them, constituted deliberate interventions to deny these populations the capacity to support themselves through difficult circumstances. Such deliberate acts of deprivation or denial, undertaken with the calculation of leading to the ultimate mass death of these populations, are the subject of this particular clause.

In terms of the facts as gathered for the case of Darfur, it is necessary to understand the notion of "physical conditions of life" in a somewhat broader vein than what the framers of the convention envisioned and rely on a mix of common sense and pattern formation to make an assessment of deliberate intent.

In the Genocide Convention, the concept of "physical conditions of life" referred to a narrow construct that to live, human beings need food, shelter, water, and protection from severe stress, such as harsh environments or grossly punishing physical activity like forced marches through forbidding terrain. Recent scholarship on livelihoods incorporates and expands on this notion of physical conditions of life, by recognizing that many populations on earth surmount difficult physical environments by developing a range of key inputs and strategies that permit them to persist in barren and harsh surroundings (Toulmin and Quan, 2000; Deininger, 2003). In rural Africa, stable access to land and enduring social relationships sustain survival of families, groups, and communities. These two parameters have been underscored in studies of livelihoods among the people of Darfur (De Waal, 2005; Young et al., 2005).

These assessments of how human beings have carved out a survivable ecological niche in even the most meager settings, by developing livelihood strategies that intertwine with resources of land and the climate, provide an analytic perspective on what is at stake in creating or destroying the physical conditions of life referred to in the Genocide Convention.

As the PHR investigators have sought to establish in their recent work on destruction of livelihoods in Darfur (PHR, in press), to survive in the increasingly dry savannah, near-desert conditions of the region has required a complex and highly evolved set of strategies around land use, livestock holdings, market interactions, savings and intergenerational transfer of wealth, and tightly reciprocal and diversified systems of social support. Without continual hard work and accumulated inputs, the land of Darfur does not provide the physical conditions of life. All environments that support human existence are a finely wrought meshing of human inputs and natural characteristics (from water holes and paths to bridges and utility grids). Darfur presents a particularly stark example of this interdependence.

All analysts and humanitarian aid workers in the region have noted the elements of livelihood destruction meted out by the attacking forces of the GOS and Janjaweed. Virtually all reports have described the extent and thoroughness of the eradication meted out in these attacks: the earth was scorched, all buildings burnt and scattered, stray cook pots were crushed, trees stood as blackened trunks. To exact this toll on one village, let alone the thousands so destroyed, requires time, planning, effort, and motivation. Further note has been made of the consistently observed follow-up assault on survivors of these attacks, the hot pursuit that forced them to abandon any goods or animals they had tried to salvage in their flight, the harassment of remnant groups attempting to hide in the barren hills and plains, and the obstruction of humanitarian aid when the international community has tried to find and reach these groups of people.

What might be the rationale? The Sudanese government knows full well the exigencies of life in the remoter reaches of this region. In Darfur, lives are tied to livelihoods. To annihilate a people does not require killing and raping the great majority, when their existence is shaped by their relationships to each other and their land and livestock. Drive them from their villages, scatter them widely, block the reach of aid groups, and many will die in the bush and many will languish in camps. As the years drag by, their options for return wither.

A sustained campaign that inflicts sweeping attacks on villages, obliteration of built structures, and forced movement of people into terrain where they cannot survive without assistance and where that assistance is subsequently impeded suggests a pattern of calculated action, deliberately imposed, in such a way that permits the application of clause (c) of the Genocide Convention.

Looking Ahead

Documentation and argument are the tools of human rights investigators and genocide scholars. Presented here is a documented pattern of devastation and death that arguably cumulates to the obliteration of physical conditions conducive to the life of a population. The epidemiological tools of the public health community linked to detailed descriptive analysis of livelihoods would suggest that what is now happening in Darfur warrants the application of Article II (c) of the Genocide Convention. To date, this argument has not proved persuasive to the international policy community (Pursuant to Security Council Resolution, 2004). The great powers are reluctant to intervene on any grounds, genocide or not, against the sovereignty of Sudan.

Although the analytic efforts of outside observers have been insufficient to thwart the killings, rapes, and forced displacement of this population, they have served to raise awareness and help sustain the humanitarian response. Relief aid from many sources and meager security efforts on the part of the African Union now shore up large remnants within Darfur. Refugees in Chad persist in some mix of hope and misery. In the fullness of time, more evidence will be unearthed and more will become known regarding the intentions of the Sudanese government and the impact of its actions on the Black Africans of Darfur. For now an open question remains as to whether historians at some later date will affirm that what we are witnessing today is some version of slow-motion genocide or a crime against humanity. It is certainly no less than one of these.

Notes

1. Sudan acceded to the Genocide Convention (the legal equivalent of signing and ratifying it) on October 13, 2003.

2. Controversy has diminished as to whether the population under attack meets the definition of a designated group in the terms of the Genocide Convention, because the preponderance of accumulating evidence continues to suggest that the Black Africans of Darfur, who belong to distinct African tribes and speak the language of these tribes as their first language and Arabic as their second, are singularly targeted for attack by the Arab Janjaweed and GOS forces and stigmatized in these attacks with derogatory terms for "black."

References

Amnesty International. 2004. *Sudan, Darfur: Rape as a weapon of war. Sexual violence and its consequences.* AFR 54/1076/2004. July 19. www.web.amnesty.org.

Berkman, L. F., and Kawachi, I. 2000. A historical framework for social epidemiology. In *Social epidemiology,* ed. L. F. Berkman and I. Kawachi, 3–12. New York: Oxford University Press.

Centers for Disease Control and Prevention (CDC). 2004. Emergency nutrition assessment of crisis affected populations Darfur region, Sudan. August-September 2004. Atlanta: CDC; Rome, Italy: U.N. World Food Programme. www.cdc.gov/nceh/ierh (accessed December 29, 2005).

Checchi, F., and Roberts, L. 2005. Interpreting and using mortality data in humanitarian emergencies: A primer for non-epidemiologists. *Humanitarian practice network paper,* no. 52. September. London: Overseas Development Institute.

Deininger, K. 2003. Land policies for growth and poverty reduction. *World bank policy research report.* Washington, D.C.: World Bank; New York: Oxford University Press.

Depoortere, E., Checchi, F., Broillet, F., Gerstl, S., Minetti, A., Gayraud, O., Briet, V., Pahl, J., Defourny, I., Tatay, M., and Brown, V. 2004. Violence and mortality in West Darfur, Sudan (2003-04): Epidemiological evidence from four surveys. *The Lancet* 364:1315–20.

De Waal, A. 2005. *Famine that kills. Darfur, Sudan.* Revised edition. New York: Oxford University Press.

Fein, H. 2001. The three P's of genocide prevention: With application to a genocide foretold—Rwanda. In *Protection against Genocide,* ed. N. Riemer, 45–66. Westport, CT: Praeger.

FEWSNET famine early warning systems network. www.fewsnet.org/ (accessed December 29, 2005).

Gillately, R., and Kiernan, B., eds. 2003. *The specter of genocide: Mass murder in historical perspective.* Cambridge: Cambridge University Press.

Gingerich, T., and Leaning, J. 2004. The use of rape as a weapon of war in the conflict in Darfur, Sudan. Report prepared for the U.S. Agency for International Development with assistance from Physicians for Human Rights, Boston and Washington, D.C., October.

Grandesso, F., Sanderson, F., Kurijt, J., Koene, T., and Brown, V. 2005. Mortality and malnutrition among populations living in South Darfur, Sudan: Results of three surveys, September 2004. *Journal of the American Medical Association* 293:1490–94.

Guha-Sapir, D., and Degomme, O. 2005. Darfur: *Counting the deaths. Mortality estimates from multiple survey data.* Centre for Research on the Epidemiology of Disasters (CRED). Brussels, Belgium: University of Louvain School of Public Health, May 26, 2005.

Harff, B. 2002. Early warning and genocide prevention. In *Will genocide ever end?,* ed. C. Rittner, J. K. Roth, and J. M. Smith, 127–30. Aegis. St. Paul, MN: Paragon House.

International Criminal Tribunal for Rwanda, Prosecutor v. Akayesu: Judgment (September 2, 1998), ICTR-96-4-T, para 688 and 731.

International Criminal Tribunal for Rwanda, Prosecutor v. Akayesu: Judgment (September 2, 1998), ICTR-96-4-T, paras 112–29.

International Development Research Centre. December 2001. *The responsibility to protect.* Report of the International Commission on Intervention and State Sovereignty. Ottawa, Ontario, Canada.

Leaning, J. 2002. Identifying precursors. In *Will genocide ever end?,* ed. C. Rittner, J. K. Roth, and J. M. Smith, 117–22. Aegis. St. Paul, MN: Paragon House.

Leaning, J. 2004. Human rights: Diagnosing genocide. The Case of Darfur. Perspectives. *New England Journal of Medicine* 351:735–38.

Leaning, J., and VanRooyen, M. 2005. An assessment of mortality studies in Darfur, 2004-05. *Humanitarian Exchange.* June 30, 2005. www.odihpn.org.

Médicins Sans Frontières Holland (MSF Holland). 2005. *The crushing burden of rape: Sexual violence in Darfur.* March 8, 2005. www.artsenzondergrenzen.nl.

Omar, S. A. S., Briskey, E., Misak, R., and Asem, A. A. S. O. 2000. The Gulf War impact on the terrestrial environment of Kuwait: An overview. In *The environmental consequences of war: Legal, economic, and scientific perspectives,* ed. J. E. Austin and C. E. Bruch, 316–37. Cambridge: Cambridge University Press.

Physicians for Human Rights (PHR). 2004. *PHR calls for intervention to save lives in Sudan: Field team compiles indicators of genocide.* June 23. www.phrusa.org/research/sudan/pdf/sudang_genocide_report.pdf (accessed December 29, 2005).

Physicians for Human Rights (PHR). January 2006. *Darfur: Assault on Survival: A Call for Security, Justice and Restitution.* www.phrusa.org/research/sudan.

Prevent Genocide International. June 15, 2004. *Convention on the prevention and pun-*

ishment of the crime of genocide. Laws against genocide. www.preventgenocide.org/law/convention/

Pursuant to Security Council Resolution 1564 of 18 September 2004. Geneva, 25 January 2005. *Report of the International Commission of Inquiry on Darfur to the United Nations Secretary-General.* www.un.org/News/dh/Sudan/com_inq_darfur.pdf.

Schabas, W. 2002. *Genocide in international law: The crime of crimes.* Cambridge: Cambridge University Press.

Staub, E. 1989. *The roots of evil: The origins of genocide and other group violence.* New York: Cambridge University Press.

Toulmin, C., and Quan, J. 2000. Evolving land rights, tenure and policy in Sub-Saharan Africa. In *Evolving land rights, policy and tenure in Africa*, ed. C. Toulmin and J. Quan. London: Department for International Development.

U.N. Doc S/1999/957. September 8 1999. Report of the Secretary General on protection of civilians in armed conflicts.

U.N. Doc A/55/985-S/2001/574. 7 June 2001. Report of the Secretary General on the prevention of armed conflict.

Westing, A. 1980. *Warfare in a fragile world: Military impact on the human environment.* Stockholm International Peace Research Institute. London: Taylor & Francis.

World Health Organization (WHO). 2004. *Retrospective mortality survey among the internally displaced population, Greater Darfur, Sudan, August 2004.* September 15. Geneva: WHO.

Young, H., Osman, A., Akililu, Y., Dale, R., and Badri, B. 2005. Darfur, livelihoods under siege. Report prepared for the United States Agency for International Development Agency. Medford, MA, and Washington, D.C.

10

Public Health Research in a Human Rights Crisis

The Effects of the Thai "War on Drugs"

Susan G. Sherman, Ph.D., M.P.H.,
Apinun Aramrattana, M.D., Ph.D., and
David D. Celentano, Sc.D., M.H.S.

Thailand's beauty and hospitality has made it one of the most desirable tourist destinations in the world. The "war on drugs," announced by then Prime Minister Thaksin Shinawatra in February 2003, is an unfortunate example of the harshness that can lie beneath the surface of Thailand's beauty. The ostensibly peaceful presentation of Thai culture covers a history of repressive military regimes, mixed policies toward ethnic minorities, and government involvement in rights violations. The war on drugs was a direct assault on some of the already most marginalized members of Thai society—drug users and ethnic minorities. And the war violated international human rights treaties and covenants to which Thailand is a signatory.

Our collaborative group had been working on HIV prevention and care research in Thailand for more than a decade preceding the abrupt change in policy that the war represented. During those years, Thailand was internationally known for its progressive response to the epidemic, and for a gradually maturing democracy and growing civil society. With our Thai colleagues, we had successfully conducted studies of HIV in sex workers, soldiers, ethnic minorities, and drug users. All of this changed abruptly after February 2003 and the launch of the war. The policy shift meant that our study participants were being threatened in the most direct way. We were forced to cease ongoing activities and to retool our effort toward understanding the impact of the war, and attempting to mitigate its harms, for our research participants. We learned a hard lesson shared by many other scientists: the context of human rights can shift quickly, and can dramatically affect the ability to conduct research. We attempt here to describe these efforts and to discuss the research methods and findings from our work.

In 2003, the "war on drugs," or the "war," had a direct impact on a joint research program of Johns Hopkins Bloomberg School of Public Health and Chiang Mai University. We were doing formative research in advance of a large behavioral intervention targeting young methamphetamine users. The war required us to essentially stop our research and shift our focus to using our research skills and extensive connections with drug users to document the effects of the war on their lives and drug use patterns. In this chapter, we describe the results of in-depth interviews and a rapid assessment, conducted in August 2004, with injection drug users to gauge how this government policy unfolded at the street level.

Conducting research with marginalized populations is challenging in many contexts. Substance use research highlights structural inequities, such as poverty and racism, in most societies and has the potential to perpetuate or dispel stereotypes about study participants. Research focusing on the causes and consequences of drug use as well as related interventions must be executed with care to protect the rights of participants. Such research is most credible when it is objective in both its conception and execution. Credibility is also derived when researchers are conscious of the implications of their work on the lives and well-being of the study participants and broader target society where they live. The very act of performing research in the context of a war against the study population—in this case, drug users—could have resulted in significant misinterpretation of our data. We describe the data and the process of doing our research to ensure that the research itself would not incur further harm on the study participants, while at the same time ensuring the safety and well-being of the study staff.

The Historical Background to Thailand's War on Drugs

The Thai government's war on drugs, announced in early 2003, was an official effort to abate the supply of and demand for drugs in the Kingdom of Thailand. It was waged against an historical backdrop of multiple interventions by successive Thai governments in the complicated socioeconomic and political environment of Southeast Asia. These actions reflected Thai interests and U.S. pressure and global interests in the midst of the Cold War (Walker, 1991); the significant level of government corruption and involvement in drug trafficking (Walker, 1991; McAllister, 2000); and larger efforts to control and reduce the autonomy of nonethnic Thai people living in the upper-north of the country.

In 1958, the Thai government bowed to U.S. pressure to make opium production and consumption illegal (Walker, 1991; McAllister, 2000). One result was a rapid rise of heroin consumption by former opium users (Westermeyer, 1976). The escalation of heroin consumption in Thailand, with its more sophisticated production methods, paved the way for the creation of drug cartels. Police protection and cooperation created deep-rooted bribery and widespread legal complicity in the drug economy, leading to a more general breakdown in the respect for the rule of law, creating a climate where human rights were frequently violated (Westermeyer, 1976).

In Thailand, as in other countries, drug use is largely left to the jurisdiction of criminal justice, with the focus on supply reduction. The approach to demand reduction through drug treatment is underfunded and has been slow to develop. The combination of a lack of drug treatment orientation with a well-articulated code of criminalization for drug possession often results in human rights violations. This is compounded in Thailand where ethnic minorities historically raised opium for traditional medicinal purposes and local use (Renard, 2001; Report of Thailand to the U.N. Human Rights Committee, 2004).

The Spread of the Use of Methamphetamine

According to Thai military officials, the foremost threat to Thailand's national security is on its northern border, a mass of "highly addictive methamphetamine pills" (Global Security, 2005). The growing methamphetamine epidemic is associated with several far-reaching political and economic factors influencing supply and demand. With the eradication of methamphetamine labs in Thailand in the early 1990s, Burma became the largest manufacturer and exporter of methamphetamine in the region. The use of methamphetamine rapidly expanded from use as a work aid by fishermen, laborers, and long-distance truck drivers into the Thai youth culture during the rapid economic expansion of the early and mid-1990s (Verachai et al., 2001). The use increased further during the 1997–1998 Asian economic crisis when many users created income by becoming small-time dealers (Phongpaichit and Baker, 2004). Sixty percent of new methamphetamine users are between 15 and 19 years old (Verachai et al., 2001), and 41.2 percent of male students and 19.0 percent of female students report ever using methamphetamine (Sattah et al., 2002). The proliferation of use in the general population was the rationale for the Thai government's 2003 war on drugs.

The Human Rights Context

Although a new democratic constitution was enacted in 1997, in part, to prevent a return to the tradition of military dictatorships in Thailand, military and police practices have been slow to change (Asian Legal Resource Centre [ALRC], 2005). Abuses are allegedly common and no external agency is charged with inspecting police torture, contravening the state's responsibility to oversee matters of human rights, according the National Human Rights Commission of Thailand (ALRC, 2005). Although the Thai National Human Rights Commission is charged with ensuring the protection of human rights in Thailand, its power has been limited. Unfortunately, the war against drug users has effectively whittled away many of the constitutional rights guaranteed to citizens, returning to the old authoritarian rule.

The War Policy

On February 1, 2003, the government of the former prime minister of Thailand, H.E. Pol. Lt. Col. Thaksin Shinawatra enacted policies that began a war on drugs (Office of the Narcotic Control Board, 2003a). The main objectives were to reduce the supply of and demand for illicit drugs throughout the kingdom. The climate of fear and eventual disregard for human rights created by these policies were encapsulated by Interior Minister Wan Muhamad Nor

Matha's January 2003 comments on the fate of drug dealers, "They will be put behind bars or even vanish without a trace. Who cares? They are destroying our country."

The war had three phases. The first phase, lasting three months, targeted drug users who were encouraged to volunteer for drug treatment in thousands of newly established rehabilitation centers located in community hospitals and health centers, as well as short-term military-style drug rehabilitation "boot camps." Drug users spent 4 to 21 days in the camps participating in physical activities and learning "life skills" that were intended to enable them to subsequently live drug-free in their communities.

Drug users who did not volunteer for drug treatment as of April 21, 2003, were targeted for compulsory treatment administered by the Thai Ministry of Justice. All known drug users and dealers who had not reported themselves to government authorities were placed on highly publicized lists and given to local law enforcement officials. Communities were pressed to turn in drug users on the lists to local police for them to be placed in the appropriate level of treatment.

Drug users were assigned to facilities by a team of public health, psychological, and probation personnel to one of four treatment modalities depending on drug use patterns and the amount of drugs in their possession on arrest: (1) in custody of probation office and sentenced to a military boot camp for four months; (2) in custody of probation office placed at an in-patient drug treatment facility; (3) retained in the custody of their local community; or (4) mandated to report on a regular basis to the probation office. Most drug users were assigned to boot camps or remanded to local probation offices where they participated in life skills training. The government also attempted to reduce supply through targeted arrests of drug syndicates and confiscation of drug supplies, drug-manufacturing equipment and chemicals, and large quantities of cash.

Based on the significant numbers of drug users who completed treatment and the large number of drug users and dealers who were arrested, the Thai government reported success in the initial phase of the war. In the first four months of the campaign, according to the Office of the Narcotic Control Board an estimated 285,200 drug users had turned themselves in to government authorities for drug treatment and a total of 55,983 people were arrested for the following charges: 353 were charged with the production of drugs;

1,729 were charged with large-scale sales; 14,585 were charged with the sale of small quantities; 19,663 were charged with drug possession; and 19,653 were charged with drug use (Office of the Narcotic Control Board, 2003c). The police confiscated an estimated 1,360 million baht (US$33.4 million) (Office of the Narcotic Control Board, 2003c).

As of April 16, 2003, a reported 2,275 drug dealers and drug users had been killed, with only 51 reportedly at the hands of the police (Office of the Narcotic Control Board, 2003c). The government blamed the remainder on large-scale drug dealers attempting to prevent underlings and users from turning their suppliers in to authorities. These latter killings are called *kha htad hton*, which translates as "cutting the links" to that person in the network. In the context of the war, the phrase refers to targeted killings along a chain of command in the drug economy, to obfuscate the identity of those above that person. In the context of human rights, virtually all of these killings are extrajudicial executions until fully investigated.

Article 6 of the International Covenant on Civil and Political Rights guarantees to individuals the right to life. In codifying this, the Thai state penal code clearly expresses that "When military and police or the officers of the administrative agencies kill a person, they are guilty of homicide under Section 288 or 289 of the Penal Code and shall be penalized accordingly like any other citizens" (ALRC, 2003). The lack of responsibility taken by the government to even investigate the extrajudicial killings grossly violates this code.

In disclaiming official responsibility for the large number of deaths, Mr. Thaksin said, "In this "war," drug dealers must die. But we don't kill them. It's a matter of bad guys killing bad guys." Few in Thailand found this explanation credible, in particular, after his subsequent statement in August 2003, that Thai security forces "would shoot to kill" when they encountered Burmese drug traffickers: "Their drugs have gradually killed our children, so we won't spare them."

This new war on drugs created tremendous pressure on many segments of Thai society, in particular, in those communities with high rates of drug use. Local leaders were forced to produce lists of resident drug users and dealers, which resulted in widespread discrimination toward all drug users, in particular, in rural areas. Coercive financial incentives were used to pressure community leaders to turn in suspects. The concept of *kha htad hton* became an opportunity for retribution and the settling of old scores.

Northern Thailand

Northern Thailand, with its proximity to drug-production areas in Myanmar, is characterized by high rates of heroin injection and methamphetamine smoking (Razak et al., 2003). Table 10.1 shows the official number of individuals directly affected by the war in northern Thailand (Office of the Northern Region Narcotic Control Board, 2003). During the first three months of the new drug policy, more than 105,000 drug users and drug dealers turned themselves in to government authorities in this region. Almost 15,000 were arrested and charged with the production of drugs and/or drug sales. In the first four months of the campaign, 533 campaign-related murders were reported in Chiang Mai, 29 of whom were drug dealers shot by police during attempted arrests, and the remaining 504 were deemed *Kha htad hton* killings (Office of the Northern Region Narcotic Control Board, 2003).

Researching Downstream Health Effects of the War on Drugs

At the outbreak of the war, our research team was conducting formative research in preparation for two large-scale intervention studies with the shared aims of HIV reduction among injection drug users (IDUs) and methamphetamine users and their social networks. The war effectively stopped our research because of safety issues for study staff and participants. We used our connections and established trust with the drug-using community and conducted several rapid assessments with IDUs and young methamphetamine users to document the effects of the new drug policies on the drug users themselves.

The methods and data presented in this chapter are derived from two separate data-collection efforts: (1) in-depth interviews with 35 IDUs that were conducted before the war and (2) a rapid assessment of 183 IDUs in August 2003, six months after the war had been declared. The current analysis compares those who reported having attended and not attended treatment camp during the drug war, a central component of the government's treatment campaign.

Determining the Study Sample

From February 2002 to February 2003, we conducted qualitative research in the northern province of Chiang Mai. A total of 263 IDUs recruited from

Table 10.1. Thai "War on Drugs" in Northern Thailand, February–April 2003

Turned themselves in to authorities under new law
   88,545 drug users arrested
   15,710 drug dealers
Arrested/charged with drug production and sales   14,080
Murdered in Chiang Mai   533
   29 claimed by police
   504 deemed killed by people in the drug trade

a variety of sources: the regional drug treatment center; a methadone clinic situated in central Chiang Mai; urban drug hot spots; and rural health centers and villages located throughout the province. The onset of the war and hostile environment delayed the initiation of our intervention trials, which had been scheduled to begin in mid-2003.

Before participating, respondents completed informed consent procedures in the Thai language. Respondents received no financial incentive for participation, but were given a project t-shirt and snack. The Thai Ministry of Public Health Ethical Committee, the Human Experiment Committee of Chiang Mai University, and the Johns Hopkins Bloomberg School of Public Health Committee on Human Research approved the formative study.

Collecting Qualitative Data

The study design included plans for collecting both qualitative and quantitative data. The semistructured interview guide consisted of questions addressing a variety of topics, including family history, drug use patterns and influences, sexual behavior, history of incarceration and arrest, drug cessation history, and drug treatment experiences in treatment camps. In-depth interviews ranging from forty-five minutes to one and a half hours were conducted in Thai and tape recorded. The recordings were transcribed and then translated into English for data analysis. Translations were reviewed for accuracy of language and meaning by project staff members fluent in both languages.

Collecting Quantitative Data

After providing informed consent, we administered a brief questionnaire to study participants. The survey was conducted in the same venues used in the formative data-collection phase, including: local health clinics; a project house in Chiang Mai city; and participants' homes. The survey examined demographic characteristics, past (the six-and three-month period before being interviewed, indicated as February and May, respectively) and current drug use patterns, past (in the six- and three-month period before being interviewed, indicated as February and May, respectively) and current drug treatment participation; history of arrest; and the effects of war on participants and their social networks. No identifying information was recorded on the survey instrument.

Analyzing the Qualitative Data

After reviewing several interviews for comprehension of interview content, we chose five interviews with particularly in-depth responses for open coding, a process of reading small segments of text at a time and making notations in the margins regarding content or analytic thought, without being constrained by existing theoretical explanations (Strauss and Corbin, 1997). The labels applied in the open coding process were then synthesized into a code list to remove redundancy and similar labels were grouped together. The resulting list was used to code another five interviews, after which the code list was refined by collapsing lower-level codes into broader thematic categories and including additional codes for emergent themes. The code list was then used to code the remaining interviews. As new themes emerged, the code list was refined and previously coded interviews were recoded as necessary. Two interviewers conducted the process and the code list was finalized after comparing their respective coding schemes. Data were entered into Atlas-ti (version 4.2), a qualitative data-management program, to organize coding and memos.

Analyzing the Quantitative Data

Univariate analyses were conducted for all variables. Data were analyzed by using Chi-square test for differences in proportions and Fisher's exact test was used for comparisons of small numbers. Multiple logistic regression techniques were used to estimate the adjusted odds ratios (AORs) and 95 percent confidence intervals (CIs) associated with having been in a treatment camp. All variables with a p-value of 0.10 or less in bivariate logistic models were included in multivariate logistic models. Manual backward stepwise regression models were used to develop the final multivariate models. All analyses were stratified by ethnicity based on a number of differences between the

Table 10.2. Sociodemographic characteristics of injection drug users in Chiang Mai, Province, Thailand, August 2003, by treatment camp status

Variable	Total (n = 183) N (%)	No treatment camp (n = 116) N (%)*	Treatment camp (n = 67) N (%)*	p-value
Male	158 (86.3)	100 (86.2)	58 (86.6)	0.95
Median age (IQR)†	32 (27–42)	30 (26–40)	39 (29–43)	0.01
Ever married	130 (71.0)	73 (62.9)	57 (85.1)	0.002
District of current residence				
Rural (vs. urban rural)	116 (64.3)	57 (49.1)	108 (88.1)	<0.0001
Thai (vs. ethnic minority)	86 (47.0)	33 (28.4)	53 (79.1)	<0.0001

*Column percent
†IQR, interquartile range

two groups. SAS 6.12 (SAS Institute, Cary, North Carolina) was used in data analysis.

These rapid assessments were the first systematic documentation of the war's effects on drug users. Although the samples are relatively small in relation to the expansive scope of the war, it provides an indication of how the war affected the lives and drug use of IDUs who live in a region particularly affected by the war's policies, northern Thailand.

Documenting Health Effects

The overall goal of the analysis was to document the effect of the Thai drug war on active drug users at the community level, a study that had not been done before. We were able to take advantage of the ethnographic work we had previously conducted as a baseline to compare the situation six months after the implementation of the war, when we conducted a rapid survey of the drug users in our studies.

Conducting a Rapid Survey

More than one-third of the study sample reported having participated in a drug treatment camp since the initiation of the drug war. The top three reasons cited for going to a treatment camp were that participants were forced to go (37%), they wanted to stop injecting drugs (20%), or they wanted to decrease their quantity of drug use (5%).

The sample's demographic characteristics are shown in Table 10.2. Study participants were predominantly male and the median age was 32 years old.

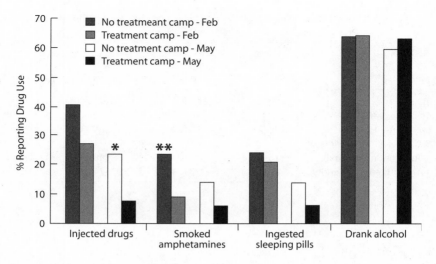

Figure 10.1. Reported patterns of drug use in February and May 2003 among 183 IDUs, Chiang Mai Province, Thailand, by treatment camp status. *p < 0.01. **p < 0.05.

There were several demographic differences between those who reported having attended treatment camp in the preceding six months and those who had not, including older age, a higher percentage having been married, a higher percentage residing in rural (versus urban) areas, and a higher percentage being ethnic Thai.

Figure 10.1 displays self-reported drug use patterns in February and May 2003, comparing those who did and did not attend treatment camps during the first six months of the war. For all four categories, the highest percentage of drug use was reported by IDUs in February 2003 who had not attended a treatment camp. Compared with those who did not attend camps, IDUs who did were significantly more likely to report injecting drugs and smoking amphetamines in May 2003. Clearly, the higher risk and more drug-involved persons participated in the treatment camps, but that participation apparently did not have the desired outcome (i.e., abstinence).

Table 10.3 shows injection and drug treatment patterns as well as the effects of the war on IDUs and their social networks. Participants who had attended treatment camps began injecting at a significantly younger age than those who had not, and were significantly less likely to report recently injecting drugs. Two-thirds of the sample reported injecting with a new syringe at their last injection, and among those who injected drugs after the initiation of the war (n = 65), 35 percent reported syringe sharing. Close to 85 percent of the sample reported "ever" having been in drug treatment, with no differences between those who were and were not in a treatment camp during the war.

A significantly higher percentage of those who did not attend treatment camp had been arrested during the war than those who had attended treatment camp. More than half of participants knew someone who was arrested during the war, 10 percent knew someone who was forced to flee from their community during the war, and more than one-fifth knew someone who was killed for drug-related activities during the war.

Results from multivariate logistic models are shown in Table 10.4. Factors that were statistically significantly associated with attending a treatment camp during the war were ever having been married (adjusted odds ratio [AOR]: 2.6; 95% confidence interval [CI]: 1.1–6.0) and being an ethnic minority (AOR: 8.9; 95% CI: 4.3–18.4).

In-depth interviews conducted with IDUs provide an insider's perspective on IDUs' experiences with the war, and provided us with an understanding of how injection practices were affected by the broader context, in particular, the constant fear of and past experiences with police.

Following Up with In-depth Interviews

We also attempted to determine the impact of the war using less-structured questioning, which allowed participants to talk about their experiences and to be less "invasive" in our approach. These data were collected to provide a more comprehensive picture of the war's effects on community residents. Ninety percent of the participants were male, all were ethnic Thais, and the median age was 38 years. Half of the 35 in-depth interviews mentioned police in relation to responses regarding where and how they inject drugs. Several themes emerged relating to effects of police on the participants' injection behaviors, including the influence of police on injection practices and fear; police crackdown effecting a change in both routes of administration and drugs of choice, namely from injecting drugs to methamphetamine smoking; and paying off police in lieu of being arrested.

The following quote exemplifies the influence of police on injection practices and fear. A 33-year-old male was responding to a question regarding if the place of heroin purchase is the same as of drug use:

Table 10.3. Injection, drug treatment history, and effects of the war on IDUs and their social networks among injection drug users in Chiang Mai, Province, August 2003, by treatment camp status

Variable	Total (n = 183) N (%)	No treatment camp (n = 116) N (%)*	Treatment camp (n = 6 7) N (%)*	p-value
Median age of injection drug use initiation (IQR)[†]	24 (19–31)	21.5 (18–26.5)	30 (23–39)	<0.0001
When was your most recent injection?				
>3 months ago	145 (79.2)	84 (72.4)	61 (91.0)	0.003
≤3 months	38 (20.8)	32 (27.6)	6 (9.0)	
In the most recent time you injected, you injected with a new syringe and needle	122 (66.7)	81 (69.8)	41 (61.2)	0.23
Among those who injected after February 2003 (n = 65):				
Shared any syringe/needle since February 2003	23 (35.4)	19 (40.4)	4 (22.2)	0.17
Ever joined a drug treatment program	155 (84.7)	95 (81.9)	60 (89.6)	0.17
Effects of the "War on Drugs" on IDUs and other drug users				
Arrested by police during the War	20 (10.9)	17 (14.7)	3 (4.5)	0.03
Knows someone who was arrested for drug-related activities during the War	95 (55.9)	64 (57.7)	31 (52.5)	0.52
Knows someone who was forced to flee from their community because of the War	16 (9.5)	8 (7.4)	8 (13.3)	0.21
Knows someone who was killed for drug-related activities during the War	36 (20.8)	19 (17.4)	17 (26.6)	0.47

*Column percent
[†]IQR, interquartile range

Table 10.4. Final multivariate model of treatment camp status—
using forward stepwise regression

Variable	Multivariate OR (95% CI)	*p*-value
Ever married	2.6 (1.1-6.0)	0.03
Ethnicity		
Ethnic minority (vs. Thai)	8.9 (4.3-18.4)	<0.0001

We have to get out as quick as possible and inject at some other places. . . . The police may come because while we are using if the police pass and see they will seize us. When probed where the participant injects drugs, he responded, At some gas stations, but there we must play [inject] very quickly because the police always come. The boys in the station inform the police. If it's in the night we would use it on a nearby road, buy one bottle of water, draw water with a syringe and put heroin into a lid. We stay at the motor-bike and inject. After injection we pull out the needle and dispose it. My friend has another needle, do it very quickly. We carry it with us, we must save it.

The police crackdown affected the participants' reported drugs of choice as well as routes of administration. In describing his social network of drug users with whom he used to inject drugs before the war, a 28-year-old male said that there are no more IDUs in his village because "they are trying to suppress drugs." When asked why, he responded, "The police eliminate addicts. They are killing and shooting them. So, they are scared of being killed or shot to dead." Instead villagers turned to using methamphetamine, which ironically was the initial focus of the war.

Police corruption was a prevalent theme among study participants. Participants described paying off police in lieu of being arrested or being charged. A 26-year-old man described paying 8,000 Baht to police on his arrest so that he could be released. When asked if this was a common amount extorted in lieu of arrest, he responded, "They wanted 20,000 baht but I told them I didn't have much enough. If they still wanted 20,000 baht, they just put me in prison. I could afford only that amount." He further described the common practice of each participating drug user paying police 5,000 Baht to use drugs in a "protected" seller's house.

Assessing Effects and Implications

These two studies provide data that examine the effects of the Thai drug war on injection drug users. Our results suggest, in accordance with the goals of the war, that IDUs significantly reduced illicit drug consumption, with more than one-third of the sample reporting having attended a treatment camp. The decrease in drug consumption was seen in both IDUs who did and did not attend treatment camp, and we saw an increase over time in the first three months of the war, between February 2003 and May 2003. IDUs did report marked decreases in drug injection, although only two-thirds of the total sample reported injecting with sterile equipment. Alcohol use continued to be high and did not decrease in either group at either time. Alcohol drinking is normative in Thai culture and alcohol is widely available; alcohol was used as a substitute for the lack of illicit drugs.

The study demonstrates that rural IDUs were more greatly affected by the war than their urban counterparts. The aggressive execution of the war in rural areas is demonstrated by the large percentage of rural IDUs attending treatment camp—most of whom were ethnic minorities. The war's effects on ethnic minorities are framed by a long and contentious history of these quasi- and illegal residents of Thailand. Their tenuous relationship with the Thai government resulted in their being forced to treatment camps at the will of the Government. Being from rural areas and being an ethnic minority were the only significant factors associated with going to treatment camps in the multivariate model.

Although these findings indicate the goals of the war were met, this begs the ultimate question: at what cost was the war successful, as deemed by whom? Drug users were arrested and jailed without trial and many were executed with no warning, trial, or justification, as documented by human rights organizations such as the Asian Legal Resource Center (2005) and Human Rights Watch (2004).

Our qualitative results indicate that fear of police was pervasive in the months preceding the war. The effect of drug users' fear of police in relation to risky behaviors is well documented in the United States. Much of this research has examined the effects of drug paraphernalia laws, which are present in many states and prohibit the possession of drug paraphernalia (in general, defined as the presence of needles and syringes on a person if stopped by the police). Similar to what was expressed by IDUs in Thailand, both ethnographic and quantitative research findings indicate that IDUs are unwilling to carry syringes in the United States for fear of being stopped by the police (Feldman and Biernacki, 1988; Koester, 1994; Gleghorn et al., 1995; Grund et al., 1995; Bourgois, 1998; Clatts et al., 1998; Bluthenthal et al., 1999). The war on drug users' HIV risk behaviors will have an impact on the risk of HIV infection and transmission and will be reduced only if meaningful HIV prevention programs, which are not punitive in nature, target IDUs.

Our study results should be viewed in light of several limitations. First, the self-reported drug use data were collected in the context of an extremely aggressive war on study participants. Self-reported data are innately subject to social desirability bias but the current study's results could have been more influenced by this bias because of the fear engendered by the war. We believe that the effect of this bias was mitigated by the trust and familiarity that participants had with our study staff as well as the anonymous nature of the survey. Social desirability could have influenced the high rates of reported opiate injection. Additionally, the data regarding drug use patterns before the war were subject to greater recall bias than more recent behaviors. There might have been systematic differences among participants in the current study with the formative research participants whom we could not contact as well as drug users who were not a part of the formative research. Therefore, these results may not be generalized to the wider community of IDUs in northern Thailand.

Our investigation provides important information from the perspective of drug users themselves toward the Thai government's war on drug policy. The voices of drug users have only rarely been heard in any discussion of the war. Although many interviewed drug users expressed their support of the war, which reflects the sentiments of the Thai population at large, the fear that has permeated the lives of such drug users cannot be underestimated in influencing their stated beliefs.

Implications of the War

The effects of the Thai drug war both on the lives of drug users and on the broader Thai society are numerous and far-reaching. Thai drug users are some of the most marginalized members of Thai society and therefore an easy target of such aggressive policies. They lack a political constituency, capital, and resources to effectively influence policy. By arresting tens of thousands of drug users without proof of drug use, the government appears to be effectively winning the fight on drugs, at least as played out in local media. The support for the war by the general population should not be underestimated, as noted by opinion polls conducted during and following the war. However, such a war effectively drives IDUs underground and limits their access to needed health, prevention, treatment, and social resources. Numerous studies in the United States (Groseclose et al., 1995; Bluthenthal et al., 1999; Aitken et al., 2002) have documented rising rates of HIV and risky behaviors among IDUs during targeted police crackdowns. The further challenges to accessing sterile injection equipment could be associated with higher rates of HIV. The climate of fear and mistrust created in such a war negatively affects access to health care services, which include HIV testing and treatment.

There are numerous ramifications of the war on Thailand as a free, civil society. Although Mr. Thaksin campaigned for political office as a modernizer, many have seen his tactics as backward steps to the dark days of military rule in Thailand. The numerous human rights violations against drug users and dealers, regardless of their guilt, did not affect the Thai public's support of Thaksin, as demonstrated by his political party's overwhelming re-election in the fall of 2004.

Thailand's War on Drugs "victory" is temporary. This campaign has dramatically reduced the drug market at the local drug trafficker and street-user level, but at an extraordinary human cost. Furthermore, there is little evidence of lasting impact on cross-border trafficking or on the drug trade's higher elements. The battle against "dark influences" has been ineffective, with few arrests of high-level operatives. Although Thaksin's war has had a major impact on Thailand's drug problem, it should be viewed as one relatively successful campaign in a long war, not as a victorious end to the war itself. Of course, at the user level, the war was anything but a "success."

Thailand's constitutional monarch, while praising the former prime minister, called him to task during the annual birthday address by requesting a full inquiry into all drug-related deaths—a request celebrated by human rights and health agencies. However, the investigation will not be conducted by an independent source, so it is widely believed that the police and governmental agencies will be exonerated. Prime Minister Thaksin accepted the admonishment as a learning tool. Thaksin has initiated talks with Burma and Laos to discuss more stringent border control measures, as Burma and Laos continue to be major contributors to Thailand's drug problem.

Thailand's war did not fare well in the international court of opinion. Numerous editorials and governments admonished the policies (Tansubhapol-Vienma, 2003). An April 23, 2003, article in the *International Harold Tribune* stated that the state-sponsored war on drugs is rapidly undermining Thailand's long struggle to become one of Southeast Asia's leading democracies—and the civil rights of Thais. The war greatly deviates from Thailand's decade-long work toward building the rule of law.

Looking Ahead

The current study exemplifies the use of epidemiological research methods in the context of a government-endorsed countrywide human rights abusive campaign. Because of our long-term research investment and connection to Thailand and its citizens, as researchers we felt nothing short of a professional obligation to use research methods in documenting the effects of the war. Through our connections with the drug-using community as well as assurances provided by local police, we felt confident that we could conduct our research without threatening the safety of our staff and our study participants. Safety of both the staff and potential participants was of paramount importance and, if it was threatened, our research would have been halted.

Several unique factors placed us in a position to collect sensitive data with drug users at such a volatile time. The most important factor was the extensive formative research that gave us connections to key informants in the drug-using community, helped establish trust with IDUs, and provided us with information about the lives and behaviors of IDUs. Second, our research team in Thailand has strong connections with both the Ministry of Public Health and the Chiang Mai District Police. These long-standing connections were established far in advance of the formative research and are useful both in protecting the safety of our staff and study participants and ensuring that our research informs public health programming.

Through scientific inquiry, researchers are in a unique position to make evidence-based public health recommendations. With this privilege, researchers are obliged to ensure that their results are used to best aid the target population. This obligation shapes the types of research that are performed, the venues in which results are presented, and the context of broader social and political realities in which the research is performed—both positive and negative. Although researchers are somewhat limited in their ability to dramatically change the structure and context, which often contributes disproportionately to the burden of disease among marginalized populations, the very act of performing research might contribute to the alleviation of this burden.

Acknowledgments

This research was supported by the National Institute of Allergy and Infectious Disease Cooperative Agreement as a part of the HIV Prevention Trials Network (1U01 AI47984). We thank the study and participants for sharing their lives. We also thank Donald Gann and Teerada Sripaipan for their support in writing this chapter.

References

Aitken, C., Moore, D., Higgs, P., Kelsall, J., and Kerger, M. 2002. The impact of a police crackdown on a street drug scene: evidence from the street. *International Journal of Drug Policy* 13:189–98.

Asian Legal Resource Centre. 2003. *Special report: Extrajudicial killings of alleged drug dealers in Thailand.* www.article2.org/mainfile.php/0203/85/ (accessed November 29, 2005).

Asian Legal Resource Centre. 2005. *Institutionalised torture, extrajudicial killings and uneven application of the law in Thailand.* www.article2.org/mainfile.php/0402/186/ (accessed November 29, 2005).

Bluthenthal, R. N., Lorvick, J., Kral, A. H., Erringer, E. A., and Kahn, J. G. 1999. Collateral damage in the war on drugs: HIV risk behaviors among injection drug users. *International Journal of Drug Policy* 10:25–38.

Bourgois, P. 1998. The moral economies of homeless heroin addicts: confronting ethnography, HIV risk, and everyday violence in San Francisco shooting encampments. *Substance Use and Misuse* 33:2323–51.

Clatts, M., Sotheran, J. L., Luciano, P. A., Gallo, T. M., and Kochems, L. M. 1998. The impact of drug paraphernalia laws on HIV risk among persons who inject illegal drugs: Implications for public policy. In *How to legalize drugs*, ed. J. Fish. Northvale, NJ: Jason Aronson.

Feldman, H. W., and Biernacki, P. 1988. The ethnography of needle sharing among intravenous drug users and implications for public policies and intervention strategies. In: *Needle sharing among intravenous drug abusers: National and international perspectives*, ed. R. J. Battjes and R. W. Pickens, 28–39. Rockville, MD: National Institute on Drug Abuse.

Gleghorn, A. A., Jones, T. S., Doherty, M. C., et al. 1995. Acquisition and use of needles and syringes by injecting drug users in Baltimore, Maryland. *Journal of Acquired Immune Deficiency Syndromes* 10:97–103.

Global Security. 2005. "Thailand's Drug War" 2005. www.globalsecurity.org/military/world/war/thai-drug-war.htm (accessed November 29, 2005).

Groseclose, S. L., Weinstein, B., Jones, T. S., Valleroy, L. A., Fehrs, L. J., and Kassler, W. J. 1995. Impact of increased legal access to needles and syringes on practices of injecting-drug users and police officers, Connecticut, 1992–1993 [see comments.]. *Journal of Acquired Immune Deficiency Syndromes and Human Retrovirology* 10 (1):82–89.

Grund, J.-P. C., Heckathorn, D. D., Broadhead, R. S., and Anthony, D. 1995. In Eastern Connecticut, IDUs purchase syringes from pharmacies but don't carry syringes (Letter). *Journal of Acquired Immune Deficiency Syndromes* 10:104–5.

Human Rights Watch. 2004. *Thailand—not enough graves: The war on drugs, HIV/AIDS, and violations of human rights.* http://hrw.org/reports/2004/thailand0704/thailand0704.pdf/ (accessed November 29, 2005).

Koester, S. 1994. Copping, running, and paraphernalia laws: Contextual and needle risk behavior among injection drug users in Denver. *Human Organization* 53: 287–95.

McAllister, W. B. 2000. *Drug diplomacy in the twentieth century: An international history.* London: Routledge.

Office of the Narcotic Control Board. 2003a. *Thailand country report.* Available online at: www.oncb.go.th/PortalWeb/urlName.jsp?linkName=emain.htm.

Office of the Narcotic Control Board. 2003b. *Three months for fighting to over come illicit drug* (in Thai), DC002–2546.

Office of the Narcotic Control Board. 2003c. A report of War on Drugs results to Office of the Narcotic Control Board by Operation Centre, Office of National Police, Operation Centre for Fighting to Conquer Drug Problems, Ministry of Interior and Operation Centre for Fighting Drug Problems, and the Royal Thai Army during February 1 to April 30, 2003.

Office of the Northern Region Narcotic Control Board. 2003. A report of the War on Drugs situations and results during February 1 to April 30, 2003.

Phongpaichit, P., and Baker, C. 2004. *Thaksin: the business of politics in Thailand.* Chiang Mai: Silkworm Books.

Razak, M. H., Jittiwutikarn, J., Suriyanon, V., Vongchak, T., Srirak, N., Beyrer, C., et al. 2003. HIV prevalence and risk among injection and non-injection drug users in Northern Thailand: Need for comprehensive HIV prevention programs. *Journal of Acquired Immune Deficiency Syndrome* 33:259–66.

Renard, R. 2001. *Opium reduction in Thailand 1970–2000. A thirty year journey.* Bangkok: U.N. International Drug Control Programme. www.unodc.un.or.th/ad/publication/opium.pdf (accessed November 29, 2006).

Report on Thailand to the U.N. Human Rights Committee. 2004. www.ohchr.org/english/bodies/hrc/hrcs84.htm (accessed November 29, 2006).

Sattah, M. V., Supawitkul, S., Dondero, T. J., Kilmarx, P. H., Young, N. L., Mastro, T. D., et al. 2002. Prevalence of and risk factors for methamphetamine use in northern Thai youth: results of an audio-computer-assisted self-interviewing survey with urine testing. *Addiction* 97 (7):801–8.

Stein, M. D., Charuvastra, A., Anderson, B., Sobota, M., and Friedmann, P. D. 2002. Alcohol and HIV risk taking among intravenous drug users. *Addictive Behaviors* 27:727–36.

Strauss, A., and Corbin, J. 1990. *Basics of qualitative research: Grounded theory process and techniques.* Newbury Park, CA: Sage Publications.

Tansubhapol-Vienma, B. 2003. UN concerned by high death toll. *Bangkok Post.* May 13, A1.

Thai Ministry of Public Health, Epidemiology Bureau, Division of Disease Control. 2003. *AIDS situation in Thailand.* Bangkok.

Urbina, A., and Jones, K. 2004. Crystal methamphetamine, its analogues, and HIV infection: Medical and psychiatric aspects of a new epidemic. *Clinical Infectious Diseases* 38 (6):890–94.

Verachai, V., Dechongkit, S., Patarakorn, A., and Lukanapichonchut, L. 2001. Drug addicts treatment for ten years in Thanyarak Hospital (1989–1998). *Journal of the Medical Association of Thailand* 84 (1):24–29.

Walker, W. O. 1991. *Opium and foreign policy: The Anglo-American search for order in Asia, 1912–1954.* Chapel Hill: UNC Press.

Westermeyer, J. 1976 The pro-heroin effects of anti-opium laws in Asia. *Archives of General Psychiatry* 33 (9):1135–39.

Wolfe, D. 2004. Condemned to death. *The Nation* 278:16–18.

11

Maps in the Sand

Investigating Health and Human Rights in
Afghanistan and Darfur

Lynn Lawry, M.D., M.S.P.H., M.Sc.

The population-level study of the health consequences from human rights violations is a dynamic process that frequently requires creative adaptation to diverse and challenging settings. The foundation for this kind of work is the use of field-based population-level methods and statistical techniques that allow for accurate assessment of the rates and risks associated with rights violations. Doing this work in conditions marked by political instability and violence makes for unique and diverse challenges for investigators, field teams, and program staff members. In these unstable and often unsafe settings, it is necessary to modify our usual research methods in what might be called "research on the fly." As senior medical researcher for Physicians for Human Rights (PHR) and now as director of evidence-based research for International Medical Corps (IMC), I have led or participated in investigations in such diverse and difficult settings as Kosovo, Pakistan, Afghanistan, Sierra Leone, Nigeria, Iraq, and Sudan. This chapter is based on those experiences—and attempts to share what we have learned about ways to adapt research designs to fit both locale-specific cultural norms and political conditions on the ground.

In 2000 Physicians for Human Rights went to Afghanistan to evaluate and put into ethnographic context issues facing women living under the Taliban regime. The Taliban's restrictions on women's right to work, to move, and to seek medical care were reported to be undermining access to health care for women across Afghanistan. But hard data on the health effect of these policies were lacking. We sought to address this information gap by conducting health care access research. The Taliban regime was not known for its openness to Western research or investigative efforts. It would not have been possible for PHR to get into Afghanistan and do this work without the assistance of many courageous Afghans. And, getting permission from the Taliban to move forward was not easy. It began by meeting their hard-line foreign minister in Jalalabad over tea in 125-degree searing summer heat. I sat with my translator, a well-known community leader, explaining to him that we would be doing a study of women and their "needs" in his town. We deliberately called the human rights issues we would be investigating "needs and freedoms" so the minister would not suspect our true intentions. Knowing he could not read in either Dari, the language of the instrument or English, I handed him our survey. It was a bluff. We knew he would not reveal his illiteracy in front of a Western woman. In addition, our translator had cleverly changed any phrase with "Taliban" or "rights" to the "financial situation." As I pushed my hand across the table to hand him the papers, he raised his hand and put it to his heart, a common show of "I trust you" and sign of respect. It was his sign of approval. He produced for us a letter of safe passage for travel that permitted us to conduct the study. We knew how to work with this minister from studying Afghan culture, discussions with Afghan leaders, advice from our local colleagues, and observations made while doing everyday things like having tea and walking in the villages and markets. After this interview, each time our data collectors came to the phrase "financial situation" in the instrument, they knew to say instead, "Rights under the Taliban regime."

Linking Rights and Health

The investigation of health consequences due to human rights violations is critical for promoting health and for closing service gaps in health delivery for populations at risk in settings of civil chaos or among those living under repressive regimes. The Universal Declaration of Human Rights (UDHR, 1948) places human rights in two categories of civil and political rights and of economic, social, and cultural rights. Civil and political rights can be considered "individual freedoms," and include freedom from discrimination, torture, and arbitrary arrest; freedom of movement; freedom to participate in government and in public expression; and the right to asylum, fair trial, privacy, life, liberty, and security. Economic, social, and cultural rights may be termed "basic needs" and include the right to employment and education; to adequate nutrition, clean water, shelter, and health; to own property; and to protect one's interests. This last set of rights comprises some of the most commonly seen violations in conflict settings where camps house refugees and internally displaced persons (IDPs). In numerous instances Physicians for Human Rights and other rights organizations have documented the health consequences of rights violations (Mann et al., 1999).

Infractions of political rights can also have marked health consequences. Under the Taliban Afghan women were denied freedom of movement that could lead to their inability to access health care services. An Afghan woman was not allowed to travel to a health clinic without a *Mahram*, a male family member acting as escort (Amowitz et al., 2001). This meant it was not uncommon for pregnant women to wait to the last minute to come for prenatal care, presenting late in pregnancy and in extremis. Many doubtless died at home. In such instances, maternal mortality can be the result of abrogating rights as broadly defined by the Universal Declaration of Human Rights. Maternal morbidity and mortality statistics are indicative of the economic, social, and cultural rights afforded to women (Amowitz et al., 2002b, 2002c). Rights violations against women in societies where they are subordinate can include early and forced marriage, and an inability to negotiate the terms of sex including the use of contraception and birth spacing. The health consequences of these conditions include malnutrition with subsequent anemia, and chronic malnutrition in childhood that can produce stunted growth including the development of a smaller than normal pelvic outlet, which increases the risk of obstructed births with devastating consequences for both mother and baby. The rate of female immunization is another important indicator of the status of women. Lack of appropriate shelter and absence of clean water or sanitation further contribute to infection and complications to pregnancy and childbirth. Women's education is one of the best predictors of women's health (Reldman et al., 1989). All these indicators may be relevant to the design and conduct of field trials undertaken to investigate links between rights and health.

Physicians for Human Rights and International Medical Corps try to go beyond previous rights-based methodologies in several ways. First is to look at multiple measures of health status as opposed to single indicators such as mortality. Second is to use population-based sampling to obtain prevalence data and generate more valid denominators for rights violations and health outcomes. And third is to frame research questions in the wide international definition of human rights described in the Universal Declaration of Human Rights. This we call "right-based" programming. The goal is to conduct research that can both document health effects of human rights violations on populations and have practical remedial uses to improve services, conduct effective advocacy, promote accountability, and give a strong public voice to people who cannot advocate effectively for their own needs.

Research Methodology

There are many places in the world where rights and health problems interact and where scientific investigation is called for. The choice of where to go may be limited by safety considerations. In Afghanistan we calculated the risk to be far less than the benefit of generating new information. This is a case-by-case determination based on hours of background research and interviews. Policy implications, timing, and funding also play a role. When money for Afghanistan in the form of a supplemental budget from Congress became available, it was imperative to have data to advocate for women's health funding. The data we obtained on maternal mortality were used to obtain $5 million for women's health programming in Afghanistan.

Initial Planning

In addition to security on the ground, the political landscape, infrastructure and logistics, funding, and potential remedies that may come out of the investigation affect where to go and what to study. They determine whether it will be possible to complete the work. Although at any time it is possible to come up with a dozen or more places in the world where conflict and rights violations exist, and where study would be desirable, this is not necessarily sufficient reason to proceed. That data *can* be obtained does not necessarily mean data *should* be. It is not ethically defensible to collect data with no policy endpoint or possible solution to issues on the ground. This is especially the case with field research in conflict zones because the nature of the setting and the work can put investigators, data collectors, and participants at risk. A first question, then, is to ask whether the potential benefits of conducting research outweigh the possible risks. Benefits to consider include heightening public awareness, fostering changes in policy and improving funding possibilities that thereby promote increased provisioning for human needs. A positive outcome of effective health and rights research includes obtaining radio, television, and print media coverage, as well as publications in professional journals. At IMC we have experienced situations in which political conditions and cultural sensitivities made it unwise to release data. In a similar vein, there have been situations in which we have planned studies that were not completed, changed the research design to account for risks and political events, and even withdrawn scientific publication of work to protect staff members, data collectors, and participants. Although it is ideal and vital to have health and rights work published in peer-reviewed journals, and thereby accepted as credible scientific work, it is more important to protect participants and in-country collaborators. Sometimes quiet diplomacy accomplishes as much as media releases, and with less risk to staff members, as the so-called name-and-shame approach common to many human rights investigations.

Survey Methodology

Both quantitative and qualitative research methods have been adapted to the task of assessing the health consequences of human rights violations (Patton, 1990). Qualitative approaches have been used for primary data collection and as formative tools to develop quantitative instruments. Quantitative studies are more highly structured approaches meant to capture specific data. Qualitative studies tend to rely on semistructured interviews with open-ended questions designed to capture testimonies and give a face to the issues on the ground. Such stories often are powerful in their ability to provoke emotional responses to situations and as such many translate into increased media and public attention, and funding for health needs.

The semistructured interviews we collected in Iraq provided poignant testimony that documented horrendous cases of torture perpetrated by the regime of Saddam Hussein against the Shia in Southern Iraq during 10 years preceding the war in 2003 (Amowitz et al., 2004). We conducted numerous interviews with torture victims and presented these findings in public reports. One such example was that of a mechanic imprisoned in Baghdad in 2002 who told us, "One afternoon, several of us were brought into a yard. Other prisoners were brought out as well. One was chained with arms outstretched to a wall and a tire was placed around his head and neck. They set it on fire. The other prisoner was brought in as the one with the tire burned. They took out a sword and cut his hands off at the wrist." While publishing this kind of testimony provides a firsthand understanding of the horrors people endured under Ba'ath rule, it does not give statistically valid numbers on how many people were similarly victimized and how widespread these abuses were. A follow-up quantitative population-based study was needed to do that and it documented that nearly every other household in Southern Iraq had a family member who suffered something similar to this account (Amowitz et al., 2004). The melding of qualitative and quantitative data is an effective way to portray the extent of rights abuses and make them real, and helps service providers better assess the medical and psychological services needs of survivors and families.

The choice of whether to seek quantitative population-based or qualitative case documentation data as a primary method is based on the feasibility of travel and access to subjects, the urgency of the situation, safety considerations for data collectors and participants, advocacy goals, resource constraints, and the timetable of programmatic needs.

Quantitative surveys should follow basic epidemiological techniques for designing instruments and conducting surveys. Instructions for local surveyors should be clear and easy to follow. After training, the survey instrument should be easy for local surveyors to administer and easy for survey respondents to understand. Developing a good survey requires extensive background research that includes a thorough understanding of the political and cultural context on the ground, including cultural sensitivities and a clear-eyed assessment of risks. For example, it was known that women in Sierra Leone that became sexual slaves to Rebels faced the horrendous practice of hand and foot amputations (Amowitz et al., 2002a). Therefore, we included questions about amputation in the sexual violence survey. In Southern Iraq, abuse, torture, and killings were rumored to have occurred within households in addition to torture centers. Based on that preliminary understanding, we included questions on this in the survey instrument. As a result we learned that more than 60 percent of abuses were reported to have occurred at home and that household members were commonly forced to witness them. This informed mental health programming to deal with an exceptionally high suicide attempt rate among household members (not just victims of the abuse) that had witnessed rights abuses of loved ones (Amowitz et al., 2004). Despite government claims of denial, preliminary investigation revealed that rape was being perpetrated against Sudanese IDPs in Darfur. Therefore, IMC felt it would be important to identify ways of improving conditions and decreasing behavior that can lead to rape and other forms of sexual violence. Because of the sensitivity of the government and the risk to humanitarian aid workers who try to investigate rape/sexual violence, we were left to identify risk patterns for sexual violence based on other reports from the field. In background research, we found that many women were raped when foraging for wood. Our survey then looked at the percent of foragers, need for fuel (wood, grass, or dung) and how best to supply this information to eliminate the risk women were taking to find fuel. The analysis showed that more than 62 percent of the foragers were women and that fuel distribution in the camps was infrequent (1%). Simply supplying fuel to the women in the camp could eliminate the need for foraging and thus decrease the risk of sexual violence (Kim et al., 2005).

The goal of a quantitative study is to credibly document the full scope of abuses, along with understanding the patterns and predictors of abuse. Good quantitative work often reveals previously hidden patterns and underlying issues, thereby identifying targets for intervention. If done properly the findings can be generalized to larger populations which case documentation does not permit. Solid quantitative research also can be a source of future leads for case documentation efforts and provide essential information for program-planning and -funding requirements. In some instances, the data may be used for prosecutions in international criminal tribunals such as the International Criminal Court. And, the data are useful for advocacy. PHR's work on rape and sexual violence during the 10-year civil conflict in Sierra Leone permitted activists to assert that each "story is but one of the more than 64,000 women who experienced such sexual violations." These numbers helped humanitarian aid agencies advocate for health services such as fistula repair and mental health programs for women who had suffered sexual violence (Amowitz et al., 2002a).

In circumstances of severe violence, it may not be feasible to conduct quantitative population-based assessments, although it is worthwhile noting that research has been completed in such challenging contexts as during authoritarian rule in Kosovo, in war-torn Sierra Leone, in Afghanistan under the Taliban, in Iraq before and during the U.S.-led occupation, and during the humanitarian disaster in Sudan. In addition to the violence and insecurity for researchers and participants, quantitative population-based surveys typically require more time and resources.

When it is not feasible or warranted to conduct quantitative research, properly designed qualitative research is the appropriate approach. Well conceived and executed qualitative studies can provide accurate and useful information, and usually can be accomplished in less time and with more limited resources than more statistically powered quantitative work.

Qualitative investigations usually consist of semistructured interviews of key informants such as victims, witnesses, religious or community leaders, government officials, military leaders, assistance providers, local and international policy makers, and other stakeholders including donors. The primary strength of the qualitative approach is that it can provide compelling, emotional, first-hand accounts of abusive practices and their consequences in the voices of victims and witnesses. This is a social sciences-based approach and attempts to elicit from those interviewed their sense of the "who, what, where, when, why, and how" of rights violations and health outcomes.

Qualitative interviews provide insight into the individual's experience of human rights abuses and thereby offer a human face and voice to the statistical numbers obtained from quantitative work. These data are most powerful when the research captures the unique words of victims and witnesses. The impact of each story is further amplified by descriptive detail, including the identity of perpetrators, graphic descriptions of events, and firsthand details not reported elsewhere. Accurate detail melded with additional sources of evidence serves to corroborate individual accounts. Sometimes qualitative data uncover events and needs not documented by quantitative survey. For example, PHR's quantitative work in Sierra Leone did not document the need for fistula repair among women victimized by sexual violence. This was uncovered during semistructured interviews (Reis et al., 2002). We have learned from our participants that qualitative and quantitative work are indeed complementary. (See Chapter 8.)

Qualitative case documentation alone does not document the prevalence of abuses, attitudes, or experiences. These data cannot be generalized to populations beyond the sample group. Because qualitative assessments are usually based on nonprobability sampling, there is an inherent potential bias to the population studied. Specific examples of this include sampling the worst cases of abuses or only those individuals willing to come forward. Sometimes the most severely victimized do not come forward or are missed because of sampling error. In other instances, the most victimized are the ones who come forward. In these cases obtaining a study population through valid sampling techniques can be necessary to generalize findings.

Qualitative data can require considerable effort to review, transcribe, analyze, and interpret, including the task of identifying exemplar themes that emerge out of diverse narrative information. This is a complicated activity requiring training and skills. Often there are language barriers to overcome that create time delay, increase costs to accurately transcribe interview material, and sometimes create difficulties in interpreting meaning in the context of cultural differences. It also is not easy to summarize these data into concise and effective reports and publications. And it may take more time to train local data collectors to do qualitative data gathering than to administer a quantitative survey. Despite the impediments and costs, the firsthand experiences of victims and witnesses can be compelling.

Survey Design

Since 1999, PHR and IMC have been developing population-based assessment tools to document the interdependence of health and human rights. The goal has been to advance strategies that may be adapted across geographic regions and political contexts. In this foundation work surveys frequently have been devised and conducted in languages other than English. These are first written in English, then translated into the relevant language(s) and then back-translated into English by one or more independent people to be proofread, edited, and finalized. When possible yet another translation is done in the field by a trustworthy translator. Working forward and back in this way ensures that the meaning of the questions in the other language(s) is the same as that in the English language version. Survey questions also must be checked carefully for switched numbers and scales. For example, we have had instances in which the scale from poor to excellent is reversed in a language that reads right to left instead of the left to right in English. Careful attention also must be paid to translating psychological terminology. In our Afghanistan survey, psychological terms were translated into neurological terminology because it is not acceptable in Afghan culture to admit one has a psychological problem. Sometimes there is no simple English equivalent for direct translation into a local language, and a question must be rewritten in the English version without changing its essential meaning or intent for it to be successfully translated back into the local language for the survey. This may be due to cultural context, such as for rape, sexual violence, and domestic violence; sometimes a local or regional term will be more effective than the legal one.

Expect that the survey instrument will undergo extensive review by numerous people for it to capture and accurately document the information needed to make change. The list of who is appropriate can include many people, but at the least it likely will need to include local partners and knowledgeable local human rights specialists. They should be given sufficient time to review and suggest changes and additions. Our experience is that some critical suggestions and changes have come from our local partners. During field testing, our data collectors have uncovered errors that would have marred the findings.

Estimating Sample Size

Quantitative studies require calculating the minimum sample size needed to ensure with some degree of confidence that the final result can be generalized to larger populations. One must consider also budget and field needs, such as the number of data collectors, sites, and transportation. To estimate sample size, one must know the size of the population you want to generalize to, such as the total refugee population in the area of interest and whether they are accessible. Bear in mind that populations at risk typically move frequently and security in these settings changes even more frequently. It is not uncommon to have to adjust sample size before or during a study.

Calculators of sample size are available on the Internet. In our recent studies, we used one on www.grapentine.com. To calculate the sample size needed for study begin estimating the relative proportion of individuals out of the entire population that are likely to be affected by the question of interest. Start by making a *best guess* of the population proportion affected by the abuse or condition of interest for which you are trying to estimate prevalence. Use input from activists in the field and partner organizations. If you do not know the proportion likely to have been affected, you can set a proportion at half, or 0.5, although this will give a quite small sample size. Next, decide on the alpha, or standard error value desired. Most researchers select 0.05, which results in conclusions with 95 percent confidence that the observations are not due to chance alone. Some studies may require values of .03 or even .01, particularly when the population under study is a guess because there are too little solid background data. The alpha selected will greatly affect the sample size needed to conduct the study. As the value goes down the likelihood of error diminishes because the sample number (N) needed to get valid results gets larger. However, increasing sample size past the required N does not result in a lower standard error and actually produces diminishing returns and increases the resources needed to conduct the study. To cut the potential error in half, it will be necessary to quadruple the sample size. For the most part, this is not practical in the situations we are considering in this chapter, which is why most researchers use .05. The point of selecting the right sample size is to be confident that the results of the work will be accurate and useful.

For example, IMC studied the prevalence of major depression among refugee households in the Darfur conflict in the Sudan. We wanted to be confident of our findings to the alpha 0.05 level. Based on an estimate of the total population in the IDP camps to be studied we came up with a sample size (N) of 1,293 households. Our goal was a 90 percent confidence level with a margin of error of ±0.01 percent (Kim et al., 2005). Study design is also a factor in determining sample size. In conducting our Iraq work our initial analysis also came up with a sample size of 1,293 households, but the study design contained two levels of clustering. To obtain results at the 95 percent confidence level and a margin of error of ±0.01 percent (10% significance) level, the sample size now had to double. Therefore, a total of 2,276 households were sampled in three governorates (Amowitz et al., 2004).

Random Sampling Technique

A random sample is a set of items drawn from a population in such a way that each time an item is selected, it has an equal likelihood of appearing in the sample. The idea is that only chance affects the selection of an item, and an item selected is replaced into the population so the next time a selection is made, the same statistical probabilities exist. Random sampling allows researchers to make valid analyses of large populations by studying much smaller sets of individuals. There is always a margin of error when one samples relatively small fractions of larger entire populations, and in general, this will be described by the confidence with which assertions from samples are described.

Simple Random Sampling

Simple random sampling involves selecting subjects by chance from a well-defined, comprehensive, and readily accessible list, for example, a study of health professionals' views of patients with HIV/AIDS (Reis et al., 2005). Accurate and easy-to-use random number generation tables and electronic programs are available to randomly sample the lists. Unfortunately, conditions on the ground in conflict, postconflict, and complex humanitarian disaster situations rarely permit simple random sampling.

Systematic Random Sampling

Systematic random sampling in general is the more practical and effective technique for conducting rights and health investigations in settings like IDP and refugee camps. Unlike cluster sampling (see below), its advantage is that each person in the sample has an equal opportunity to be selected. This is important when studying refugee and IDP camps, where subgroups of people often reside in pseudovillages within the camp that have important characteristics different from those of the larger population in the camp with regard to important factors such as duration of exposure to the conflict, arrival time, and sociodemographics. These differences need to be researched and understood before determining the sampling frame. The primary disadvantage of doing effective systematic random sampling is that it requires accurate mapping of the entire camp or village before conducting the study. This may take additional days of planning in the field and acquiring satellite, satellite-based, and publicly available maps. When no map is available, it may be necessary to construct a map of an entire village or camp with the help of village elders (Box 11.1). Once we drew our map in the sand.

The most useful maps available for setting up this kind of survey now are the U.S. satellite maps at a 1:100,000 or 1:50,000 resolution that may be obtained from the U.S. Department of State. Getting them is likely to take time and patience. These maps permit accurate counting of huts, homes, neigh-

Box 11.1. Guidelines for constructing accurate and reliable maps for random sampling

1. Obtain maps from camp administrators or humanitarian assistance groups. The World Food Program is involved in camp distribution and may have either satellite-based or other maps.
2. Check the accuracy of the map by walking through the camp or viewing from a vantage point. Be sure that there are adequate landmarks on the map, such as camp clinics, schools, roads, and markets.
3. If a map is not available, create one. (a) Try to view the camp from a high elevation, by standing on top of a vehicle or on a hill overlooking the camp, and represent each household. (b) Include roads and landmarks so data collectors can easily retrace your steps. Use roads and other landmarks to break down the camp into survey areas that are easily demarcated for data collectors.
4. Review the map with data collectors before they sample households, and make certain they are sampling accurately and understand the area boundaries.
5. Determine the average number of households/domiciles (could be tents or huts). If this is not known, it will be necessary to sample some number (approximately 20) of each type of domicile and inquire about the number of households or families in each domicile.
6. Each data collector should have a map and receive instructions on the area for which he or she is responsible. In addition, the data collector should have a plan for the following: (a) starting point, (b) sequence for counting domiciles, (c) method for skipping uninhabited domiciles or domiciles that do not meet the selection criteria, and (d) method for identifying where one left off at the end of the day without making notations that could link data to individuals. Data collectors should not make marks on huts/tents with pens or leave any other identifiable notations.

borhood blocks, and the like. It is also possible to do this with global positioning system (GPS) coordinates when maps are unavailable (Committee on Population, 2002).

Cluster Sampling

Cluster sampling is simple or systematic random sampling performed in a randomly selected area of a camp, village, or town. It is particularly useful for sampling large populations, as done in the urban areas of southern Iraq (Amowitz et al., 2004). This approach assumes homogeneity among the areas being sampled. It is important to hold the number of sampling levels to a minimum. Cluster sampling should be used in cities where it is impossible to do a systematic random sample.

Stratified Random Sampling

Stratified random sampling is random sampling in subgroups of a population. In most cases of human rights investigations, it cannot be used because the available baseline data are insufficient to characterize the population subgroups to be studied.

Nonprobability Sampling and the Population-based Survey

Intentional, nonprobability sampling (for example, snowball chain sampling) should be considered when the primary concern is not to generalize from the sample to the larger population, or when it is simply not possible (due to security or conflict concerns among others) to use a more randomized sampling frame. Selection of a specific sampling technique will depend on a number of factors and will be driven most by security conditions on the ground.

Protecting Human Participants

In the United States and many other countries, research designs involving human participants must go for approval to an independent institutional review board (IRB) or ethical committee made up of scientists, doctors, nonscientists, and community members. The IRB reviews the research methodology and its risk to participants and decides whether the risks are reasonable when compared with the potential benefits. The IRB also reviews the consent form to ensure that it accurately and intelligibly describes for participants the research protocol, including benefits and risks. An IRB is guided by relevant provisions of several codes and regulations that include, but are not limited to, Title 45 of the U.S. Code of Federal Regulations and the Declaration of Helsinki (U.S. Department of Health and Human Services). IRBs may be based in university and hospital settings, or institutionally independent, like the Western Institutional Review Board located in Olympia, Washington.

The IRB process involves submitting a research proposal in a standardized form that addresses the ethical issues relating to the proposed research and survey instruments. The IRB will review and discuss the proposal, and may request additional information either by phone or, in the case of a federally funded project, in a teleconference with the data collectors. The final step is to approve or reject the research plan with or without changes to the consent statement, surveys, and, or protocol.

Sometimes issues and specific nuances involved in health and human rights research may not be well understood by an Institutional Review Board. In general the panel participants will not have firsthand experience conducting research in the context of civil strife or under repressive regimes. The educational gap, including basic literacy, between human subjects in developed nations and the developing world is likely to be enormous so the kind of signed informed consent employed by researchers in developed nations is not likely to be appropriate in human rights-challenged situations. And, even the implications of signing an informed consent is different in these two kinds of settings. We have found that once a thumbprint or signature is put on a form an expectation often exists that special assistance will follow, especially if the research is administered by a known humanitarian aid organization. To deal with this we substituted verbal informed consent for the signed informed consent. The purpose of the informed consent statement is to provide human subjects or their legally authorized representative information on risks and benefits of participating in a research study. This includes an accurate description of the research protocol. In addition to being informed, the human subject must not be under coercion or threat. The language of the informed consent must be fully understandable to the subject or the subject's representative and there must be sufficient time to consider whether to participate.

Unfortunately, individuals who participate in studies designed to document the health effects of rights violations rarely will benefit directly or immediately from the research, because the research likely will be used to guide policy only. And, there may be negative consequences from members of their community and the government in power. To comply with the Declaration of Helsinki, as revised in 2000, every effort must be made to ensure protection and confidentiality, and to minimize potential adverse consequences to participants (World Medical Association [WMA], 2000).

We have worked assiduously to ensure that data from participants are kept anonymous and rely on verbal informed consent to minimize a paper trail that might put participants at risk. In most cases, participants do not receive material compensation and are informed of this in the consent process. Many studies have had changes made in the research questions at the last minute because of insecurity on the ground, population movements, and new conflict or new background information. For example, in 2005, an IMC study in Sudan was changed less than 24 hours before departure because of the arbitrary arrest and incarceration of aid workers accused of assessing sexual violence violations in Darfur. The local police had interrogated data collectors and even IDPs in and around the IDP camps in Darfur. The protocol and survey were changed immediately to ensure the safety of the staff on the ground and the participants to be interviewed. Fortunately, the IRB understood the complexity and emergent nature of the changes and responded within less than 48 hours (Kim et al., 2005). The point is that any and all changes on the ground must be brought back to the IRB and approval obtained before beginning study in the field.

Appropriate IRBs or their Ethical Committee equivalents can be difficult to identify in some countries. In some settings, these are government entities, and so may be unwilling to approve studies, which would identify government collusion in rights violations. In others, it may be unsafe to notify a national committee of in-country investigators' participation, so other forms of human subjects review may be necessary. In some contexts ethical reviewers may even use bribery to approve the study instead of seeing that their primary responsibility is to protect human subjects. It is incumbent on researchers, and most especially those investigating rights violations, to be familiar with international ethical standards and apply them in the best way possible to the situation at hand, meeting the spirit of the guidelines and being flexible to context.

Building a Research Team

Team members must be committed to the goals of the research. It is essential to work with impartial, nonpartisan data collectors in countries that have extremely volatile political issues. Where possible, it also is important to assign local staff members to roles like staff or research coordinator, and to have one person be the leader or principal investigator. A coordinator or research assistant should be assigned to keep track of surveys and assure completeness.

Overseeing the local staff is important. Keep in mind that local staff members may have been subjected to the abuses that one is investigating. In such instances personal agendas and motives can cloud impartiality and in some instances put others at risk or bias data collection, especially with qualitative data. Working effectively and respectfully with colleagues and peers and with the varied people encountered in the field, including local government officials, survivors of atrocities, representatives of other international agencies, and members of the local population including translators and drivers can make or break an investigation. Under the extremely stressful situations that may exist in the field, small disagreements can explode into major conflicts. Participants should be aware of this and take extra care to resolve disagreements in a productive and respectful manner. Each member of a team must be committed to the functional integrity of the team and dedicated to the success of an investigation. Data collectors must be able to address and be flexible in the face of conflict, logistical obstacles, and other problems, while maintaining priorities and focus, and flexibly adjusting the research plan in the field. It is not uncommon for the plan envisioned before the study to fall apart just before the study starts.

Team members should have a grasp of the historical, political, and cultural context of the place and situation they are researching before they arrive in the country. This includes classic history, as well as ethnic, language, and religious background and context. Informants often expect (and they deserve the consideration of having) team members to know seminal events both in their immediate and distant past. Familiarization with covenants such as the International Covenant on Civil and Political Rights, the International Covenant on Economic, Social, and Cultural Rights, the Convention on the Rights of the Child, the Convention on the Elimination of All Forms of Discrimination against Women, the Convention against Torture, and the Geneva Conventions, and additional protocols is important in the context of the research (Mann et al., 1999).

Finally, where feasible, the data collection team should include local people. Training them effectively is essential for the study to be successful. Over the years, PHR has developed training guidelines (see below) that continue to be used and modified to local norms of education, for example, relatively high in Iraq and low in Afghanistan.

Cultural Context

Proper understanding of cultural context will determine the validity and reliability of the data collected and the ease with which a study can be conducted. It also is essential for getting the community to buy in so the study can be completed. For example, researchers in Muslim countries must wear appropriate modest clothing and women must cover their heads. It is imperative to use the right words, such as "Dauya" to describe an untrained birth assistant in Afghanistan. And, to take the time to fit in, like stopping for tea in households, even with time constraints. Similarly, it is important to make an effort to meet and court village elders, camp Sheiks, and regime leaders to gain access to the communities of interest. It takes time, but it may be necessary to spend a day or more having tea with local leaders, graciously accepting gifts and being respectful. Translators and local drivers often are the best resources for learning to navigate cultural rules.

Female data collectors usually are more effective than males for interviewing women or mixed groups of men and women. In some countries, men cannot sit with a female they are not related to. However, cultural norms sometimes can be bridged. In the Shia areas of southern Iraq, we were unable to recruit enough female data collectors and so had to include males. The protest that "it was impossible" for men to interview women did not pan out. After extensive training on gender sensitivity and developing strategies for having men interview women without ignoring local culture, male data collectors were able to interview women independently and ask questions about rape and sexual and domestic violence. When the data were analyzed, it seemed clear that male and female interviewers produced similar results. Still, doing this required understanding and attending to the nuances of social norms.

Training Data Collectors

Over the years, PHR has developed a standardized protocol for training data collectors that could be used in and adapted to a variety of settings (Reis et al., 2002). Because effective research depends on the quality of interviews by local interviewers, training locally based interviewers is a key component. Qualified individuals should train locally hired interviewers in a coordinated program of classroom teaching and experimental role play followed by several days of field observation. Expect training to take three to eight days. At IMC we have had to deal with government oversight of and interference with the selection and training of local data collectors. In Sudan, local government officials oversaw the hiring of local data collectors. Several data collectors were "given to us" by local authorities. This was not negotiable. These individuals were unqualified obvious "minders" who fed information back to the local authorities. They could not be fired. Data from these "minders" that appeared incongruent with that from other data collectors was either cleaned or not included in our final analysis. This was unavoidable for the work to go forward.

Evaluate data collectors on the basis of education, language skills, and their experience and knowledge about the specific topic under study. Data collectors should be fluent in English, and at least one other language. Where this is not possible, it will be necessary to have a translator present throughout training. Data collectors should at least be literate and where possible have at least a high school level of education. Experience with survey instruments and methodology is preferable, but clearly not always possible in settings where the infrastructure is limited with regard to rights and health. In Sudan and Afghanistan it was particularly difficult to find educated female data collectors. Not all could read Arabic well and even fewer were versed in speaking and writing in regional languages and dialects. It is desirable to have two to four field supervisors on a project to oversee and provide training for data collectors. They may be assigned other jobs, as well. It is to be hope d that each supervisor will bring a slightly different specialized set of skills and experience to the team, even experience in academic settings.

Box 11.2 shows a five- to seven-day basic training schema, which includes classroom teaching and experiential role play followed by field observation. The style of the program is participatory and interactive with the trainers. At the end of the seventh day, trainees are tested on content and their ability to conduct an interview using a mock survey that incorporates difficulties they may encounter in the field. The survey is printed in the local *Lingua Franca* (most commonly used language); data collectors may have to learn to administer the survey in other local languages, if necessary. If they thoroughly understand the meaning and intent of each item in local languages, they are likely to be able to translate it into other languages they may be using with the respondent. The survey instrument may be revised during the training process, as the prospective data collectors point out cultural issues and mistakes in the instrument. Questions can be restated for easier reading and understanding. A good training curriculum enhances the future data collector's understanding of the survey and ability to translate it into any language they will be using.

- *Training day 1.* Training begins by introducing participants, trainers, and local partners to each other and an overview of the project and the train-

Box 11.2. Schedule for training data collectors

Day 1 Training
　Introductions
　Introduction to research organization and local partner
　Purposes and overview of the project
　Confidentiality and conduct agreement discussion
　Training plan, field work plan, and logistics
　Mock interview and recording exercise
　Survey review and questions
Days 2–4 Training
　Summary of previous day's activities
　Overview of HIV/AIDS
　Definitions
　Informed consent
　Interview skills
　Role-play
　Feedback
　Discussion of feedback and interview skills
Days 5–6 Training
　Continue practice
　Role-plays in groups of 3, feedback, switch roles
　Discussion with entire group for common issues and problems
　Instrument revisions and instruction
　Test
Day 7 Training
　Review tests with individual data collectors
　Observe individually in role-plays, review documentation
　Using maps and systematic random sampling in field sites
　Identification, assistance, referral for serious problems and severe cases
Day 8 Survey
　Begin survey and individual observation by supervisors
　Nightly team meetings to discuss issues encountered and recording errors

ing course. It includes providing basic understanding of confidentiality and expectations for data collectors' conduct, including professional integrity and dignity, reporting accuracy, and adhering strictly to rules for sharing information. The main part of the day introduces the survey in a role-played mock interview that includes filling out responses on the survey. Data collectors review the survey, give feedback, ask questions, and suggest changes in the instrument. Marked surveys are reviewed for recording errors that need to be corrected. An initial assessment is made of the data collectors' capabilities.

- *Training days 2–4.* Each day begins with a summary of the previous day's exercises followed by a question and answer period. The first major topic is informed consent along with a discussion of cultural, traditional, and societal myths. Technical terms are defined so that all data collectors will be working with the same definitions and concepts. Interview skills are taught through exercises in which trainers act out both poor and good interview techniques. Data collectors are given instructions on how to introduce themselves, present themselves with positive body language (such as open posture), and avoid negative body language (such as eye rolling), ask questions without leading respondents, and maintaining privacy and confidentiality. The final part of each day involves role playing in the interview setting. Data collectors break down into groups of three where one is the interviewer, one is the participant, and the other observes and takes notes on how to improve the interviewer's skills. The last exercise is a feedback session. During the role-playing exercises trainers circulate among the groups observing, giving feedback, and gathering information. Common problems are highlighted and addressed; from time to time, trainers call the group together to discuss and clarify issues. Closing each day includes addressing common problems.

- *Training days 5–7.* During these three days, trainers became familiar with each data collector's strengths and weaknesses. At the end of day 7, a test is administered to all data collectors. The test includes the researcher, two trainers to evaluate the interview, and a mock participant with a scripted answer to the survey. The test is intended to test the skill and ability of the data collectors using a mock survey that incorporates all of the difficulties the survey may bring with it and his/her ability to quickly and accurately record answers. A standardized scoring sheet is used to grade the test. Supervisors for the field are identified as those who show exceptional surveying ability, organization, and leadership.

- *Training day 7.* On the last day, trainers distribute a test to each data collector and discuss individually errors and areas of concern; each data collector focuses on their own weaknesses and ways to improve. Mapping and sampling are explained at the end of the day. The field supervisor's role is discussed. Data collectors are encouraged to bring up problems to the supervisor. Data collectors proceed to the field site and are observed at least once while conducting a complete interview; supervisors provide feedback on problems observed and, in particular, evaluate:

– appropriate and accurate introduction and explanation of the survey's purpose
– complete and accurate questioning and corresponding documentation
– ability to elicit information about private, shameful, and traumatic events in a warm and respectful manner
– correct and simple explanation of terms
– appropriate requests to interview other household members
– complete and accurate closing statement
– ability to accomplish the above in rapid fashion while maintaining warmth and respect. Primary interviews are expected to take no more than one hour, while secondary interviews should take at most 40 minutes.
– accurate counting and selection of households in accordance with sampling method at each field site
– ability to find and maintain privacy for interviews in crowded settings

By the end of day 7, supervisors should be thoroughly aware of each data collector's strengths and weaknesses. On day 8, data collection begins with supervisors continuing to provide guidance, review, and advice to data collectors. A supervisor should review each completed survey and give immediate feedback for errors or items left blank. In our experience, data collectors can become completely familiar with an instrument and able to complete a survey after a week of training. Most documentation errors are simple careless omissions that are readily correctable with immediate feedback. By the end of a project, the average length of a primary interview typically is 20 to 40 minutes.

Entering and Cleaning Data

Wherever possible, data entry should be done in the field by either the researcher or trained volunteers. Sometimes this is not possible because of time constraints, security, or lack of electricity. It is possible to use a number of different databases. However, we have found that the basic spreadsheet is the easiest data entry format with the variables running across the top. Configure the database after the survey is completed to ensure that questions are not missed. After entering the data, pull a random sample of questionnaires and compare the data entered in the database with the data on the primary collection forms. A good rule is to check about 10 percent of the total surveys collected.

It is essential to clean the data in the database before attempting data analysis. In Sudan, it was discovered that food units were entered in many forms: cups, cans, and *Melawas* (tin cans from international food distribution that were used as a measure in the market). Each *Melawa* was approximately 9 cups, but the amount sold could vary significantly from merchant to merchant. Because of this, we had to consider this as a dichotomous variable (i.e., meat present in household or not) (Kim et al., 2005). In Afghanistan, women do not commonly know their age, and stated age may vary from actual age by 5–15 years, so during the maternal mortality study one woman reported being 20 years old and having 12 children (Amowitz et al., 2003). Based on an average age of 15 at menarche, this was, to say the least, highly unlikely, so we had to delete her age from the data. Here again was an example of research on the fly. The point is that meticulous data cleaning is necessary.

Data Analysis

Structured surveys to assess the prevalence and nature of human rights violations, and attitudes and opinions of respondents, typically are useful for descriptive analysis only, not for testing hypotheses. Descriptive statistics include measures of central tendency (i.e., mean, median, and mode) and variability (range, variance, and standard deviation). Sometimes percentiles, quartiles, and percentile ranks are useful. Data analysis must conform to the intended study design. Therefore, hypothesis testing is not appropriate unless specifically integrated into the research design.

Looking Ahead

There is general agreement in the public health community that forcibly displacing populations and violating their rights can have significant health consequences that can be measured as excess morbidity and even mortality. It is critical to thoroughly investigate and document the abuses that lead to adverse consequences and demonstrate these links. As we move forward, this will be crucial for promoting health, filling gaps in services needed for populations at risk, and informing the world community about conditions that marginalized and vulnerable populations face. We also can expect that changing trends in international conflicts and funding priorities will also affect what, where, and how we conduct population-based health and rights research. Regardless, it will be necessary to have accurate numbers based on reliable data. This chapter has provided a basic overview of the field methods for doing this work in the context of maintaining high research standards and emphasizing that researchers have to be inventive and adaptive in their work.

In retrospect, the data collected helped to make modest but important changes for the populations we studied. After the data showed that 99 percent of women in Herat Province in Afghanistan gave birth alone or with an untrained traditional birth attendant (TBA), the U.S. Congress approved funding to train TBAs (Amowitz et al., 2003). These data convincingly documented a paucity of educated women in the country available to be trained as midwives or even obstetricians in a reasonable amount of time, due to years of civil war, cultural prohibitions, and the destructive effect of Taliban rule on the education of women. Data from work in Sierra Leone documented the need to improve funding for rape-related health consequences, such as fistula repair, a previously unmet need, and for holding the perpetrators of abuse accountable after ten years of civil war (Amowitz et al., 2002a; Reis et al., 2002). While no one advocacy argument always works, creative research efforts clearly will have their place in making broad and powerful arguments against the forces of government-sponsored violence, negligence and inaction, and discrimination.

References

Amowitz, L. L. 2003. Afghanistan. In *Pocket Guide to Cultural Assessment*. 3rd ed. Ed. C. D'Avanzo. Philadelphia: WB Saunders, 1–6.

Amowitz, L. L., Iacopino, V., Burkhalter, H., Gupta, S., and Ely-Yamin, A. 2001. *Women's health and human rights in Afghanistan: A population-based assessment.* Boston: Physicians for Human Rights.

Amowitz, L. L., Kim, G., Reis, C., Asher, J., and Iacopino, V. 2004. Human rights abuses and concerns about women's health and human rights in Southern Iraq. *Journal of the American Medical Association* 291 (12):1471–79.

Amowitz, L. L., Reis, C., Hare-Lyons, K., Vann, B., Mansaray, B., Akinsulure-Smith, A., Taylor, L., and Iacopino, V. 2002a. A letter from Sierra Leone: Prevalence of war-related sexual violence and other human rights abuses among internally displaced persons in Sierra Leone. *Journal of the American Medical Association* 287 (4):513–21.

Amowitz, L. L., Reis, C., and Iacopino, V. 2002b. Maternal mortality in Herat Province, Afghanistan in 2002: An indicator of women's human rights. *Journal of the American Medical Association* 288 (10):284–91.

Amowitz, L. L., Reis, C., and Iacopino, V. 2002c. *Maternal mortality in Herat Province, Afghanistan: The need to protect women's rights.* Boston: Physicians for Human Rights.

Kim, J., Torbay, R., and Lawry, L. (formerly Amowitz). 2005. Basic needs, mental health, and women's health among internally displaced persons in Nyala District, South Darfur, Sudan. www.imcworldwide.org/pdf/SouthDarfurAssessment.pdf (accessed December 5, 2005).

Mann, M., Gruskin, S., Grodin, M., and Annas, G. 1999. *Health and Human Rights.* New York: Routledge.

Committee on Population. 2002. Demographic Assessment Techniques in Complex Humanitarian Emergencies: Summary of a Workshop (2002). Washington, DC: National Academies Press. www.nap.edu/books/0309084970/html/18.html (accessed December 5, 2005).

Patton, M. Q. 1990. *Qualitative Evaluation and Research Methods.* Newbury Park, CA: Sage Publications, 169–283.

Reis, C., Amowitz, L. L., Hare-Lyons, K., and Iacopino, V. 2002. *The prevalence of sexual violence and other human rights abuses among internally displaced persons in Sierra Leone: A population-based assessment.* Boston: Physicians for Human Rights.

Reis, C., Amowitz, L., Heisler, M., Moreland, R., Mafeni, J., Anyamele, C., and Iacopino, V. 2005. Assessment of discriminatory clinician attitudes and practices toward patients with HIV/AIDS in Nigeria. *PLoS Medicine* 2 (8):e246.

Reldman, J., Makuc, D., Kleinman, J., and Cornoni-Huntly, J. 1989. National trends in educational differentials in mortality. *American Journal of Epidemiology* 129: 919–33.

United Nations. 1948. *Universal Declaration of Human Rights,* adopted and proclaimed by U.N. General Assembly Resolution 217A (III) (December 10, 1948) www.udhr.org/UDHR/default.htm (accessed December 5, 2005).

U.S. Department of Health and Human Services. 2003. Title 45 CFR Part 46: Protection of human subjects. Available at: http://ohsr.od.nih.gov/mpa/45cfr46.php3 (accessed December 5, 2005).

World Medical Association. 2000. *Declaration of Helsinki: Ethical principles for medical research involving human subjects.* 5th rev. Edinburgh, Scotland: World Medical Association.

Civil Conflict and Health Information

The Democratic Republic of Congo

Chris Beyrer, M.D., M.P.H., Arpi Terzian, M.P.H.,
Sara Lowther, M.H., John A. Zambrano, M.H.S., Noya Galai,
Ph.D., and Mwandagalirwa Kashamuka Melchior, M.H.S.

Political instability, social disruption, and the chaos of conflict and war have profound effects on the health of populations (Foege, 1997). An additional consequence of social disorganization can be the interruption of health research and the destruction of the existing scientific infrastructure for conducting future work, making both the measurement of adverse health outcomes and responses to these threats more difficult in unstable social contexts. As we demonstrate in this chapter, there are some key lessons for health information to be learned from the past two decades of corrupt and repressive government, and the civil war and social chaos that followed its demise, in the Democratic Republic of Congo (DR Congo). A result of DR Congo's long period of disruption has been a paucity of health information with which to understand health effects on its population. Another has been the dispersal of a once-thriving research community. Both are features of what we call *stability bias:* the systematic undersampling of populations and health threats in contexts of conflict and instability in favor of more stable settings where health research can more easily be conducted. In this chapter we examine the effect of governmental neglect and repression, and of the resulting civil war, in the Congo (formerly called Zaire under the rule of dictator Mobutu Sese Seko) on health research, in specific the initiation of new studies and the publication of peer-reviewed research papers on malaria and HIV/AIDS. In addition to systematically reviewing study starts and publications, we have developed a human rights and political timeline for the same period, which we bring to bear on the research effort. We chose to look at the effects of instability and rights violations on research in these two diseases because they were and remain important public health problems in the DR Congo and were under active investigation before the outbreak of civil war. Additional chapters in this volume describe innovative strategies for conducting epidemiological studies and adapting methodologies to settings of social unrest, such as the DR Congo. (See Figure 12.1.)

Documenting the Impact of Civil Strife on Research

To assess the potential impact of civil strife on the ability to conduct research, we looked at the initiation of new studies and the publication of peer-reviewed research on HIV/AIDS and malaria during the time of civil unrest in Zaire/Congo, beginning just before the recognition of HIV/AIDS in the early 1980s, and continuing through the peace accords of 2004. We chose this setting as a model for study, because even though poor and beset by a repressive regime, Zaire/Congo had an active public health research infrastructure that was actively engaged in biomedical investigation and was one of the leading HIV/AIDS research partners in Africa, due in large part to the groundbreaking Projet SIDA collaboration. We decided to look at the two domains of HIV/AIDS and malaria, because these two infectious diseases are of worldwide importance and because infectious diseases are widely accepted to have ancient yet still relevant relationship to civil strife, war, and postwar periods (Foege, 1997). Recent examples of the interaction of infectious diseases, civil conflict, and settings of rights violations include the dramatic increases in population levels of Kala azar (visceral leishmaniasis, a parasitic infection that is generally fatal if left untreated) in ethnic conflict areas of Sudan (Das, 2002); increased malaria attack rates among Afghan civilian refugees fleeing war (Rowland et al., 2002); malaria outbreaks among peacekeeping forces in East Timor (Kitchener, 2002); malaria in Liberia associated with civil war

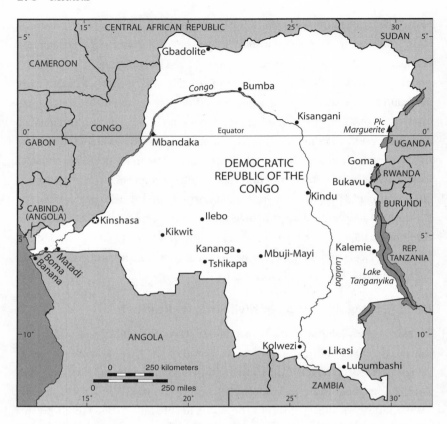

Figure 12.1. Congo, Democratic Republic. After map from the University of Texas at Austin Libraries, Perry-Castañeda Library Map Collection (available at www.lib .utexas.edu/maps/cia05/congo_demrep_sm05.gif)

(Massaquoi and Kennedy, 2003); and increases in HIV/AIDS rates and vulnerabilities associated with civil conflicts and/or their aftermaths in Cambodia (Beyrer, 1998), Burma (Beyrer, 1998), El Salvador (Wollants et al., 1995), Pakistan (Strathdee et al., 2003), Mozambique (Cossa et al., 1994), Rwanda (McKinley, 1998), and DR Congo (Mulanga et al., 2004). The two-decade timeline we selected is designed to uncover impacts before, during, and in the aftermath of civil conflict. Note that the aftermath of conflict can be a vulnerable time for populations, even when human rights conditions improve. For example, the return to relative peace in Cambodia (Beyrer, 1998) was accompanied by an upsurge in infectious diseases, such as HIV/AIDS and tuberculosis, because of the return of refugees and new high rates of population mobility and mixing. A similar postconflict surge in disease spread has been documented in Mozambique, following the reestablishment of peace and population mobility after years of war (Foreit et al., 2001).

Before its fall into social chaos, Zaire had a strong tradition of conducting population-based research in tropical and infectious diseases. From 1984 to 1991, Projet SIDA was one of the most important international collaborators in the field of HIV/AIDS. Project investigators, like expatriate alumni Jonathan Mann, Peter Piot, currently director of UNAIDS, Thomas Quinn of Johns Hopkins University, Henry Francis of the Fogarty International Center, and Robert Ryder of the University of North Carolina School of Public Health, went on to play key leadership roles in the global response to HIV/AIDS. Congolese investigators with Projet SIDA, such as Bila Kapita, Nzilambi Nzila, Frances Lepira, and Kashamuka Mwandagalirwa made major contributions to understanding AIDS in Africa. Because DR Congo played such a prominent role in the early years of African HIV/AIDS research, and because it has faced such marked political and social instability in recent years, we felt it would be a useful model for assessing the impact of instability on public health research in general.

The regional war in the DR Congo began in earnest in 1996 with the collapse of the long-standing dictatorship of Mobutu Sese Seko, its "president for life." The Mobutu decades (1965–1996) were marked by repression, corruption, a political system described as a *kleptocracy* in which ruling elites stole from the nation state for their personal enrichment (Hochshild, 1999), as well as widespread poverty and a grossly inadequate social and economic infrastructure. After Mobutu, living standards and political conditions declined further. From 1998 to 2002, the nation fell into civil war. Estimates of the loss of life during this period range from 3.0 to 4.7 million persons, mostly among civilians (International Rescue Committee, 2003). This is the largest civilian death toll in war recorded in Africa, and the largest worldwide since World War II. An estimated 1.8 million Congolese were internally displaced by the conflict, and another 300,000 forced to flee as refugees to neighboring countries (International Rescue Committee, 2003). Congo's conflict spread beyond its borders to and from the neighboring states of Uganda, Rwanda, Angola, Namibia, Chad, South Africa, Zimbabwe, and Sudan (U.S. Central Intelligence Agency, 2004). It involved battles over resources, ethnicity, and political power. The competing parties fought over diamond revenues, control of coltan, a Congolese mineral resource used in the manufacture of cell phones (U.S. Department of State, 2004), and there was an attempt to destroy Hutu militia remnants in the aftermath of the conflict in Rwanda. Already devastated by authoritarian military rule and mired in poverty under Mobutu, during the civil war Congo plunged into even more extreme levels of civil mortality, violence, and rape. By any standard, the peoples of the DR Congo have faced some of the worst human rights abuses of our time (U.S. Department of State, 2004). At this writing, the latest rights allegations to emerge from this catastrophe were the use of Congolese women and girls as sexual slaves by U.N. peacekeeping forces in the Ituri conflict zone (Human Rights Watch, 2005).

Bibliometric Analysis

We began our study of the impact of civil strife on research by conducting a bibliometric analysis of new studies initiated and papers being published as a result of investigative work performed in the DR Congo from 1980 to 2004. As indicated previously, this period was selected because it covers the years before, during, and after the fall of the Mobutu regime, and because we felt it was sufficient to demonstrate mid- to long-term trends. A bibliometric analysis is a review performed through measures of publications, citations, and the like. In this instance, we focused on published peer-reviewed papers and other literature available to the academic community. We chose HIV/AIDS and malaria because both conditions are clearly of importance to the health of the population in general and the Congo had been an important center for work on these infectious diseases before the civil war. We felt it was important to include malaria studies to avoid overestimating the potential impact of closing Projet SIDA, Zaire's single largest research group whose work was focused on HIV/AIDS. After amassing the data on research, we constructed a timeline of national political turmoil and human rights abuses from news reports, additional published accounts, and reports from human rights organizations, the U.S. Department of State, and the U.S. Central Intelligence Agency (Box 12.1).

The bibliometric analysis started with a database search of Index Medicus (U.S. National Library of Medicine), Excerpta (MEDLINE and EMBASE), PubMed, ISI, and all the databases available through the Cochrane Library (Cleveland, 1979). Our search used *Mesh* terms and, or keywords including:

Malaria, HIV, Acquired Immunodeficiency Syndrome, HIV/AIDS, Zaire, and Democratic Republic of Congo for the period January 1, 1980, through June 1, 2004, unrestricted by language. We did not restrict the search to types of articles, types of studies, or other publication features. Potentially relevant articles from PubMed, ISI, MEDLINE, and EMBASE databases were combined and duplicates removed. Potentially relevant articles were examined and, based on review of title, abstract, and keywords, were categorized as articles to retrieve or not retrieve. Articles were not retrieved when abstracts clearly stated that they were not about the disease of interest, were not about the DR Congo or Zaire, were clearly not original reporting and collecting of data, such as review articles, editorials, and opinion pieces.

Retrieved articles were then examined and included or excluded from this systematic review. Retrieved articles were excluded if the diseases of interest (malaria and HIV/AIDS) were not the primary focus of the publication, if the articles did not involve original data collection, or were organizational or planning reports only. Studies were also excluded if the dates of data collection could not be ascertained or if the research itself was concluded before 1980, which was the case with malaria studies, but not HIV. Studies were included that had a primary focus on the diseases of interest, were the result of original data collection, and for which dates of study implementation were available. We reviewed the introduction, methods, and results sectors to ascertain the dates during which the research was conducted and data collected in Zaire/Congo, and ascertained the "publication delay" between the completion of research and publication. Reference Manager Citation software was used to create a database of publications for studies conducted on malaria and HIV/AIDS from 1980 to 2004 in Zaire/Congo.

Findings

The overall temporal trend in the number of initiated studies was described using a nonparametric lowess smoothed curve (Cleveland, 1979). Lowess smoothed curves are statistical techniques to account for variances within distribution data sets that cannot be analyzed with standard approaches due to small numbers of events. To estimate the change in rates of initiated studies over time, Poisson regression models were applied separately to the malaria and HIV data. Poisson regression was used because this statistical approach to analysis is well suited to estimating change rates for rare events. Time was

Box 12.1. Key events in the history of Democratic Republic of Congo/Zaire

1885	King Leopold of Belgium is granted ownership of new colony, the Belgian Congo, at Berlin Conference of 1884–1885.
1959	Riots against Belgian rule erupt in Leopoldville (later Kinshasa).
1960	Patrice Lumumba leads new country, Republic of the Congo, to independence after abrupt departure of the Belgians. Lumumba subsequently assassinated.
1965	Marshal Mobutu Sese Seko seizes power in a coup d'état, renames state Zaire.
1977	Uprising against Mobuto's rule by Angola-based Congolese rebels reaches deep into Zaire; repelled when Mobuto seeks foreign assistance.
1980	Mobutu continues to enforce one-party rule. Opposition parties are increasingly active. Mobutu's attempts to quell these groups draw international criticism.
1984	Mobutu elected president without opposition in highly controlled elections.
1986	Rising corruption and economic mismanagement bring Zaire's foreign debt to more than US$6 billion, inflation at 1,000% per year.
1987	National Population Policy is drafted with the aim of improving the quality of life and living conditions. Policy never adopted by Mobutu regime.
1989	Zaire defaults on loans from Belgium; cancellation of many development programs and increasing economic decline.
1990	United States and International Monetary Fund (IMF) suspend aid. Under pressure at home and abroad, Mobutu agrees to end ban on multiparty politics, appoints transitional government, but retains substantial executive powers.
1991	Riots by unpaid soldiers in Kinshasa against regime, followed by widespread looting and social unrest. Mobutu agrees to coalition government with opposition leaders, but retains control of security apparatus and important ministries. In September 1991, CDC, NIH, and Belgian Institute of Tropical Medicine expatriate staff leave Zaire. Projet SIDA suspends operations.
1992	One million Zairian Christians join "March of Hope." Mobutu forces kill at least 30, and hundreds are wounded. Political tensions rise. Mobutu accused of inciting ethnic violence to retain power.
1993	Rival pro- and anti-Mobutu governments created. Social unrest continues.
1994	Mobutu agrees to the appointment of Kengo Wa Dondo, an advocate of free-market reforms, as prime minister. The presidents of Rwanda and Burundi are killed after their plane is shot down over Kigali. In Rwanda, extremist Hutu militia and elements of the Rwandan military begin systematic massacre of Tutsis. Within 100 days, some 800,000 Tutsis and moderate Hutus are killed; Hutu militias flee to Zaire, taking with them some 2 million refugees. Refugee camps in Zaire fall under the control of the Hutu militias responsible for the genocide in Rwanda.

continued

1995	Extremist Hutu militias and Zairean government forces attack local Zairean Tutsis; Zaire attempts to force refugees back into Rwanda. Fighting in Zaire between rebels and government forces cause 875,000 refugees to return to Rwanda. Tutsi rebels capture much of eastern Zaire while Mobutu is abroad for medical treatment. Rwandan troops invade and attack Hutu militia-dominated camps in Zaire to drive home the refugees.
1997	Rebel leader Laurent Kabila seizes power in May 1997. Kabila's coalition of Tutsi and other anti-Mobutu rebels, aided by Rwanda, captures Kinshasa; Zaire is renamed Democratic Republic of Congo (DR Congo). Kabila pledges elections by April 1999.
1998	Regional war begins in August between Congolese government, Uganda, and Rwanda-backed Congolese rebels. Rwanda and Uganda-backed rebels rise up against Kabila and advance on Kinshasa. Zimbabwe and Namibia send troops to repel them. Angolan troops side with Kabila. Rebels control much of eastern Congo. War leaves 1.8 million Congolese displaced in DR Congo and 300,000 refugees.
1999	Lusaka peace accord, a ceasefire, signed by DR Congo, Zimbabwe, Angola, Uganda, Namibia, Rwanda, and Congolese armed rebel groups. Uganda soon backs formation of a rebel group and takes control over the northern third of DR Congo.
2000	U.N. Security Council authorizes a 5,500-strong U.N. force to monitor ceasefire, but fighting continues.
2001	Laurent Kabila is assassinated. His son, Joseph Kabila, becomes head of state ten days later. Rwanda withdraws from eastern DR Congo and Uganda agrees to withdraw. United States says war killed 2.5 million Congolese directly or indirectly. U.N. panel says warring parties are deliberately prolonging the conflict to plunder gold, diamonds, timber, and coltan, which is used in the making of mobile phones.
2002	Peace talks in South Africa. Interim government formed.
2003	President Kabila signs a new constitution, under which an interim government will rule for two years, pending elections. Last Ugandan troops leave eastern DR Congo as reports emerge of bloody clashes between rival militias in Bunia area. Thousands of civilians seek asylum in Uganda. United Nations warns of possible genocide unless peacekeeping force is deployed. In June, French peacekeepers arrive in Bunia, spearheading a U.N.-mandated rapid-reaction force.
2004	Ceasefire is considered fragile, but holding.
2005	Allegations of rape and sexual abuse in the Ituri region, involving militias and U.N. peacekeeping forces.

Table 12.1. Rates of initiation of malaria and HIV/AIDS studies, DR Congo, 1980–2003*

Years	Malaria studies initiated		HIV/AIDS studies initiated	
	No. of studies/year	rate ratio (P)	No. of studies/year	rate ratio (P)
1980–1982	1	1.0 (Ref)	—	—
1983–1985	4.7	4.7 (0.07)	7.5	1.0 (Ref)
1986–1988	7.3	7.3 (0.02)	16	2.1 (0.05)
1989–1991	4.3	4.3 (0.09)	7.3	1.0 (0.96)
1992–1994	1.7	1.7 (0.60)	0.3	0.0 (0.07)
1995–1997	1.3	1.3 (0.78)	1.3	0.2 (0.05)
1998–2000	1	1.0 (1.00)	0.3	0.0 (0.07)
2000–2003	0.3	0.3 (1.00)	0	0.0 (0.00)

*Based on Poisson regression model using iterative least-squares methods and allowing overdispersion

included in the model as a series of indicator variables and the results are presented in terms of rate ratios and corresponding p-values (Table 12.1). The Poisson model parameters were estimated using iterative least-squares methods and scaled on deviance to allow for overdispersion (McCullagh and Nelder, 1989). All analyses were done using STATA 8. We divided the timeline into three-year intervals to improve estimates of stability.

We identified 146 potentially relevant articles through the initial searches for the period from January 1, 1980 to June 1, 2004 in malaria research. Of these, 46 were determined to be not relevant, and 100 were retrieved. Among retrieved articles, 66 were included in the final analysis, and 34 excluded. Of excluded articles, 13 were not primarily malaria focused; 6 did not involve data collection in Zaire/Congo; 11 had indeterminate or not reported dates of field research; 4 were published after 1980 but had concluded data collection before 1980. In all 228 articles were identified as potentially relevant to HIV/AIDS publications from DR Congo/Zaire for the period 1982–2004. The first publication identified was from 1984, shortly after identification of the disease in the country. Of the 228 articles, 175 were retrieved. Of retrieved articles, 68 were excluded from the final analysis, and 107 were included. Of excluded articles, 25 were letters or correspondence, 17 were newspaper articles, 11 were historical articles or secondary data analyses, 12 were conducted outside the DR Congo, 1 was unrelated to HIV/AIDS.

This study has some important limitations. First, because we systematically searched the scientific literature for published research, we may have failed to identify newly initiated research studies either that never published results or

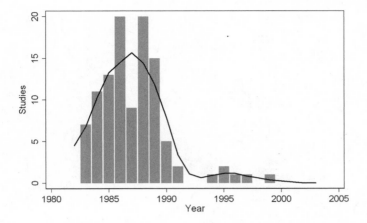

Figure 12.2. HIV/AIDS studies initiated, DR Congo, 1982–2004 (lowess smoothed curve with bandwidth 0.3)

whose results are awaiting publication. This is most likely to be the case for studies begun in the past few years, and especially since the 2002 accords, which have not yet generated publications. Nevertheless, given the long time frame of this study, and the profound instability of the 1994–2002 period, it is unlikely that many research studies have been missed. Second, although the Cochrane Library does include so-called gray literature publications such as reports from nongovernmental organizations (NGOs) and other non-peer-reviewed publications, it is almost certain that our systematic review did not capture some information sources, including government and NGO reports. Still, the trends for start up of research studies argue that activities, and not only publications, were adversely affected by the political context.

Assessing the Impact of Civil Strife on Research and Researchers

The results of our bibliometric analysis show a clear relationship between increasing political and social disorder and the reduction of scientific output. By the time the 1998–2002 war had begun, the research infrastructure had already been essentially shut down, and the impact of the conflict on the diseases in question could no longer be assessed, at least in the context of ongoing research studies. Figure 12.2 shows the distribution of HIV/AIDS studies initiated and published from 1982 to 2004, and Figure 12.3 shows the trend for malaria research studies. The number of newly initiated research studies

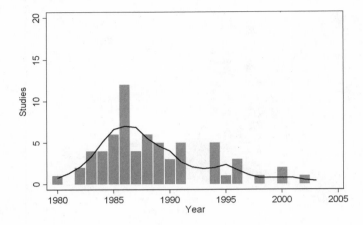

Figure 12.3. Malaria studies initiated, DR Congo, 1980–2004 (lowess smoothed curve with bandwidth 0.3)

increased significantly during 1980–1988 for both diseases, peaked for both between 1986 and 1988, and then drops markedly.

Using 1980–1982 as our baseline measure (one study initiated per year), the relative rates of malaria studies were elevated through 1991 with a significant peak in 1986–1988 ($p = 0.02$). After 1991 the rate of new studies being initiated was similar to the baseline. The baseline average rate for HIV/AIDS was 7.5 studies initiated per year during 1983–1985, doubles during 1986–1988 ($p = 0.05$), and then decreases to the baseline rate during 1989–1991. After 1992, the number of new studies drops to levels significantly lower than the original baseline rate ($p < 0.001$).

Along with fewer new studies being initiated, there was a reduction in the number of papers published in this area. Figure 12.4 shows the distribution of HIV/AIDS publications between 1980 and 2004 for DR Congo. Figure 12.5 shows malaria publications during the same period. For both diseases, there is a rise in the number of publications through the 1980s that peaks slightly later than the new study initiatives, but which falls off precipitously after 1993 for malaria, and after 1994 for HIV/AIDS. The median publication delay from completion of data collection to date of publication was 2.7 years.

We considered also whether factors other than civil unrest might account for the significant reduction in research activity. For example, perhaps global funding for research was reduced or the prevalence of HIV/AIDS and

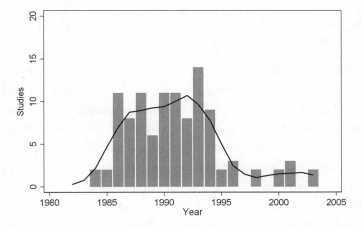

Figure 12.4. HIV/AIDS studies published, DR Congo, 1982–2004 (lowess smoothed curve with bandwidth 0.3)

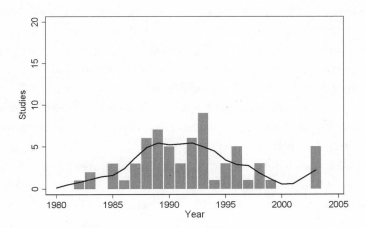

Figure 12.5. Malaria studies published, DR Congo, 1980–2004 (lowess smoothed curve with bandwidth 0.3)

malaria decreased, thereby eliminating the need for research. Neither is the case. During this time, increased funding became available for HIV/AIDS work worldwide and other countries in the region stepped up their research efforts. Meanwhile, HIV/AIDS and malaria became more widespread in Sub-Saharan Africa. It would thus appear that the primary cause for reduced scientific investigation was that researchers were unable to conduct their work because of Mobutu's political repression and widening civil conflict.

Looking Ahead

Research is a special category of health information. Biomedical research, in general, and human participants research, in particular, have high degrees of oversight and review. This work is labor intensive, is costly to perform, and requires a high level of skill. Many, if not most, biomedical research projects are collaborative in nature and require the assistance of governmental agencies, funding entities, and training institutions. Typically, there are a host of complex operational issues and ethics concerns. Because of these factors, biomedical research is arguably a more sensitive indicator of the impact of instability on information than census data, vital statistics reports, mortality measures, and other forms of public health information. Repressive regimes and civil conflicts can inhibit and interrupt research projects, making it unsafe for researchers and staff members to go into troubled areas. To date, surprisingly little attention has been paid to the divergence between what we know about the transmission of disease in stable social settings and what transpires in regions and periods of social instability. Might there be a systematic bias inherent in public health research that favors social and political stability over instability? Does the fact that conducting research in adverse conditions is hazardous and complicated make it less likely that research will be completed and more likely that adverse consequences on the health of populations will tend to be underreported?

The clear correlation between increased political instability and diminished research activity in Zaire/Congo is a valuable model for understanding what can be expected to occur in similar settings. This cannot be said for other repressive governments, such as the military dictatorship in Myanmar (Burma), where the last national census of Burma's population was done by the British more than 50 years ago (Smith, 1996). From 1980 to 1989, the Mobutu regime retained dictatorial power, the economy faltered, social and political tensions rose, and human rights violations were widespread. Still conditions were seemingly stable enough during the latter part of this period, from 1986 to 1988, for new studies of malaria and HIV/AIDS to be initiated at a relatively brisk rate. New HIV/AIDS studies peaked in the years 1986–1988 at 16.0 per year and declined significantly thereafter. Malaria research activity and outputs during the 1980s were also impressive and also peaked in the 1986–1988 period. Although Zaire/Congo was poor and beset by increasingly repressive governance, there was relative political stability during the 1980s.

Then, in 1989, the financial excesses of Mobutu's regime reached a breaking point and Zaire defaulted on its loans from Belgium. International financial and political support for the regime ended. Social and political tensions increased from 1989 to 1991 and then accelerated rapidly from 1990 to 1994, leading to economic and social collapse. Threats to the regime's political power in the form of rising demands for change from the people of Zaire were met with increasing state-sponsored ethnic tension and street violence. Around 1991, as the situation became increasingly unsafe, the country's educated elites, including its researchers, began to leave. With the exodus of research talent from 1992 to 1994, there was a marked decline in the number of new studies of malaria and HIV/AIDS. Starting in the early 1990s, the number of publications declined. No new HIV/AIDS or malaria research studies that later would yield publications were identified during 1992 or 1993, although there were some studies begun in 1994 among refugees. In 1990, there were 17 publications in the peer-reviewed literature reporting on HIV/AIDS research in DR Congo. By 2002 there were none. The picture for malaria studies and publications is only slightly less grim. Nearly all of the post-1998 malaria studies are on Congolese refugees and displaced persons. The Rwandan genocide that began in 1994 was a regional watershed that affected Congo/Zaire. The Rwanda conflict led to a regional war in 1998 that precipitated the fall of the Mobutu government. The period of extreme social chaos ended in 2002, but to date the research infrastructure has not fully recovered and there has been only a modest upswing in research activity.

If the initiation of new work and its publication is a reasonable indicator, effective research activity stopped five years before the 1998 regional conflict. It appears the tensions of the late 1980s took a toll that took several years to observe. By the time the government collapsed, there already was little or no human investigative capacity and hence no way to assess the effect of events on the health of the population. Does this demonstrate a systematic bias in health information favoring the collection of information in stable settings over unstable ones? Is there a bias against collecting information when it is most needed and is this likely to mean there will be an underreporting of the adverse effects of conflict on the health of vulnerable populations? The findings of this work suggest that there has been, indeed, a marked decline in research activity in DR Congo as a result of instability. When one considers how many other African states have endured similar kinds of conflict, and how few have been consistently stable, the potential impacts of this finding are considerable.

Instability has continued to make biomedical research challenging in the DR Congo, but there have been several recent initiatives, including that of the Fogarty International Center of the National Institutes of Health, to restart the research effort.

The shutdown of the Congo's research capacity starting in the later years of the Mobuto dictatorship, well in advance of the war, are important for current debates about the purported impact of war on HIV/AIDS. The DR Congo has recently been used as an example of an HIV epidemic that may not have been worsened by a huge and bloody conflict (Spiegel, 2004). One interpretation of our findings is that it is impossible to assert with any confidence *any* suggested impact of the regional war on either HIV or malaria in the Congo, because the capacity to assess such impacts, once so strong, had already been destroyed when the war began. Did the political chaos produce a similar difficulty with regard to investigating human rights abuses as it did for HIV/AIDS and malaria? Many human rights and international organizations, including Human Rights Watch, Africa Watch, and others, have decried the limited media and diplomatic attention paid to the war in Congo. Definitive reckonings of the impact on the Congolese people lie, it is hoped, in the future. The example of the Truth and Reconciliation Commission in South Africa, and of the U.N. War Crimes Tribunal for Rwanda now underway in Arusha, Tanzania, suggest there may be ways to shed light on the past that can be helpful for states and peoples emerging from social disruption and conflict.

Population-based research should start with reliable baseline population statistics; lacking these data poses a formidable problem for investigators. Other contributors to this volume discuss strategies for providing services and conducting research in difficult settings, such as along the Thai-Burma border, and in Afghanistan, Iraq, Sudan, and Sierra Leone. After 1993, estimates of HIV/AIDS and malaria in the DR Congo should be treated with caution, and in doing so implications for the larger region should be considered because of the country's huge geographical size and its population comprising roughly 15 percent of Sub-Saharan Africa. One must also consider the impact of lacking trained and experienced scientific observers, such as medical personnel, relief workers, journalists, and clergy. These individuals may have been forced out of conflict areas because of safety concerns or harassment by government, or they may be working in such adverse conditions that their access to populations is too restricted to perform solid investigation. In 2004 Médecins sans Frontières voluntarily left Afghanistan after 24 years of relief efforts there (Anonymous, 2004). Observers who stay in conflict zones may be unable to function objectively, a problem discussed by the Lebanese American researcher Harout Armenian, who described the political pressures epidemiologists faced during the Lebanese civil conflict of the 1980s (Armenian, 1986, 1989). North Korea is a repressive state not at war, but where unbiased observers are routinely denied access to populations and government data have little credibility (Natsios, 2003). The point is that reliable information is likely to be unavailable during times of civil conflict and under repressive and hostile governments. Births, deaths, and outbreaks of disease may go unrecorded and underreported, thereby affecting both the numerators and denominators of vital statistics. The implications are of great importance to the health of populations: we know much more about health in stable settings, where it is likely to be better, than in unstable and repressive ones, where what we do know suggests that health and rights threats are more common, more dire, and more likely to have an impact on the lives of individuals, families, and communities trying to survive through times of strife.

References

Armenian, H. 1986. In wartime: Options for epidemiology. *American Journal of Epidemiology* 124 (1):28–32.

Armenian, H. K. 1989. Perceptions from epidemiologic research in an endemic war. *Social Science and Medicine* 28 (7):643–47.

Beyrer, C. 1998. Burma and Cambodia: Human rights, social disruption, and the spread of HIV/AIDS. *Health and Human Rights* 4:85–97.

Cleveland, W. S. 1979. Robust locally weighted regression and smoothing plots. *Journal of the American Statistical Association* 74:829–36.

Cochrane Library. 2004. Issue 3. Chichester, UK: John Wiley & Sons. www.cochrane .org.

Cossa, H. A., Gloyd, S., Vaz, R. G., Folgosa, E., Simbine, E., Diniz, M., and Kreiss, J. F. 1994. Syphilis and HIV infection among displaced pregnant women in rural Mozambique. *International Journal of STD & AIDS* 5:117–23.

Das, P. 2002. Infectious disease surveillance update: Severe outbreak of Kala Azar in Sudan due to civil war. *Lancet Infectious Diseases* 2 (12):716.

Foege, W. H. 1997. Arms and public health: A global perspective. In *War and Public Health*, ed. B. Levy and V. Sidel, 3. New York: Oxford University Press.

Foreit, K. F., Barreto, A. T., Noya, P. A., and Nhatave, I. 2001. Population movements and the spread of HIV/AIDS in Mozambique. *Journal of Health and Human Services Administration* 24 (3):279–94.

Hochshild, A. 1999. *King Leopold's Ghost.* New York: Mariner Books.

Human Rights Watch. 2004. Democratic Republic of the Congo: Confronting impunity. Human Rights Watch Briefing Paper, January.

Human Rights Watch. 2005. Seeking Justice: The Prosecution of Sexual Violence in the Congo War. March 2005. Vol. 17, no. 1(A). http:://hrw.org/reports/2005/drc0305.

International Rescue Committee. 2004. Mortality in the Democratic Republic of Congo: Results from a nationwide survey. IRC Special Report, April-July. www.theirc.org/resources/DRC_MortalitySurvey2004_RB_8Dec04.pdf.

IRIN News Agency. 2004. Afghanistan: MSF pulls out of country. Ankara, July 28.

Kitchener, S. 2002. Malaria in the Australian defence force associated with the Inter-FET peacekeeping operation in East Timor. *Military Medicine* 167 (9):iii–iv.

Massaquoi, M. B., and Kennedy, S. B. 2003. Evaluation of chloroquine as a potent anti-malarial drug: issues of public health policy and healthcare delivery in postwar Liberia. *Journal of Evaluation in Clinical Practice* 9 (1):83–87.

McCullagh, P., and Nelder, J. A. 1989. *Generalized linear models.* 2nd ed. London: Chapman and Hall.

McKinley, J. C., Jr. 1998. Ravaged by war and massacre, Rwanda faces scourge of AIDS. *New York Times*, May 28, sec. Foreign Desk.

Mulanga, C., Bazepeo, S. E., Mwamba, J. K., Butel, C., Tshimpaka, J. W., Kashi, M., Lepira, F., Carael, M., Peeters, M., and Delaporte, E. 2004. Political and socioeconomic instability: how does it affect HIV? A case study in the Democratic Republic of Congo. *AIDS* 18 (5):832–34.

Natsios, A. S. 2003. Life inside North Korea. Testimony before the Subcommittee on East Asian and Pacific Affairs, Senate Foreign Relations Committee, Washington, D.C., June 5.

Rowland, M., Rab, M. A., Freeman, T., Durrani, N., and Rehman, N. 2002. Afghan refugees and the temporal and spatial distribution of malaria in Pakistan. *Social Science and Medicine* 55 (11):2061–72.

Smith, M. 1996. *Fatal Silence: Freedom of Expression and the Right to Health in Burma.* New York: Article 19, 19–29.

Spiegel, P. B. 2004. HIV/AIDS among conflict-affected and displaced populations: Dispelling myths and taking action. *Disasters* (3):322–39.

Strathdee, S. A., Zafar, T., Brahmbhatt, H., Baksh, A., and ul Hassan, S. 2003. Rise in needle sharing among injection drug users in Pakistan during the Afghanistan war. *Drug and Alcohol Dependence* 71 (1):17–24.

Stroup, D. F., Berlin, J. A., Morton, S.C., et al. 2000. Meta-analysis of observation studies in epidemiology: A proposal for reporting. *Journal of the American Medical Association* 283 (15):2008–12.

U.S. Central Intelligence Agency (CIA). 2004. The World Fact Book: Democratic Republic of Congo. www.odci.gov/cia/publications/factbook/geos/cg.html.

U.S. Department of State, Bureau of Democracy, Human Rights, and Labor. 2004. Democratic Republic of Congo: Country reports of human rights practices. February 25.

Wollants, E., Schoenenberg, M., Figueroa, C., Shor-Posner, G., Klaskala, W., and Baum, M. K. 1995. Risk factors and patterns of HIV-1 transmission in the El Salvador military during war time. *AIDS* 9:1291–92.

PART III

Policy

13

From Human Rights Principles to Public Health Practice

HIV/AIDS Policy in Brazil

Varun Gauri, Ph.D., Chris Beyrer, M.D., M.P.H., and
Denise Vaillancourt, B.A., M.I.P.P.

In 2005 Brazil recently refused a $40 million grant to fight AIDS because the donor government, the United States, stipulated that grant recipients must sign a pledge condemning prostitution (*Wall Street Journal,* May 2, 2005). The head of Brazil's National AIDS Program, Pedro Chequer, was outspoken: "Our feeling was that the manner in which the USAID funds were consigned would bring harm to our program from the point of view of its scientific credibility, its ethical values and its social commitment" (*International Herald Tribune,* July 25, 2005). To followers of the AIDS program in Brazil, the action was not surprising. For more than a decade, Brazil has implemented an AIDS program that has aggressively provided prevention and treatment, and taken steps to minimize the stigmatization of HIV-affected populations. Principles of nondiscrimination and the right to health care have been included in what is widely regarded as one of the most successful responses to HIV/AIDS in the developing world.

The Political and Social Context

It is impossible to understand the social, political, and public health response to AIDS in Brazil without reference to two events that coincided with the emergence of the epidemic: the transition from military to civilian democratic rule and the development of the government health system, the Sistema Único da Saúde, or SUS. (See Box 13.1.)

Brazil's military government that ruled from 1964 to 1985 weakened the peasant movement, suppressed workers' strikes, manipulated opposition political parties, undercut basic civil liberties, infiltrated all levels of government with its secret intelligence service, and was implicated in thousands of instances of torture and political assassination (Mainwaring, 1986; Skidmore, 1989). When the military and its allies finally lost important gubernatorial elections in 1982 and then the presidency in 1985, it was due in no small part to the remobilization of Brazilian civil society that had begun in 1978 (Stepan, 1989). As a result, when the AIDS epidemic emerged in the early 1980s, activists had recent experience with successful social mobilization, and they grafted the methods and objectives of the democracy movement onto their struggle to compel a forceful response to the epidemic on the part of the government. Several individuals, who would contract HIV and then become leading figures in the AIDS movement, including Herbert Daniel and Herbert de Souza (Betinho), had been exiled during the period of military rule. For them it was evident that the military era had demonstrated the relationship of secrecy and the centralization of power to lethal consequences, and that the same associations characterized the democratic government's early responses to AIDS (Galvão, 2000).

Most health care services provided under the military government were administered by the social security institute (INAMPS), and were restricted to formal sector workers who contributed payroll taxes. INAMPS contracted private hospitals and physicians to provide the majority of health care services for its beneficiaries, reinforcing already large regional and class inequalities in access. The movement to restore democracy to Brazil spun off a movement to provide health care to underserved groups and regions (*movimiento sanitarista*), based in some of the largest cities, including São Paulo (Weyland, 1995). It advocated universal access to publicly funded health care and a strategic decentralization of authority over health care to the states and municipalities to weaken the political ties between INAMPS and the private facilities, which had resisted reforms. The movement partly achieved its objectives only after the return of civilian democratic government. The 1988 Constitution called health care a "right of all and the duty of the state" and guaranteed universal and equal access to health care, interpreted to mean that the government would make health care available free of charge. The 1990 law that created the SUS reaffirmed those principles, and also established the principles of decentralized management and wide consultation in the health sector through representative national and state conferences. The mechanisms for decentralization were only clarified with regulations in 1996 and 2002. Together, they transferred responsibility and minimum financing for primary care to municipalities *(piso ambulatorial básico,* or PAB), established criteria by which states and municipalities could qualify to manage higher-level care and receive direct funding for that purpose, and created a series of incentives for localities to adopt specific health care initiatives, such as the family health and basic medicines programs. A constitutional amendment in 2000 set floors for expenditures on health care on the part of the federal government (an increase over the previous year's expenditures equal to the growth in GDP), the states (12% of revenues), and the municipalities (15% of revenues). Currently, the federal government negotiates health sector responsibilities with the states, and the states with municipalities, on a case-by-case basis, resulting in wide variation in the extent and structure of local management. Some practices, though not codified in law, have become standard nationwide: for instance, generally speaking, the federal government takes responsibility for purchasing antiretroviral (ARV) drugs for HIV/AIDS, and the states and municipalities share responsibility for drugs for opportunistic infections and for sexually transmitted infections (STIs).

These two events, regime transition and the development of the SUS, had four important consequences for the directions that AIDS policy took in Brazil. First, the legacy of the struggle against the human rights abuses of the military regime informed and motivated activism toward AIDS policies. The important role of nondiscrimination, the right of access to treatment, and civic consultation in Brazil's AIDS policies followed in part from this historical connection. The extent of social mobilization around AIDS was unprecedented in health care, and was responsible for the visibility, political strength, and stability that the national program would achieve (Galvão, 1997;

Box 13.1. Timeline of key events: Brazil

		Brazil			
Year	National events	State/municipal events	HIV/AIDS events and data	Bilateral donors and multilateral agencies	World Bank
1981					Northwest Region Integrated Development Program–Health: Loan 2061-BR approved.
1982		Military and its allies lost key gubernatorial elections. A popularly elected governor led São Paulo for the first time since 1964.	7 AIDS cases among MSM diagnosed.		
1983		São Paulo state health secretariat established an AIDS program in the Division of Leprosy and Dermatological Health, mandated notification of AIDS cases, and launched public awareness campaigns for and with HRG.	Newspapers called AIDS the "gay cancer."		

continued

1984	Outro Coisa (NGO) distributed informational AIDS pamphlets in São Paulo.		10 AIDS cases among hemophiliacs diagnosed.		National Health Policy Studies Loan 2448-BR approved. São Paulo Basic Health Care: Loan 2447-BR approved.
1985	Military lost presidential elections, ending nearly two decades of military rule. INAMPS declared AIDS a public health, not medical, problem for state health secretariats to address despite their lack of facilities. Portaria No. 236 (May 2) established the National AIDS Program.	Eleven states have AIDS programs. GAPA established in São Paulo. The cardinal-archbishop of Rio de Janeiro called AIDS a divine punishment.	14 IDU, 15 heterosexual, and 16 blood transfusion AIDS cases diagnosed.		
1986	Federal government mandated notification of AIDS cases.	São Paulo state assembly passed a law mandating HIV testing of all blood supplies.		WHO, through PAHO, began to provide substantial financial and technical assistance.	Northeast Basic Health I: Loan 2699-BR approved.

Box 13.1. Timeline of key events: Brazil *continued*

Brazil

Year	National events	State/municipal events	HIV/AIDS events and data	Bilateral donors and multilateral agencies	World Bank
1987	Federal Council of Medicine passed resolution urging doctors to notify blood donors of their HIV status. National AIDS Program began to coordinate and lead activities of state health secretariats.	Medical Council of São Paulo passed resolution urging against dismissal of workers as a result of their HIV status.	26 perinatal HIV cases diagnosed.		
1988	New constitution declared that "health is a right of all and a duty of the state," guaranteeing universal and equal access to health services, provided for free by the government. National AIDS Program consolidated within Ministry of Health (MOH).	Demonstrators placed AIDS Solidarity banner on Cristo Redentor statue in Rio de Janeiro. São Paulo state established its own AIDS reference and treatment center, launched "day hospital" programs, and began to track unused beds in public			Northwest Region Integrated Development Program Health: Loan 2061-RR approved Northeast Endemic Disease Control: Loan 2931-BR approved.

continued

			Adult Health in Brazil: Adjusting to New Challenges published (November).
hospitals for AIDS patients to use. Serological testing required for all national public and private blood banks. Congress passed Law No. 7649 (January 25) granting rights guaranteed to workers with incapacitating or terminal illnesses for people living with HIV/AIDS. Congress rejected a proposed law to limit entry of HIV-positive foreigners. National AIDS Commission formed and included representatives from the Ministries of Health, Labor, Justice and Education, Order of Lawyers, Federal Council of Medicine, and other civil society groups.			
1989	Inflation reached 1,862% per year. Major national businesses launched prevention	Municipality of Santos launched its first needle exchange program, but a court ruling halted it.	

Box 13.1. Timeline of key events: Brazil *continued*

Brazil

Year	National events	State/municipal events	HIV/AIDS events and data	Bilateral donors and multilateral agencies	World Bank
	campaigns in the workplace. Ministry of Armed Forces launched HIV prevention program among enlisted personnel.	First meeting of Brazilian NGOs working on AIDS occurred in Belo Horizonte.			National Health Policy Studies: Loan closed (December). Northeast Basic Health II: Loan 3135-BR approved. Amazon Basin Malaria Control: Loan 3072-BR approved.
1990	Sistema Unico de Saúde (SUS) established, reinforcing the principles of decentralized management and constitutional right of access to health service. Collor elected president and mentioned AIDS in a public speech. The federal government communicated to the	São Paulo state launched a needle exchange program. Municipal AIDS commissions began to coordinate activities without input from the state health secretariats.			

	Bank that it would "no longer borrow for social sectors." National AIDS Program dismantled; MOH established a decentralized AIDS response mechanism, launched a publicity campaign emphasizing the danger of AIDS to uninfected people, refused to participate in WHO anti-HIV vaccine trial, and began to isolate itself from civil society groups.				
1991	MOH began to acquire and distribute free AZT, Ganciclovir, and Pentamidina to AIDS patients.		One study estimated that 700,000 Brazilians were infected with HIV.	DKT do Brasil launched a condom social marketing campaign.	*Women's Reproductive Health* published (August)
1992	Fifth health minister in two years assumed command. Portaria No. 291 (June 17) passed for the national health secretariat to reimburse treatments for	At least 67 state and municipal laws on HIV/AIDS passed.	One study forecasted that 1.2 million Brazilians will be infected by year 2000. World Bank estimated 300,000-400,000 PLWHA in Brazil.	USAID launched the first 5-year strategy.	São Paulo Basic Health Care: Loan closed (June).

continued

Box 13.1. Timeline of key events: Brazil *continued*

Brazil

Year	National events	State/municipal events	HIV/AIDS events and data	Bilateral donors and multilateral agencies	World Bank
	AIDS patients provided by private philanthropic hospitals. Portaria No. 7750 (July 14) passed for INAMPS to certify hospitals, day facilities, and laboratories to provide AIDS care and services. Portaria No. 869 (August 11) passed for the Ministries of Labor, Health, and Administration to prohibit HIV testing in physical examinations of public sector workers. President Collor impeached and his last minister of health accused of corruption.				

continued

National AIDS Program reconstituted with its former director; it reestablished contact with civil society and GPA and began policy dialogue with the Bank for an HIV/AIDS project.

The government began to import and distribute AZT for free through SUS.

NGOs began to provide services in addition to their advocacy role after receiving AIDS I funds.

1993 The government began to produce its own AZT and introduced a 14-month tax holiday for imported condoms.

Ibero-American Health Ministerial Meeting held and endorsed needle and syringe exchanges and bleach distribution for IDU HIV prevention.

ANRS launched a 2-year study on the neurological impact of HTLV-1 infection.

AIDS I: Loan 3659-BR approved (November).

Box 13.1. Timeline of key events: Brazil *continued*

Brazil

Year	National events	State/municipal events	HIV/AIDS events and data	Bilateral donors and multilateral agencies	World Bank
1994	Plano Real cut inflation to 3% per month in the second half. Cardoso elected president. National AIDS Program adopted harm reduction as an explicit policy. FNC approved a six-site pilot harm-reduction program proposed by MOH.			ANRS sponsored bilateral seminars on vaccines, HIV/TB, adolescent HIV prevention, HIV patient care, and quality control.	*The Organization, Delivery and Financing of Health Care in Brazil: Agenda for the 90s* published (June). AIDS I: Loan 3659-BR became effective (June).
1995	Congress passed Decreto Legislativo No. 56 (April 19) approving the San Salvador protocol for economic, social, and cultural rights.	São Paulo state secretary of health openly endorsed harm-reduction approaches and outlined key strategies for incorporation into state programs. Municipality of Santos launched its second needle exchange program but it was halted by police		ANRS carried out a study of sexual behaviors in Brazil and Southern Cone countries.	Northeast Basic Health I: Loan closed (December).

seizures and later moved to São Vicente.

Salvador do Bahia launched its first needle exchange program.

| 1996 | A regulation clarified the mechanisms of decentralizing SUS. Decree No. 1904 (May 13) passed to establish the National Program on Human Rights under the Ministry of Justice; four of the short-term goals related to HIV/AIDS. Congress passed Law No. 9313 (November 13), stating that "all carriers of HIV and AIDS patients will receive, free of charge from the SUS, all medications for that treatment." Congress passed patent law. Nationwide, an estimated 600 NGOs working on AIDS. | A regulation established per-capita payments to municipalities for primary care management and initiated transfer of management responsibilities of secondary and higher facilities to some states/municipalities. | AIDS I: Midterm review (September). Northeast Endemic Disease Control: Loan closed (June). Amazon Basin Malaria Control: Loan closed (June). *Addressing Nutritional Problems in Brazil* published (October). Health Sector Reform (REFORSUS): Loan 4047-BR approved. |

continued

Box 13.1. Timeline of key events: Brazil *continued*

Brazil

Year	National events	State/municipal events	HIV/AIDS events and data	Bilateral donors and multilateral agencies	World Bank
1997	Portaria No. 874 (July 3) passed to specify that ARV drugs be provided to AIDS patients and treatment protocols be developed according to CD4 counts and viral loads. MOH created a national, computerized scheme to track use of ARV drugs. Three national AIDS reference centers established. HIV surveillance system revamped with AIDS I funds.			UNAIDS Theme Group established in November, with UNICEF as its first coordinating agency.	AIDS first appeared in the CAS, which called for "the control of traditional and emerging communicable diseases, i.e., dengue fever and malaria, and AIDS, respectively" and the reduction of "the growth rate of the AIDS epidemic" among its goals. Northeast Basic Health II: Loan closed (December).
1998	Floating Real-US$ exchange rate established. Despite a balance-of-payment crisis and shrinking			USAID launched the second 5-year strategy, with $8.4 million for FY2001-2002.	*The Brazil Health System: Impact Evaluation Report* published (June). AIDS I: Loan closed

	budget expenditures for HAART increased.	UNDCP launched a 4-year, $2.5 million drug abuse and STD/HIV/AIDS prevention project. UNESCO and UNDCP contracted by the Bank to carry out AIDS II activities.	(June); ICR completed (December). AIDS II: Loan 4392-BR approved (September). Disease Surveillance and Control (VIGISUS): Loan 4394-BR approved.
1999	National AIDS coordination council established a unit for external cooperation Laws passed to create a new category of public-interest civil society groups with a more favorable tax status.	UNESCO replaced UNICEF as the UNAIDS Theme Group chair.	AIDS II: Loan effective (February). Assistance Strategy for the Health Sector in Brazil mentioned AIDS briefly in the context of communicable disease prevention. *Public Policies in the Pharmaceutical Sector: A Case Study of Brazil* published (January). CAS excluded AIDS except in project list. Health Sector Reform (REFORSUS): Loan closed (December).
2000	Parliamentary Group on AIDS created. Forum 2000 held in Rio de Janeiro to convene the Latin American and Caribbean members of the Horizontal Technical Co-operation on HIV/AIDS Group.	DFID launched a 5-year, £1 million project to support the Horizontal Technical Cooperation on HIV/AIDS Program. UNAIDS appointed the first Country Program Adviser for Brazil. UNDCP replaced	

continued

Box 13.1. Timeline of key events: Brazil *continued*

Brazil

Year	National events	State/municipal events	HIV/AIDS events and data	Bilateral donors and multilateral agencies	World Bank
	Constitutional amendment passed to set health care expenditure floors for the federal, state, and municipal governments.			UNESCO as UNAIDS Theme Group chair.	
2001	The government expressed an intent to issue a compulsory license on an AIDS drug held by Roche.			USAID designated Brazil as an "intensive-focus" country. UNAIDS launched a 1-year project to assist Brazil in implementing the Horizontal Technical Cooperation on HIV/AIDS Program for Angola, Mozambique, São Tome and Príncipe, and Guinea-Bissau. WHO/PAHO launched a 1-year project to establish a data bank for	AIDS II: Midterm review completed (May). CAS Progress Report noted that "in recent years, the Brazilian HIV/AIDS program has reached for worldwide recognition of its achievement in preventing and treating HIV/AIDS."

continued

2002   Another regulation further clarified the mechanisms of decentralizing SUS; with the 1996 regulation, it transferred primary care financing and delivery to municipalities. Minister of Health signed a law to establish transfer of funds from federal to state/municipal governments for HIV/AIDS/STI activities; to qualify for funds, states and municipalities must have program of actions and goals

AIDS drugs in Brazil. In WTO Ministerial Meeting, representatives from developed countries agreed that developing countries can override patents under TRIPS in public health emergencies. ANRS launched a $1.4 million HIV vaccine trial. GTZ launched a 2-year, €1 million project to re-equip six national reference laboratories and improve STD diagnoses.

Maternal and Child Health published (February). *The Potential Demand for an HIV/AIDS Vaccine in Brazil* issued by DEC (December). AIDS appeared in CAS Progress Report in context of millennium development goals.

Box 13.1. Timeline of key events: Brazil *continued*

Brazil

Year	National events	State/municipal events	HIV/AIDS events and data	Bilateral donors and multilateral agencies	World Bank
2003	(PAMs) with performance benchmarks and targets.	PAMs from 14 states and 158 municipalities approved (May).		ANRS invested €10 million to build a research center. CDC opened a Brazil office as part of its Global AIDS Program with $1.3 million for FY2003. GTZ launched a 2-year, €0.5 million project to support the Horizontal Technical Cooperation on HIV/AIDS Program. USAID launched a 6-year strategy, with up to $48 million for the entire project.	*Decentralization of Health Care in Brazil: A Case Study of Bahia* issued (May). AIDS II: Loan closed (June). Disease Surveillance and Control: Loan closed (December).

GAPA, Support Group for AIDS Prevention; UNDCP, United Nations Drug Control Programme; CAS, Country Assistance Strategy; MDGs, Millennium Development Goals

Teixeira, 1997). Although there were sixteen different ministers of health during the period 1985–2003, there were only four different national AIDS coordinators. Although most government programs suffered budget cuts following the financial crisis in 1998, the street protests on the part of activists ensured, according to several observers, that the AIDS program did not. The law that authorized the provision of ARV drugs to AIDS patients in 1996 enjoyed the support not only of the political left, which had traditionally been associated with the *sanitarista* movement, but also right-of-center parties, one of whose members, ex-president José Sarney, authored the legislation and guided it to congressional approval.

Second, localities were the site of the earliest government response, and some of them, in particular, São Paulo, retained influence throughout the development of official policies. In the crucial period between 1982 and 1988, popularly elected opposition parties controlled several important state governments, including São Paulo, for the first time in nearly twenty years. These states responded to the epidemic before the federal government did, and their approaches, which emphasized substantial collaboration with civil society for preventive activities and a human rights orientation, became a model for future activities at the national level.

Third, the principles of universal and equal access to health care, enshrined in the constitution and the SUS, established the legal and moral basis for the management of opportunistic infections and provision of zidovudine (AZT) monotherapy to AIDS patients through the mid-1990s, and then combination ARV therapy beginning in 1996.

Fourth, once established, the national AIDS program could not effectively decentralize activities to the states and municipalities because the legal and regulatory bases for decentralization were not consolidated until the late 1990s. As a result, outside of the most affected states, interventions remained centralized; and even in those states, AIDS interventions were isolated from other health care services, which were being slowly decentralized.

The Role of Civil Society

Collaborations of the Brazilian government with civil society organizations in the formulation and implementation of HIV/AIDS policy began early. Two nongovernmental organizations (NGOs), *Somos* and *Outra Coisa*, participated in the state of São Paulo's AIDS outreach and prevention programs for gay men in 1983. By 1986, several NGOs were involved in the federal government's policy working groups. In 1988, four NGOs (*Associação Brasiliera Interdisciplinar de AIDS, Grupo Gay da Bahia, Associção Brasiliera de Entidades de Planejamento Familiar,* and *Centro Corsini de Investigação Imunológica*) were given a formal role in the interministerial National AIDS Control Commission (Teixeira, 1997). A web of collective actors, including preexisting organizations, such as *Grupo Gay de Bahia* and *Atobá,* as well as new organizations such as GAPA (Support Group for AIDS Prevention) emerged to deliver services, advocate, and influence government policy (Parker, 1994). In the early years, while NGOs were collaborating with the National AIDS Program, including distributing prevention materials to vulnerable populations, many NGOs were also protesting the government's delay in regulating the national blood supply and its failure to provide information and resources for AIDS control.

The influence of civil society organizations has been striking. NGOs were vocal in their opposition to AIDS policies under the administration of President Fernando Mello de Collor (1990–1992) and influential in the government's decision to reappoint the former leader of the national AIDS program after Collor was impeached (Teixeira, 1997; Galvão, 2000). Civil society organizations demonstrated and lobbied successfully so that condoms would be included (along with beans, pasta, and rice) in the "basket of necessities" that large Brazilian corporations provided their workers, and in the simultaneous decision in 1998 to exempt condoms from taxes, so that the price of the condom would fall an estimated 30 percent (*A Folha de São Paulo,* 1998a). Brazilian civil society and AIDS NGOs played a role in lobbying Congress and the President's office to overcome resistance within the Ministry to the World Bank loans for AIDS, and launched simultaneous street demonstrations in sixteen states in 1999 to secure additional funding for AIDS treatment despite the recent devaluation and financial crisis. Although several government programs had suffered budget cuts in 1998, and although in the original proposal from the Ministry of Finance the largest cut was to fall on health care, the AIDS budget was not cut and, in fact, was listed in the "essential" programs to be protected. While the final proposal from the Ministry of Finance for 1999 increased the budget for AIDS drugs to R$314 (US$176 million, using average exchange rates for 1999), the Ministry of Health managed to reallocate resources internally so that the ARV budget was R$500 million (US$80 million), and then in September (partly in response to the street protests) an additional R$157 million (US$88 million) was appropriated for ARVs (whose domestic prices had risen as a result of the devaluation) (*A Folha de São Paulo*, 1998b, 1998c, 1999a, 1999b; interviews with Brazilian policy makers).

The number of Brazilian AIDS NGOs multiplied after a first World Bank loan earmarked a stream of money to civilian organizations for outreach, support, and prevention efforts; and their numbers in turn increased the visibility and political strength of the AIDS community in Brazil (the number of registered NGOs working on HIV/AIDS increased from 120 to 480 between 1993 and 1997; see Galvão, 2000). A review conducted for the World Bank in 2003 found 798 different NGOs working on HIV/AIDS in Brazil. After the return of the previous director of the National AIDS Control Program in 1992 and the beginning of the first World Bank loan in 1993, the government began to transfer resources to NGOs for HIV/AIDS prevention, outreach, treatment, and support projects. Between 1993 and 2003, $25.5 million was transferred to NGOs for activities related to HIV/AIDS outreach and support (World Bank, 2004). More than $10 million was budgeted for transfer to NGOs in 2004, and the government now plans to allocate 15 percent of the HIV/AIDS programmatic budget to NGOs (Programa Brasiliero de DST/AIDS, 2004). To promote sustainability on the part of NGOs, current procedures require NGO funds to be matched with private contributions raised by the NGOs.

The Early Policy Response

As in most countries, the first reports of AIDS in Brazil were received with denial, stigmatization, and blame on foreigners. A columnist in the leading newsmagazine speculated that AIDS might be the consequence of estrogen consumption on the part of homosexuals (*Veja*, 1982). Although some clergy, such as the Cardinal of São Paulo, counseled support for AIDS patients, others, such as the Cardinal of Rio de Janeiro, viewed the disease as divine retribution: "When the love of God, manifested in obedience to his teachings, is disparaged, whippings from a new threat to life awaken the recalcitrant." Even within the Ministry of Health in Brasília, some officials argued that AIDS did not satisfy the epidemiological criteria of "transcendence," "magnitude," and "vulnerability" necessary to warrant a response from public institutions. As late as 1985, INAMPS argued that AIDS was a "public health problem," not a medical concern, and therefore an issue for the state health secretariats, even though the latter had few health facilities available to them at the time (Teixeira, 1997).

The response of health sector officials in São Paulo was more aggressive. In 1983, under a popularly elected governor for the first time since 1964, the state government of São Paulo established an AIDS program in its Division of Leprosy and Dermatological Health, made AIDS notification compulsory, and initiated public awareness campaigns among and with the support of "high-risk groups," which consisted almost exclusively of men who have sex with men (MSM) at that time. Public funds for prevention were limited, so the state health authorities collaborated with gay rights NGOs and the gay and bisexual community, universities, the press, and community groups. The participation of physicians with long experience in treating leprosy and who belonged to the *sanitarista* movement sensitized health policy makers in São Paulo to issues of discrimination and stigma. A study of HIV/AIDS knowledge and awareness in 1987 in São Paulo State showed that 88 percent of MSM believed themselves to be "well informed" or "reasonably well informed" about AIDS in contrast to 65 percent of young people and only 49 percent of commercial sex workers (Bond, 1989). The study, conducted by the newspaper, *A Folha de São Paulo*, asked respondents to assess their own perceived knowledge about HIV/AIDS. It did not ask respondents about their understanding of specific modes of HIV transmission. The sample sizes in São Paulo were relatively small: 292 young people; 199 MSM and 103 commercial sex workers. It is not known whether this was a representative sample. In a larger sample of the general population of Brasilia and seven state capitals (n = 4,436), 64 percent rated themselves "well informed" or "reasonably well informed." Misconceptions among commercial sex workers in São Paulo and in the general population in Brasilia and seven state capitals were common, with roughly 49 percent of commercial sex workers and 23 percent of the general population believing that HIV could be transmitted through casual contact. Most respondents had received their HIV messages through the Ministry of Health and mass media (Bond, 1989).

The São Paulo state assembly passed legislation in 1986 requiring serological testing for all blood transfusions in the state. The state health secretariat coordinated a pilot AIDS education program in schools, but the program did not continue once the state education secretariat took control. In a joint initiative, the state health and justice secretariats recommended combating AIDS in prisons with education and made the case against isolating HIV-positive prisoners. However, in practice in the early years prison authorities implemented compulsory serological testing and isolation throughout the country. In 1988 the state established its state reference and treatment center (CRT) for AIDS and launched programs of "day hospitals" and the tracking of unused beds in public hospitals for use by AIDS patients. The CRT would become a leading national institution in treatment, support, prevention, and research.

The National AIDS Program was established at the federal level in 1985 (Portaria No. 236, 1985). This program changed its name several times during its history. (See Galvão, 2000, for a list of names.) For simplicity, it is called the National AIDS Program (NAP) throughout this document (whatever its legal name at any given point in time, with the exception of bibliographic references). Financial and technical support from the World Health Organization (WHO) and Pan American Health Organization (PAHO) began in earnest in 1986 and the NAP was consolidated. The importance attached to nondiscrimination, human rights, and NGO participation on the part of the São Paulo program, as well as many of the eleven other state programs in existence in 1985, informed the organization of the national program. In 1987 the national program began coordinating and leading the activities of the state health secretariats, which until then had led the AIDS response.

It was not until 1988 that Congress passed laws requiring serological testing for all blood banks and granting persons living with AIDS the rights guaranteed to workers with incapacitating or terminal illnesses (Law No. 7649, 1988). That same year a multisectoral council that reported to the Ministry of Health, the National AIDS Commission, was established and mobilized support for the AIDS program across the political spectrum. The NAP launched several activities in collaboration with other ministries, such as the AIDS in the work place program in conjunction with the Ministry of Labor, but over time most programs fell to the Ministry of Health alone. In 1989 the Ministry of the Armed Forces initiated a program for AIDS prevention among enlisted personnel (Portaria No. 1, 1989). Annual meetings of Brazilian NGOs working on AIDS began in 1989 in Belo Horizonte.

Voluntary counseling and testing services for those who do not know their HIV status, a cornerstone of prevention programs, were limited in this period. AIDS testing was done in clinical settings and to confirm suspected AIDS cases, not as a tool for surveillance and prevention. Nationwide, condom sales were relatively flat and at low levels (fewer than 10 million male condoms per year) from 1987 to 1992.

AIDS policies in Brazil entered a new and difficult phase in 1990 following hyperinflation and the election of a controversial new president. The NAP was dismantled and, in a pattern consistent with President Collor's effort to govern with the support of the media and public opinion and without the support of some of the traditional party alliances, the Ministry of Health set up an alternative structure for organizing the response to AIDS. Municipal AIDS and Commissions would coordinate activities in the field without input from the state health secretariats, which had been leading the response since 1983. These Municipal AIDS Commissions frequently lacked the expertise to develop and manage HIV/AIDS policies. Conflict with state secretariats and confusion regarding the direction of policies occurred throughout the country. At the same time, the Ministry of Health launched a publicity campaign that emphasized the danger of AIDS to the uninfected and isolated itself from the NGOs and community groups that had been active for almost a decade. Declaring, "Brazil will not be a guinea pig" and impugning the expertise of the World Health Organization, the Minister of Health refused to participate in WHO-led HIV vaccine trials, which resulted in the virtual isolation of the Brazilian AIDS program from the international community.

Nevertheless, President Collor did mention AIDS in a public speech in 1990 (a first), the government began to purchase and distribute some AIDS drugs, offering AZT monotherapy free of charge, and it continued to advance the rights of AIDS patients. The national secretariat for health care (the former Secretaário Nacional de Assistência à Sáude) began to reimburse treatments for AIDS patients provided by private philanthropic hospitals in 1992 (Portaria No. 291, 1992). INAMPS also initiated the first of several ministerial decrees credentialing hospitals, day hospitals, and laboratories for providing AIDS care and services (Portaria No. 7750, 1992). The Ministries of Labor, Health, and Administration approved a decree prohibiting the use of HIV tests in physical examinations of public sector workers (Portaria No. 869, 1992). By the end of 1992 at least 67 local laws and resolutions regarding HIV/AIDS had been approved at the state and municipal levels. These included requirements that motels and hotels provide condoms, guarantees of non-discrimination for public sector workers and students, legal recognition and incorporation of AIDS NGOs, the reservation of hospital beds for AIDS patients, incorporation of information on HIV prevention into public and private school curricula, and compulsory HIV testing of prisoners.

By the early 1990s, a Brazilian strategy toward HIV/AIDS had emerged— an approach embracing prevention among high-risk groups, universal access to treatment, and respect for human rights. After the resignation of the president under corruption charges in September 1992, the new government reconstituted the NAP and invited back its previous director. The program recommitted itself to previous relationships with NGOs, the state health secretariats, and the international AIDS community. Among the first important steps of the program was to begin discussions with the World Bank regarding the possibility of a loan for combating HIV/AIDS.

Explicit Human Rights Protections

The establishment of legal protections, especially legislation guaranteeing nondiscrimination in the civil sphere, has been an important way in which governments have acted to support HIV-positive individuals. These measures protect the well-being and dignity of persons living with HIV/AIDS, and they also promote public health efforts by encouraging previously stigmatized individuals to come into contact with formal institutions. In the United States, for instance, people living with HIV/AIDS gained enormous protections when their status was included under the Americans with Disabilities Act (Public Law 336 of the 101st Congress, July 26, 1990). The Department of Justice's Regulations for Title II (*Federal Register.* July 26, 1991) included HIV in the list of diseases and conditions covered by the protections under this act. The Brazilian Congress passed a law similar to the U.S. law in 1988, guaranteeing workers the same rights afforded to those with other incapacitating illnesses. In addition, in Brazil, the National AIDS Commission in 1988 rejected a provision that would have limited the entry of HIV-positive foreign nationals into the country; and a regulation in 1992 prohibited the use of serological tests before admission into civil service and during periodic health testing of civil servants (Pimenta and Veriano, 2002). In 1995, the Brazilian Congress passed a legislative decree that approved the San Salvador protocol for economic, social, and cultural rights (Decreto Legislativo no. 56, 1995). In 1996, an executive decree established the National Program on Human Rights under the Ministry of Justice (Decreto no. 1904, 1996). An annex to the latter decree enumerated the administration's short- and medium-term goals, and of the thirteen short-term goals under the heading of equal protection under the law, four were related to HIV/AIDS.

Prevention Programs in the 1990s

Brazil's epidemic primarily affected members of vulnerable and stigmatized groups and later the urban and rural poor, so providing services to these groups required leadership, innovative programs, and political will. The engagement of NGOs and civil society in the organization and delivery of targeted interventions strengthened the position of these often-marginalized stakeholders, helping to sustain commitment for prevention among the populations most likely to contract HIV.

Over the course of the decade, Brazil sharply increased the number of interventions targeted at MSM, commercial sex workers, and injection drug user (IDU) populations. (See Figure 13.1.) During the period 1999–2003, the program implemented 547 projects, which covered an estimated 899,386 commercial sex workers, 631 projects reaching some 145,807 IDUs (an estimated 18.2 percent of that population), and 486 projects covering some 3,074,980 MSM reaching a reported coverage of 96 percent of that population. Coverage rates are in need of further substantiation and should be interpreted with caution. These figures include both public-sector- and NGO-executed projects.

Harm Reduction

Harm reduction seeks to reduce the spread of HIV associated with injection drug use through outreach, education in safer practices, needle and syringe exchange programs, access to counseling and drug treatment, and non-judgmental approaches to working closely with individuals and communities. Harm-reduction programs are supported by an extensive body of evidence to show that they are cost-effective, can reduce HIV and other blood-borne pathogen transmission, and can serve as effective bridges to drug treatment and health care (Des Des Jarlais and Friedman, 1998). They do not encourage young people to initiate drug use, as is often feared. Yet they remain controversial, politically challenging, and resisted by many countries. The United States, for example, continues to have a ban on federal funding for needle and syringe exchange programs and to regulate access to injection equipment.

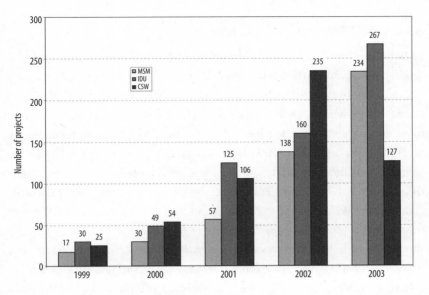

Figure 13.1. Growth in targeted interventions for high-risk groups, 1999–2003.
Source: Beyrer, Gauri, and Vaillancourt, 2004

By 1988, the linkages between injectable drugs, shared needles, HIV infection, and HIV transmission to partners of drug users were becoming known. The municipality of Santos and the state of São Paulo launched "harm-reduction" programs that included needle exchanges in 1989 and 1990, respectively. However, the Federal Narcotics Council (FNC) intervened to halt the program in Santos and the political leadership in the secretariat of health put an end to the initiative in São Paulo. Over time, however, political support for harm reduction grew. A meeting of the Ibero-American Health Ministers in 1993 endorsed needle and syringe exchanges and bleach distribution to prevent HIV among IDUs. The National AIDS Program adopted harm reduction as an explicit policy in 1994. The FNC approved, in 1994, a six-site pilot harm-reduction program proposed by the Ministry of Health. In 1995 the São Paulo state secretary of health openly endorsed harm-reduction approaches and outlined key strategies to be incorporated into state programs. The original pilot project in Santos was eventually implemented in Salvador, and by 1997 some 5,000 needles had been exchanged (Inciardi et al., 2000).

Behavioral Effect of Prevention Efforts

Behavioral studies in Brazil have used a number of standard measures to assess risk, including the proportions of men and women reporting multiple and/or casual sex partners in the past year, using a condom with the most recent sexual act, using a condom with regular partners and casual partners, using a condom when having sex for the first time, and reporting of male same-sex behaviors. Table 13.1 provides an overview of the limited information available on key trends in prevalence and behaviors among high-risk groups. Between 1999 and 2001, the use of condoms among IDUs increased from 42.1 percent to 62.9 percent and the proportion of IDUs ever tested for HIV increased from 52 percent to 66.4 percent. In addition, needle sharing among this group decreased over this same period from 70 percent to 59.4 percent (Universidade Federal Minas Gerais/National AIDS and STDs Control Program [NASCP], 2001). A study of 3,000 commercial sex workers conducted in 2001 revealed that 73.8 percent of this group (composed of program participants) used condoms with their clients (versus 60 percent of commercial sex workers not participating in the program) but only 23.9 percent of them used condoms with their regular (nonpaying) partners. Almost half of the commercial sex workers studied (49.2%) had been tested for HIV versus 36 percent of those not participating (Universidade de Brasília/NASCP, 2003). Trends in behavior over time among commercial sex workers are not available. Use of condoms among MSM in 2001 was reported to be high at 81 percent with regular partners and even higher at 95 percent with casual partners (Projeto Bela Vista, 2003). Without baseline data to indicate levels of condom use among MSM, it is difficult to assess trends over time. Testing history among MSM was reported to be significant, with 73 percent of urban men reporting having been tested in 2001 (Projeto Bela Vista, 2003).

Brazil's AIDS program also increased efforts to broaden prevention messages to the general population. The project procured condoms that were made available to the public through targeted interventions, social marketing initiatives, and distribution through the Ministry of Health. Male condoms distributed through the Ministry of Health more than tripled between 2000 and 2003 from 77 million to 270 million and those sold through the commercial sector increased from 228.4 million in 1997 to 427.1 million in 2003 (Ministry of Health/NASCP, 2003). Between 1997 and 2003, the sale

Table 13.1. Prevalence of HIV and risk indicators for high-risk populations, Brazil, 1999-2002

Indicator	IDU 1999[a]	IDU 2001[b]	CSW 2001[c]	MSM 1994–1999	MSM 2001[d]	MSM 2002[e]
HIV prevalence	52%	36.3%	6.5%	10.8%		
HCV prevalence	60%	56.4%	4.5%			
Condom use	42.1%	62.9%	73.8% with clients; 23.9% with regular partners		81% with regular partners; 95% with casual partners	70% in all anal intercourse in past 6 months
Ever HIV tested	52%	66.4%	49.2%		73%	69%
Needle sharing	70%	59.4%				
Sample size	287	869	3,000	1,082	800	1,200
Location	5 cities	7 cities	5 cities	unknown	7 capital cities	10 capital cities

Source: Ministry of Health/NASCP, 2003, compiled from the following studies: Federal University of Minas Gerais and NASCP (a, b); Federal University of Brasilia and NASCP (c); Opinion polls carried out by Instituto Brasileiro de Opinião Publica e Estatística (d,e).
Note: All these data must be interpreted with caution. The first study on IDUs was of dubious quality and included only program users. The data on commercial sex worker (CSW) condom use and HIV testing refer only to the CSWs who participated in the project. Use of condoms with clients by nonparticipating CSWs is less than that for participating CSWs (60% versus 74%) as is the percentage of those ever tested for HIV (36% versus 49%). Data on MSM for 1994–1999 rely on a very biased sample, given that there was considerable sample attrition.

of condoms rose significantly (from 228.4 million to 427.1 million condoms) and the mean price of condoms fell from US$0.57 per condom to US$0.28 in 2001 (see Figure 13.2), largely because of the reduction/elimination of duties and taxes. (Before the first loan in 1993, the World Bank urged Brazil to develop a plan to eliminate taxes on condoms. Condoms were made exempt from taxes in 1998.) According to Ministry of Health statistics, between 1986 and 2003, use of condom in first sexual encounter among the general population increased from 4 percent to 55 percent. A 2003 poll reported that 65.2 percent of persons aged 14–19 reported using a condom in their first sexual encounter.

The Ministry of Education, Ministry of Justice (Special Secretariat for Human Rights), National Anti-Drugs Secretariat, and Ministry of Labor undertook additional prevention activities. A 2001 survey of schools carried out

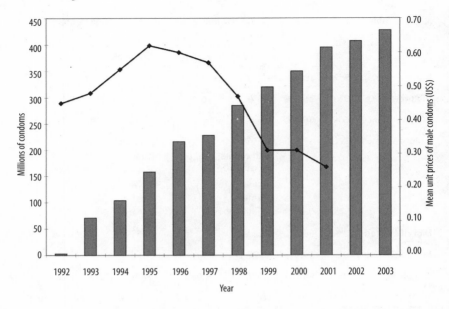

Figure 13.2. Annual sales and unit prices of male condoms in Brazil, 1992–2003. *Source*: Brazil Ministry of Health

by the Ministry of Health with support from the U.N. Educational, Scientific, and Cultural Organization (UNESCO) revealed that 70 percent of the schools carried out prevention activities with students; 97 percent of all students had correct information on how AIDS was transmitted; and 90 percent of students with active sex lives changed their behavior regarding STD and AIDS after intensive exposure to school prevention activities (Ministry of Health/ NASCP, 2003).

A population survey conducted in 2003 showed a significant increase in the proportion of persons who spontaneously cited the use of condoms as a method for protecting themselves, from 50 percent in 1998 to 88.9 percent in 2003 (Centro Brasiliero de Análise e Planajamiento, 2000; Instituto Brasiliero de Opinião Pública e Estatística/MS, 2003). The proportion of sexually active military conscripts that reported using a condom in their most recent sexual encounter was 68 percent in 2003, a slight increase from 1998 data that indicate proportions of 51.2 percent in the north and central west, 66.6 percent in the south, and 67.7 percent in Rio and São Paulo. In its final report on AIDS II, the Ministry of Health reports that use of condoms among the general population in all sexual encounters declined between 1998 and 2003 from 63.7 percent to 57.8 percent with casual partners and from 21.0 to 11.4 percent with long-term partners. (The Ministry of Health does caution in its report that this trend is questionable, as the earlier study (Centro Brasiliero de Análise e Planajamiento, 2000) documented behaviors of an urban-only population (which typically registers higher condom use) and the 2003 population poll included both urban and rural populations.)

In addition, public policies have been attempting to encourage the adult population to be tested for HIV, to enhance both prevention and treatment programs. A large body of evidence suggests that not knowing personal HIV status is an indicator of poor uptake of prevention information (Sweat et al., 2000). A 1998 randomized population survey found that 20.2 percent of the adult population had been tested at least once; rates were higher in the south (25 percent) and lower in the north-northeast (9.6 percent) (Fonseca et al., 2003). Among 3,000 female sex workers interviewed in 2001, nearly half (49.2%) had ever been tested (Universidade de Brasília/NASCP, 2001). Testing history was even more common among MSM, with 73 percent of urban men reporting having been tested in 2001 (Instituto Brasileiro de Opinião Pública e Estatística/MS, 2001).

Treatment Programs

Brazil's public health system began to provide free AZT to all patients with clinical AIDS in 1991. The national secretariat for health care began to reimburse treatments for AIDS patients provided by private philanthropic hospitals in 1992. Between 1993 and 1996 Brazil created 190 new treatment facilities for AIDS patients and 31 publicly financed home care services. Shortly after the efficacy of highly active antiretroviral therapy (HAART; or triple-drug antiretroviral therapy) for improving survival and quality of life of AIDS patients was established internationally in 1996, the Congress passed a law (that same year) specifying that ARV drugs would be provided to AIDS patients, and Brazil began to provide HAART for patients with clinical AIDS late that year. The law stated that "all carriers of HIV and AIDS patients will receive, free of charge from the Unified Health System, all medications necessary for that treatment." (Law No. 9313, 1996). A 1997 Ministry of Health decree established the treatment protocols related to CD4 counts and viral loads (Portaria No. 874, 1997). To support the HAART program, Brazil upgraded more than sixty laboratories nationwide to monitor the viral loads of patients on HAART or to conduct T CD4+ lymphocyte testing. In 2003, there were 140,000 individuals on HAART in Brazil (World Bank, 2004).

Reported deaths from AIDS rose steadily from approximately 6/100,000 persons in 1990, to more than 11/100,000 in 1994. AIDS deaths peaked in 1995 at just over 12/100,000 persons. AIDS deaths declined thereafter, to 10/100,000 in 1996, 8/100,000 in 1997, and 6.3/100,000 in 2000. The number of AIDS deaths has remained stable since 1998, with no further declines and in fact a slight increase. Survival after diagnosis has increased from a median of 5 months for those diagnosed in 1986 to 58 months for those diagnosed since 1996 (Marins et al., 2003).

At the time that the policy of universal free access to HAART was introduced in late 1996, the cost of antiretroviral treatment in Western countries was already on the order of $10,000–20,000 per patient per year. Bringing down the cost of drug treatment has been a major focus of the AIDS program, and the government has fought for flexibility in the international intellectual property regime on human rights grounds. As a result, there have been significant drug price declines since the start of the ARV program, and these have been dramatic since the universal access policy in 1997. The cost of the 076 AZT regimen for prevention of mother-to-child transmission of HIV fell from US $660 in 1997 to US$170 in 2001. The costs for two-drug regimens fell from $3,810 in 1996 to $630 per patient/year in 2001. For triple therapy the costs declined 66 percent per patient per year, from $4,500 in 1998 to $1,540 in 2001. By 2001, all ARV treatment costs per patient per year declined by 48 percent and these declines appear to be ongoing. Costs have been reduced through a two-pronged strategy: (1) Local formulation and distribution of seven antiviral drugs including zidovudine (AZT), Didanosine (ddI), Lamivudine (3TC), Estavudine (d4T), Endeavor, Ritonavir, and Nevirapine; and (2) for those drugs Brazil does not manufacture, generic purchases or bulk purchase at reduced prices on the international market. Drugs in this category include Abacavir, Saquinavir, Nelfinavir, Amprenavir, Efavirenz, and Lopinavir, and most of the more difficult-to-manufacture and expensive protease inhibitors are in this category. Nevirapine, for example, declined in cost from US$3.04 to US$1.25 per capsule from 1999 to 2001 (NAP, 2003).

The HAART policy reduced, in the short run, the incidence of opportunistic infections requiring hospitalization, invoking a cost savings in terms of avoided admissions estimated at US$76 million per year in 1997, climbing to nearly $360 million per year in 2001 (calculations from NASCP statistics, 2003). (The number of yearly admissions per AIDS patient declined from 1.7/year in 1996 to 0.28/year in 2001. Because the long-term prognosis for patients receiving HAART remains uncertain, patients receiving antiretrovirals might well require hospitalizations in the future. Thus, the estimates of hospitalization costs avoided might be more accurately treated as estimates of costs deferred.)

Surveillance as of 2004

AIDS surveillance is well established in Brazil, but HIV surveillance and incidence are important in measuring and tracking the evolution of this epidemic and in measuring the effect of a program. Although Brazil's HIV surveillance system has been strengthened in recent years, in 2004 it still fell short of a fully functional system that is able to generate a continuous stream of reliable and representative data that permit monitoring of the epidemic geographically and among different population groups. During the three-year period 1997–1999, sentinel surveillance data were reported twice a year from the three types of sentinel site: maternities, emergency rooms, and STD clinics. The number of sites reporting has fluctuated with each reporting period, making the data difficult to interpret and also making it difficult to determine the number of fully functional sentinel sites. In October 1999 reports were received from 39 STD clinics, 64 maternities, and 46 emergency rooms. HIV testing was done on randomized patients of these clinics producing statistics per semester on about 7,000 STD patients, 12,000 pregnant women, and 8,600 emergency room patients nationwide. In 2000 Brazil introduced significant changes to its surveillance system because it was perceived that hospital surveillance sites had become reference centers for HIV/AIDS and thus were providing biased estimates. The Brazilian surveillance system now selects a random sample of 150 hospital maternities, which have more than 500 deliveries per year to test women delivering in that hospital for a more representative measurement of HIV prevalence. A different random sample of hospitals, which may include some of the same hospitals, is used for each measurement. As of 2004, only two measurements had been taken since this change: one in 2000 with data from 128 hospital maternities (15,426 pregnant women tested) and from 25 STD clinics (4,636 STD patients tested) and one in 2003, for which data are not yet available. The program subsequently decided to drop the STD clinic sentinel sites, because the quality of the data from these sites was considered too unreliable. The Brazilians have opted for less-frequent surveillance measurements because it is considered too expensive to conduct every year.

HIV surveillance is still limited to pregnant women and to military conscripts (the latter through annual surveys). (These data are now being supplemented by an information system established to support routing reporting of epidemiological and behavioral data on Center for Testing and Counseling [CTA] clients by the network of CTAs.) High priority, high-risk groups that are a primary focus of prevention efforts (MSM, IDUs, commercial sex workers) have not been systematically included in routine HIV sentinel surveillance efforts. Special studies on HIV among these groups undertaken with project support have been carried out to supplement sentinel system data, but they lack a systematic methodology that would have allowed the tracking of trends over time or cross-regional analysis. With Centers for Disease Control and Prevention (CDC) support, in 1998 the NASCP initiated efforts to strengthen its capacity to estimate the incidence of HIV based on cross-section studies of prevalence. (This support involves the application of the serological testing algorithm for recent HIV seroconversion (STARHS) strategy, developed by the CDC, which allows for the determination of whether people with newly reported cases of HIV were infected within the past year.)

With the exception of annual surveys of military conscripts, there has been no surveillance system in Brazil for routinely collecting data on behaviors of segments of the general population or of high-risk groups. In the absence of a viable system for evaluating program performance and impact, the numerous studies and supervisions carried out by a multiplicity of actors, covering a range of methodologies, indicators, geographical areas, populations, implementers, and time frames, have been almost impossible to consolidate to provide a coherent overview of program performance or impact on behaviors. NAP recently launched an effort to collect systematic behavioral and biological data.

The Current State of the Epidemic

As of 2000, an estimated 600,000 Brazilians were living with HIV infection, down from PAHO's estimate of 750,000 in 1992. (As part of the preparation of a third World Bank loan to support Brazil's HIV/AIDS program (AIDS III), the bank estimated that about 800,000 Brazilians were infected in 2002.) As of March 2002, 237,588 AIDS cases and 110,651 deaths from AIDS had been reported since the beginning of the epidemic. In the absence of adequate HIV surveillance data, the population prevalence of HIV has been reliably estimated at 0.65 percent through national probability sampling of pregnant women in 2002. The study (Szwarcwald, 2002) included 132 sentinel sites and anonymous blood collections from 15,426 pregnant women. Overall, 0.47 percent of women (95% confidence interval [CI] 0.36, 0.58) were HIV infected. Using a gender ratio derived from recent AIDS reporting, rates in men of reproductive age were estimated at 0.84 percent (95% CI 0.65, 1.04). This gave a combined population prevalence of 0.65 percent (95% CI 0.51, 0.80) for the population aged 15–49 years nationwide. This well-done study is likely to be the best estimation available of the HIV infection rate in Brazil in 2000. Using wider (68%) confidence intervals and census data on the national population generates total numbers of HIV infections at 597,000 with a lower limit of 548,000 and an upper bound of 647,000. This study generated the widely used figures of 0.65 percent HIV prevalence and the estimate of 600,000 people living with HIV in 2000, and there is little reason to think that these estimates are substantially lower or higher than the 68 percent confidence intervals. Whereas the history of HIV/AIDS suggests complacency is always a danger, the characterization of a still concentrated epidemic seems, on the whole, correct, well below the 2 percent rate UNAIDS has suggested for describing generalized epidemics (Szwarcwald, 2002). Brazil's HIV epidemic in 2004 can thus be characterized as concentrated, still largely limited to individuals and groups engaging in high-risk behaviors for HIV: commercial sex workers, heterosexuals with multiple partners, and female partners of IDUs and bisexual men. While transmission doubtless continues to occur in persons at risk (and an increasing proportion of persons at risk are women, especially partners of IDUs and bisexual men), there is no evidence of acceleration or increasing rates of new HIV infection. Rather, HIV infections are stable or slightly declining, while HIV/AIDS survival times are significantly increasing.

The modes of transmission of the epidemic, the prevalence and behaviors of high-risk groups, and the prevalence by region of the country have evolved since the early 1980s. From 1980 to 1990 sexual transmission accounted for

63.8 percent of AIDS cases and this has gradually increased to 74.4 percent of AIDS cases in 2000. Within this category, transmission through MSM decreased by more than half from an estimated 47.4 percent of all AIDS cases during the 1980s to 20.3 percent in 2000, and the share of cases attributable to heterosexual transmission more than tripled from 16.4 percent to 54.1 percent. Heterosexual transmission is still limited to high-risk groups (partners of IDUs and bisexual men and people with multiple partners). Transmission through intravenous drug use rose from an estimated 18.5 percent of total cases in the 1980s to a high of 24.8 percent in 1992 and subsequently declined in the ensuing years to 11.4 percent in 2000. Transmission by transfusion has decreased as a share of reported AIDS cases from 5.3 percent in the 1980s to 0.2 percent in 2000 and perinatal transmission rose from 1.8 percent in the 1980s to 2.5 percent in 2000. (See Table 13.2.)

Studies on the HIV prevalence of the highest-risk groups reveal prevalence levels of 36.3 percent among IDUs, 10.8 percent among MSM, and 6.5 percent among commercial sex workers (see Table 13.1) for recent years in various samples, most of them non-national. As noted in Table 13.1, these data must be interpreted with caution. Trend data on HIV prevalence over time are not available for these groups.

The incidence of AIDS in Brazil, as measured by year of diagnosis, increased from 8.2/100,000 in 1991 to a high of 18.2/100,000 in 1998 with a decline to 12.0 recorded in 2002, but patterns across regions vary. In 2002 the south surpassed the southeast as the region with the highest incidence; and incidence rates in the north and northeast, while showing slight decline in 2000, are still of concern (see Table 13.3). Again, trends in AIDS cases reflect levels of transmission that occurred some 10 years before.

PAHO estimated that 750,000 persons were living with HIV in Brazil in 1992 and that this number would be more than 1 million within 18 months. This did not happen. HIV infections are well under a third of expected cumulative totals. The extent to which Brazil's lower rates were due to prevention is difficult to quantify, and the spread was likely overestimated in the early 1990s. Few, if any, of the countries with similar rates in 1990 mounted anything like Brazil's targeted and progressive prevention response, however. This vigorous HIV prevention response almost certainly played an important role in making later commitments to universal treatment more feasible—by de-

Table 13.2. Reported cases of AIDS, by mode of transmission and year of diagnosis (%)

	Cumulative 1980–1990	Annual					Cumulative total 1980–2002
		1992	1994	1996	1998	2000	
Sexual	63.8	59.2	60	61.5	70.2	74.4	65.6
MSM	47.4	33.5	26.9	21.8	22.4	20.3	26.6
Hetero	16.4	25.7	33.1	39.7	47.8	54.1	39
IDU	18.5	24.8	21.4	17.9	13.3	11.4	17.2
Transfusion	5.3	2.4	1.8	1.7	0.2	0.2	0.5
Perinatal	1.8	2.8	3.4	4	3.3	2.5	3
Unknown	10.7	10.8	13.3	15	13	11.6	12.4
Total	100	100	100	100	100	100	100

Source: Brazil Ministry of Health, 2002

creasing the number of Brazilians needing AIDS care through averting HIV infections.

Looking Ahead

The incidence of HIV in Brazil appears to have stabilized, discrimination against people living with HIV/AIDS has declined, Brazil is providing state-of-the-art treatment to individuals with clinical AIDS, and the National AIDS Program appears to have the requisite political strength to maintain an aggressive response. Nevertheless, Brazil's AIDS response will face three significant challenges in the years ahead. First, equity remains a problem. Of the 600,000–800,000 estimated to have HIV, some 175,000 either are receiving ART or are on active follow-up. Many of the remaining individuals probably are not aware of their HIV status, and many in all likelihood have limited contact with the health care system. In more isolated parts of the country, nutrition and access to water exacerbate the consequences for HIV for poor individuals. Second, the AIDS treatment program remains a relatively well-functioning enclave in a poorly integrated health care system of mixed quality. Many people with AIDS who require specialist care do not receive appropriate referrals. The quality of health care service in many facilities is poor, and many individuals in the health care system do not receive appropriate diagnosis, testing, and counseling. Third, Brazil will face financing challenges as new, and probably expensive, AIDS treatment medications become available, and as the population of AIDS patients receiving chronic, long-term care

Table 13.3. Reported cases of AIDS (number) and incidence (per 100,000), by region, 1980–2002

Region	Cumulative 1980–1990 cases	Annual 1992 Cases	Annual 1992 Inc.	Annual 1994 Cases	Annual 1994 Inc.	Annual 1996 Cases	Annual 1996 Inc.	Annual 1998 Cases	Annual 1998 Inc.	Annual 2000 Cases	Annual 2000 Inc.	Annual 2002 Cases	Annual 2002 Inc.	Total 1980–2003[†] cases
North	221	185	1.8	317	2.9	455	4	644	5.4	663	5.3	606	4.5	5,992
Northeast	1,637	1,039	2.4	1,405	3.2	2,005	4.5	2,773	6.1	2,692	5.8	2,383	4.9	25,905
Center west	760	653	6.8	925	9.2	1,243	11.8	1,330	12.1	1,349	11.8	957	7.9	13,824
Southeast	20,723	11,918	18.8	14,067	21.5	17,803	26.6	19,295	28	16,299	23	11,861	15.9	203,537
South	1,831	1,523	6.8	2,517	11	3,813	16.2	5,327	22.1	5,470	22.1	5,089	19.8	48,190
Brazil	25,172	15,318	10.3	19,231	12.5	25,319	16.1	29,370	18.2	26,474	15.9	20,897	12	297,468

Source: Ministry of Health, 2003

*Inc., incidence

[†]Includes preliminary data through September 2003

swells. Maintaining political support in the context of sharply rising costs could pose a potential problem.

Acknowledgments

Sections of this chapter have appeared in Varun Gauri, Chris Beyrer, and Denise Vaillancourt, Brazil's Response to HIV/AIDS: Policies and Politics, 1983–2004 (under review); and Chris Beyrer, Varun Gauri, and Denise Vaillancourt, *Evaluation of the World Bank's Assistance in Responding to the AIDS Epidemic: Brazil Case Study.* OED, World Bank, October 2004.

References

A Folha de São Paulo. July 6, 1998a.

A Folha de São Paulo. September 18, 1998b.

A Folha de São Paulo. September 23, 1998c.

A Folha de São Paulo. September 2, 1999a.

A Folha de São Paulo. September 9, 1999b.

A Legislação sobre HIV/AIDS no Mundo de Trabalho. In *ILO, HIV/AIDS no Mundo do Trabalho: As Ações e a Legislação Brasileira.* Brasilia, 2002.

Americans with Disabilities Act, Public Law 336 of the 101st Congress, July 26, 1990.

Beyrer, C., V. Gauri, and D. Vaillancourt. 2004. Evaluation of the World Bank's assistance in responding to the AIDS epidemic: Brazil case study. Case Study for the OED evaluation of the Bank's HIV/AIDS assistance. Washington, DC: World Bank, Operations Evaluation Department.

Bond, L. S. 1989. Public information about AIDS in Brazil, the Dominican Republic, Haiti, and Mexico. *Bulletin of the Pan American Health Organization* 23:86–94.

Brazil Ministry of Health. 2002. *Epidemiological Bulletin.* March.

Centro Brasiliero de Análise e Planajamiento. 2000. Comportamento Sexual da População. Brasileira e Percepções do HIV/AIDS. São Paulo, Brasil.

Decreto Legislativo No. 56, April 19, 1995.

Decreto No. 1904, May 13, 1996.

DesJarlais, D. C., and Friedman, S. R. 1998. Fifteen years of research on preventing HIV infection among injecting drug users: What we have learned, what we have not learned, what we have done, what we have not done. *Public Health Report* 113 (Suppl. 1):182–88.

Fonseca, M. G., Travassos, C., Bastos, F. I., Silva Ndo, V., and Szwarcwald, C. L. 2003. Social distribution of AIDS in Brazil, according to labor market participation, occupation and socioeconomic status of cases from 1987 to 1998. *Cadernos de Saúde Pública* 19:1351–63.

Galvão, J. 1997. As Respostas Religiosas Frente à Epidemia de HIV/AIDS no Brasíl. In *Políticas, Instituições e AIDS: Enfrentando a Epidemia no Brasil,* ed. Richard Parker. Rio de Janeiro: Jorge Zahar Editor/ABIA.

Galvão, J. 2000. *AIDS no Brasil: A Agenda de Construção de Uma Epidemia.* Brasil, Editora 34.

Inciardi, J. A., Surratt, H. L., and Telles, P. R. 2000. *Sex, Drugs, and HIV/AIDS in Brazil.* Boulder, CO: Westview Press.

Instituto Brasileiro de Opinião Pública e Estatística/MS. 2001. Pesquisa sobre homosexualismo.

Instituto Brasiliero de Opinião Pública e Estatística/MS. 2003. Pesquisa com a População Sexualmente Activa.

International Herald Tribune. July 25, 2005.

Law No. 7649, January 25, 1988 (Brazil).

Law No. 9313, November 13, 1996 (Brazil).

Mainwaring, S. 1986. The transition to democracy in Brazil. *Journal of Interamerican Studies and World Affairs* 28:149–79.

Marins, J. R., Jamal, L. F., Chen, S. Y., Barros, M. B., Hudes, E. S., Barbosa, A. A., Chequer, P., Teixeira, P. R., and Hearst, N. 2003. Dramatic improvement in survival among adult Brazilian AIDS patients. *AIDS* 25:1675–82.

Ministry of Health Epidemiological Bulletin. March 2002.

Ministry of Health/National AIDS and STDs Control Program (NASCP). 2003. Rélatorio de Implementaçao et Avaliaçao, 1998 a 2003. Accordo de Emprestimo BIRD 4392/BR-Projeto AIDS II, Versão Preliminar, Brasilia-DF.

National AIDS Program (NAP), HIV/AIDS Surveillance Data. 2003.

Parker, R. B. 1994. A AIDS no Brazil, 1982–1992, Calecão História social de AIDS; no. 2. Rio de Janeiro, RJ: ABIA:IMS-UERJ:Relume Dumará.

Pimenta, M. C., and Veriano, T. Jr., 2002. As Ações Brasileiras de Combate ao IV/AIDS e o Mundo do Trabalho, and João Hilário Valentime, A Legislação sobre HIV/AIDS no Mundo de Trabalho in *ILO, HIV/AIDS no Mundo do Trabalho: As Ações e a Legislação Brasileira.* Brasilia.

Portaria No. 236, May 2, 1985.

Portaria No. 1, April 27, 1989.

Portaria No. 291, June 17, 1992.

Portaria No. 7750, July14, 1992.

Portaria No. 869, August 11, 1992.

Portaria No. 874, July 3, 1997.

Programa Brasiliero de DST/AIDS. 2004. *Resposta: A experiência do Programa Brasileiro de AIDS.*

Projeto Bela Vista. 2003. *Estudo Sócio-comportamental e Determinação da Incidência de Infecção por HIV em uma Coorte de Homens que Fazem Sexo com Homens, em São Paulo, Brasil.*

Skidmore, T. E. 1989. Brazil's slow road to democratization, 1974–1985 (Chap. 1). In *Democratizing Brazil: Problems of Transition and Consolidation,* ed. A. Stepan. New York: Oxford University Press.

Stepan, A. 1989. *Democratizing Brazil: Problems of transition and consolidation.* New York: Oxford University Press.

Sweat, M., Gregorich, S., Sangiwa, G., Furlonge C., Balmer, D., Kamenga, C., Grinstead, O., and Coates, T. 2000. Cost-effectiveness of voluntary HIV-1 counseling and testing in reducing sexual transmission of HIV-1 in Kenya and Tanzania. *Lancet* 356:113–21.

Szwarcwald, C. L. 2002. Oportunidades perdidas na detecção precoce do HIV na gestação: Resultados do Estudo Sentinela-Parturiente, Brasil. (Unpublished report, used with permission of the author.)

Teixeira, P. R. 1997. Políticas públicas em AIDS. In *Políticas Instituições e Aids*, ed. Richard Parker. Rio de Janeiro: Jorge Zahar, Editor.

U.S. Department of Justice's Regulations for Title II. *Federal Register.* July 26, 1991.

Universidade de Brasília / National AIDS and STDs Control Program (NASCP). 2001. *AIDS e Profissionais de Sexo em Brasíl.*

Universidade Federal Minas Gerais / National AIDS and STDs Control Program (NASCP). 2001. *O Projeto AjUDE Brasil: Avaliação Epidemiológica dos Usuários de Drogas Injetáveis dos Projetos de Redução de Danos.* Brasilia: Ministério da Saúde.

Universidade de Brasília / National AIDS and STDs Control Program (NASCP). 2003. *AIDS e Profissionais de Sexo em Brasíl.*

Wall Street Journal. May 2, 2005.

Weyland, K. 1995. Social movements and the state: the politics of health reform in Brazil. *World Development* 23:1699–1712.

World Bank. 2004. *Project performance assessment report: Brazil first and second AIDS and STD control projects.* Report no. 28819. Washington, D.C.: World Bank, Operations Evaluation Department.

14

Seeing Double

Mapping Contradictions in HIV Prevention and Illicit Drug Policy Worldwide

Daniel Wolfe and Kasia Malinowska-Sempruch

There are common wisdoms that people committed to HIV prevention repeat like mantras. One of these is that two decades of HIV have taught the world some clear lessons on how to successfully contain the virus. We note that effective HIV prevention includes not only the provision of tools such as condoms and clean needles to help block HIV transmission, but also mechanisms that involve the people directly affected—whether sex workers in Thailand, gay men in the United States, or women in Uganda or Brazil. We emphasize that treatment and prevention are complementary, not in competition. In a trend coincident with the new dominance of corporate-based philanthropies (Bill & Melinda Gates Foundation) and "private-public partnerships" (The Global Fund to Fight AIDS, Tuberculosis, and Malaria) in setting the global AIDS agenda, we underscore the importance of "evidence-based" approaches, "proven effectiveness," and "value added." We hope that appeals to science and corporate efficiency will transcend the moralism that has made condoms, clean needles, and methadone, and the programs that provide them, the subject of so many years of conflict. (See Box 14.1.)

All these assertions, however correct, must be measured against other, less discussed truths. As with the work of Sir Isaac Newton, whose age-of-reason breakthroughs coincided with alchemical experiments he conducted in a private laboratory, HIV prevention is in some important sense a project divided: exalting scientific principles even as it leaves other less-than-rational beliefs unquestioned. Indeed, for all the talk of evidence-based approaches, there is an insidious alchemy at work—a process by which certain people with HIV, or those at risk, are transmuted into something less than human, and thus deserving of something less than human rights. AIDS stigmatization is widely condemned when expressed in its crudest incarnations, as when Gugu Dlamini was beaten and stoned to death in KwaZulu Natal after disclosing her HIV status in 1998. Less examined are the more subtle acts of violence, common in national parliaments or multilateral institutions with headquarters in New York, Vienna, or Geneva, by which certain people are sentenced to death simply by being deemed unworthy of particular attention.

With AIDS, whose rise has been irrevocably twinned with that of the increasingly globalized economy, the distance between the world's informational-financial capitals and the people suffering most from the epidemic is instructive in understanding how the human costs of HIV and the humanity of those infected come to be eclipsed. Given the high rates of HIV infection among African Americans, fewer than twenty miles from the New York Stock Exchange, or the phenomenon that finds HIV infection skyrocketing among drug users in one St. Petersburg neighborhood at the same time as foreign investment explodes in another, this distance is best understood as economic, rather than geographic. Sociologist Manuel Castells, describing the rise of financial and informational networks linking new elites across cities and nations, has noted the parallel emergence of what he terms "black holes," areas with no access to key nodes on the network. Subject to sharp reductions in government services as the state redirects resources in the service of new economic priorities, people in these regions—whether in certain neighborhoods, or in entire provinces, countries, or continents—turn instead to informal or "perverse" economies (Castells, 1991): arms or drug dealing, smuggling, selling of sex, blood, children, or even body organs. As anthropologist Richard Parker (2000) noted, where underground economies develop, epidemics of

---

Box 14.1. Harm-reduction timeline

2001   At a special session of the General Assembly in June, the United Nations
        endorses the "Declaration of Commitment" on HIV/AIDS. Member states
        unanimously pledge support for increased access to sterile syringes and
        other harm-reduction measures to prevent the transmission of HIV among
        injection drug users.

2004   After a visit from U.S. Assistant Secretary of State Robert Charles in Novem-
        ber, head of the U.N. Office on Drugs and Crime Antonio Mario Costa pledges
        to be "even more vigilant" in removing mention of harm reduction from
        UNODC website and publications. Later in the month, a senior UNODC staff
        member reminds regional offices to "ensure that references to harm reduc-
        tion and needle/syringe exchange are avoided in UNODC documents, publi-
        cations and statements."

2005   In February, U.S. Congressional representative Mark Souder convenes a
        hearing against harm reduction. Ignoring seven federally funded studies that
        showed needle exchange to reduce the transmission of HIV without encour-
        aging illicit drug use, Souder labels the approach "ideological" and ineffec-
        tive. In March, U.S. representatives oppose all mention of needle exchange
        or the human rights of drug users in resolutions proposed at the U.N. Com-
        mission on Narcotic Drugs. One Latin American delegate says negotiations
        with the United States are "like taking a beating." In May, Russia's state
        drug control authorities propose a return to mandatory criminal sentencing
        for "large" and "extra large" doses of heroin. Under the old law, the heroin
        residue in a used syringe was classified as a "large" dose and punishable
        by up to seven years imprisonment. In June, the program coordinating board
        of UNAIDS, whose members include Russia and the United States, adopt a
        policy paper on HIV prevention. Recommendations include increased access
        to sterile syringes and protection and promotion of the human rights of
        drug users.

HIV and sexually transmitted infections often follow. Equally importantly, those engaged in perverse economic activity are frequently labeled as morally perverse: suspicious or criminal elements seen as a threat to, rather than a part of, the public imagined by "public health."

This chapter examines some of the political mechanisms that transform injection drug users (IDUs) into something less than human. Specifically, it argues for the importance of "seeing double": that is, of examining the parallel policies that seek, on the one hand, to use the best methods to protect people from HIV, and, on the other hand, to treat drug users like drugs, as something to be controlled or contained. We take the policies of various agencies and programs of the United Nations as a case in point. Long after the scale and speed of HIV transmission through contaminated injection equipment has become clear, the United Nations continues to pursue contradictory recommendations regarding drug users and the prevention of HIV. The discordance is echoed at the national level, where drug control and HIV prevention entities rarely communicate with each other, plan independently, and often pursue conflicting aims.

The price of failure to clarify and coordinate policy responses to injection-driven epidemics, already high, will only grow higher. Although routinely viewed by law enforcement as a deviant minority, drug users are more appropriately seen, in many parts of the world, as a majority in need of treatment and support. Five countries in the former Soviet Union and Asia—whose combined populations approach 2 billion—are already reporting extensive HIV epidemics (>50,000 registered cases per country) in which the majority of cases are due to injection drug use. Like injection-driven HIV epidemics more generally, these—in China, Malaysia, Russia, Ukraine, and Vietnam—have grown at rates unprecedented in sexually transmitted epidemics. In Russia, where infections are increasing faster than anywhere else, as many as 1.2 million people were living with HIV in 2004—as many as in Canada and the United States. Nearly all registered infections have occurred in the past ten years, and 87 percent of them are due to injection drug use (Joint United Nations Programme on HIV/AIDS [UNAIDS], 2004). In China, where the first cases of HIV were reported in 1985, the government estimated that as many as 650,000 were infected at the end of 2005—with the largest share of registered cases, 44 percent, among IDUs (International Harm Reduction Development Program [IHRD], 2006; UNAIDS, 2005). Outside observers suggest that actual numbers of HIV cases, fueled by blood-collection practices that have infected hundreds of thousands in the country's central provinces, may be much higher (Human Rights Watch, 2003). (See Figure 14.1.)

If current trends continue, mega-epidemics among IDUs are likely to be documented in dozens more nations—including those that have recorded only a handful of AIDS cases and those that have successfully reduced infections among non-drug users. Although registered cases of HIV in Indonesia and Iran have not yet passed the 50,000 mark, both countries are estimated to have HIV epidemics that are at least that large, with IDUs accounting for the largest share of infections in both countries (UNAIDS, 2004; *Jakarta Post,*

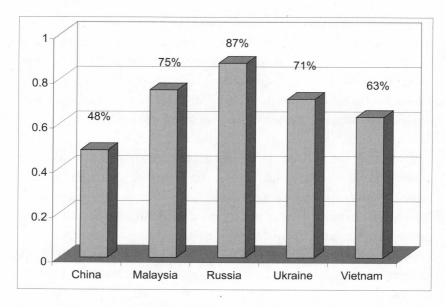

Figure 14.1. Intravenous drug users as a percentage of all registered cases of HIV in countries with established HIV epidemics (>50,000 cases). *Source*: Aceijas et al., 2006

2005). IDUs are the majority of those infected in the Baltic States of Lithuania, Latvia, and Estonia and the Central Asian Republics of Tajikistan, Kazakhstan, and Uzbekistan, all of which report rapidly growing epidemics (Central and Eastern European Harm Reduction Network [CEEHRN], 2002). IDUs constitute the majority of new infections in Western Europe, North Africa. and parts of the Middle East, Latin America, India, and Burma. Overall, the number of countries reporting HIV among IDUs has more than doubled in the past decade, from 52 in 1992 to 114 in 2003 (Strathdee and Poundstone, 2003). Outside of Africa, just under one in three of all HIV infections now comes from a contaminated needle.

The good news, we commonly tell ourselves, is that interventions to stem HIV and other harms among IDUs—particularly syringe exchange and methadone maintenance treatment—have proven easy to implement and highly effective in trials from Australia to Thailand to Belarus. The bad news is that evidence of effectiveness has so far proved a poor match for ideology. Years after gold-standard research has shown how swiftly injection drug use can spread HIV and the approaches most effective in containing that explosive growth, most countries with injection-driven epidemics continue to emphasize criminal enforcement and demand for abstinence over the best practices of public health. If current epidemiological trends are any indication, the result may be one of the most tragic missed opportunities of the new millennium: the creation of an HIV crisis in Asia and the former Soviet Union that could clearly have been averted.

Seeing Double: Competing Frameworks for Drug and HIV-Prevention Policy

The tension elicited in most listeners by the phrase "the human rights of drug users"—and its absence in the vast majority of U.N. documents or national government plans—suggests the limits of general appeals for stigma reduction and rights of people with HIV. When it comes to the problem of injection drug use and related HIV infection, human rights claims have been less prominent than two other frameworks in shaping national and international responses. The first of these is a law enforcement framework that seeks to track, restrict, or eliminate illicit drugs, and those who sell or buy them, from social circulation. In this framework, emphasis rests on the supply of and demand for drugs; drug users are understood and responded to primarily or exclusively as participants in illegal patterns of exchange. Emphasizing criminalization and containment, this framework identifies police action, interruption of trafficking, and penal institutions such as prisons as pivotal to effective response. When drug treatment is offered by the state, it is cast in the mold of punishment: coercive, lacking in almost all supportive services save the "service" of intense discipline and forced labor without compensation, and carrying severe penalties for relapse. Not surprisingly, relapse is the experience of the vast majority.

The second approach emerges from the best practices of public health—or, more specifically, the brand of public health that recognizes drug users as a deserving part of the public. This approach focuses on risks rather than on the drugs themselves, considering both adverse health effects and the range of people affected. These include drug users as well as their sexual partners, their children, and their extended families or communities. Unlike the law enforcement approach, this one prioritizes epidemiological analysis, recognizing that not all illegal drugs carry equal risks, and identifying mediating factors that increase drug risk and related disease, including those risks that result from drug policies rather than the use of illicit drugs themselves. A public health approach also seeks to identify the tools and interventions that best contain adverse health effects among the largest number of people. These necessarily include interventions for those drug users who are outside correctional or drug treatment systems or those who have returned to drug use after a period of abstinence. In all countries, the majority of drug users remain outside treatment or penal systems.

The criminal enforcement and public health frameworks used to shape policy responses to drug use have not been equally endowed or emphasized. Historically, far greater resources have flowed to the enforcement approach, which in turn has directly and indirectly shaped the capacity of health care workers, nongovernmental organizations, and treatment programs to offer services to drug users without suspicion of undermining public order, violating moral norms, or contributing to antisocial behavior. In low- and middle-income countries, public health measures that do not require drug users to relinquish all claims to autonomy before receiving help, or those that recognize that abstinence is not the only desirable outcome—such as needle exchange or overdose prevention—have been illegal, unfundable, or insufficiently supported at the national level. Substitution treatment programs that offer medically prescribed substitutes to block craving for opiates, thus reducing injection, crime, and other risks and costs associated with opiate addiction, are similarly absent or insufficient. Many governments have kept substitution treatment and needle and syringe exchange in a state of perpetual "pilot program," effectively delaying for years the comprehensive approaches that can contain injection-related HIV transmission.

Disunited Nations: Competing Approaches in the International System

Despite the rhetoric of unity epitomized by recent U.N. emphasis on the "three ones" (one national HIV/AIDS plan, one national coordinating authority, and one monitoring and evaluation system), law enforcement and public health approaches to drug use sit in an uneasy relation to each other within multilateral institutions and at the national level. The Global Fund to Fight AIDS, Tuberculosis, and Malaria, proposed by U.N. Secretary General Kofi Annan in 2001 and operational by 2002, has greatly enhanced the possibilities for those seeking to reach injection drug users with HIV prevention and treatment interventions: in 2005, for example, the fund directed more than 3 million U.S. dollars to HIV prevention among drug users in the former Soviet Union alone. Global Fund support has also begun to force consideration of how IDUs are integrated into efforts to "scale up" antiretroviral therapy for those with HIV. In the case of injection drug use, as with other drivers of the global HIV epidemic, Global Fund expenditures have focused more on creating parallel structures for care and prevention than on reforming the policies that render IDUs vulnerable to HIV in the first place. Because the Global Fund's approach is one that grows out of the directions provided by the national representatives who dominate its board, this limitation is best understood as hereditary: National governments with the most serious injection-driven epidemics are among those least likely to implement policy reform to contain them. On questions of illicit drug abuse and HIV prevention, the ostensibly United Nations has been a house divided for too long.

U.N. Drug Control Conventions in Theory and Practice

The unusual policy status of drug abuse is made clear because it is one of the few public health issues to be governed by international agreements that direct signatories on how to regulate and respond to the problem. Three U.N. protocols known collectively as the U.N. drug conventions—the 1961 Single Convention on Narcotic Drugs as amended in 1972, the 1971 Convention on Psychotropic Substances, and the 1988 Convention against Illicit Traffic in Narcotic Drugs and Psychotropic Substances—guide the global, and in many cases, national regulation of illicit drugs. Licensing for legal production of substances scheduled by the treaties, as well as monitoring efforts to prevent their diversion to illegal markets, is the responsibility of a "quasi-judicial" body known as the International Narcotics Control Board (INCB), a 13-member group of law enforcement professionals, psychiatrists, pharmacologists, and other experts empowered by the 1961 convention (as amended in 1972) to assess how well countries were complying (INCB, 2003a).

In theory, the language of the conventions is flexible enough to accommodate a range of public health responses to illicit drug use, and to allow countries to tailor responses to national realities (Bewley-Taylor, 2002; Room, 2003). The 1971 convention requires that parties not only act to discourage drug use, but also that they take all practicable measures "for the early identification, treatment, education, aftercare, rehabilitation, and social integration" of those who use illicit drugs (United Nations, 1971). Although requiring criminalization of drug possession for personal use, the 1988 convention does not specify what penalties must be attached, leading some to suggest that counseling instead of police action, or issuing of citations that are not recorded in permanent police records, would fulfill the letter of the law (Krajewski, 1999; Room, 2003). In addition, the 1988 convention specifies the primacy of efforts to minimize human suffering related to drug use, and reiterates that treatment, education, aftercare, and rehabilitation are acceptable alternatives to punishment (United Nations, 1988). A 2002 analysis by U.N. legal experts concluded that these provisions, and the fact that HIV prevention measures were not undertaken with the goal of inciting drug use, were likely to make such interventions as syringe exchange, substitution treatment, and safer injection sites to prevent the transmission of HIV and hepatitis C virus legally justifiable under the conventions (INCB, 2002).

In practice, however, the entities charged with interpreting the conventions have routinely emphasized enforcement and interdiction as the primary outcomes of importance. The INCB, whose members are appointed to "serve the interests of the international community," issues pointed criticisms of countries perceived to be doing too little to regulate drug diversion or production; quality and availability of drug treatment, by contrast, goes largely unmonitored and unmentioned. Western European measures to reduce criminal penalties for cannabis use, now adopted in Spain, Portugal, the Netherlands, and part of London, for example, have been criticized by the INCB as sending the wrong message and "endangering all eradication efforts, including those outside of Europe" (INCB, 2000). Two decades of HIV infection had little impact on INCB analysis: the board in 2000 expressed regret that harm reduction had "diverted the attention (and in some cases, funds) of Governments from important demand reduction activities such as primary prevention or abstinence-oriented treatment" (INCB, 2002). The INCB has also been sharply critical of medical prescription of heroin in Switzerland and England, and threatened to revoke Australia's ability to cultivate opium for medical purposes on learning of plans to implement safer injection rooms to reduce risk of HIV and hepatitis C (Fazey, 2003).

Language is a critical tool in the transmutation of the person who uses drugs to less-than-human status, and the INCB's own words are carefully chosen. They refer only to drug abuse, emphasizing that any illicit drug use, by virtue of its legal status, is de facto abuse. They describe those lost to addiction as "casualties," suggesting that active drug users are in important ways as good as dead. They condemn "normalization" of any illicit drug, thus reinforcing the idea that drug abusers must be regarded per se as abnormal (INCB, 2000). Recognizing that these are contested claims, Board members preemptively challenge experts who might differ, using quotation marks around phrases such as "medical marijuana" and "harm reduction" (INCB, 1997, 2002b). Their rhetoric often links policy proposals that in context may be unconnected into a seamless, threatening whole: syringe exchange is routinely paired with safer injection rooms, safer injection linked to drug decriminalization, and decriminalization to drug legalization and incitement of others to abuse drugs (INCB, 1997, 2000; Schaepe, 1999; Room, 2003).

More recently, HIV has forced some nuance into INCB analysis. The INCB report issued in 2004, for example, acknowledged that "governments need to adopt measures that may decrease the sharing of hypodermic needles" and that the implementation of substitution treatments "does not constitute any breach of treaty provisions" (INCB, 2003). The board, however, sought to ensure that these concessions were not mistaken for endorsement: the press release the INCB sent out to accompany the report was entitled "INCB Cautions on 'Harm Reduction' Measures in Drug Control." The report also reiterated opposition to safer injection rooms (which it termed "drug injection rooms"), without explication of the legal grounds for the position, and despite the ruling by U.N. lawyers finding that such efforts might indeed fall within the umbrella of activity permitted by the conventions (INCB, 2002, 2004).

Whereas INCB members are accountable only to themselves, governments find voice through the U.N. Commission on Narcotic Drugs (CND). Meeting annually to issue a variety of declarations and resolutions, the CND has also seen a marked increase in nuance in consideration of harm reduction. At the 2005 session, the first to focus on HIV prevention as a theme of debate, seventeen of thirty representatives who participated in the debate expressed support for or interest in learning about harm reduction and needle exchange. Those in favor included country representatives from China, Morocco, and Iran. Even Sweden, a major donor to U.N. drug control and a country known for its emphasis on abstinence, allied itself with an European Union (EU) statement in support of harm reduction. Only the United States labeled harm reduction a "term best avoided," though Japan expressed concern that needle exchange might encourage drug abuse.

At the CND, one dissenting voice—in particular, when it is that of the world's largest donor to U.N. drug control—is sufficient to shape the outcome of the entire session. In the drug war, as in other conflicts, the United States has had notable success in convincing the world that the only strong response is a strongly punitive one. Drug politics make strange bedfellows, and the coalition of the prohibitionists in the drug war has often included Russia, Malaysia, and Japan. Although substances have been added to those scheduled by the conventions, the CND has left the conventions themselves unchallenged and unchanged.

The entity responsible for coordination of drug supply and demand reduction programs on the ground, the U.N. Office on Drugs and Crime (UNODC, formerly UNODCCP), turns uncomfortably between the poles of law enforcement and disease prevention. On the one hand, the agency annually dispatches millions of dollars and a wide range of scientific, military, and police experts to assist in international counternarcotics efforts. High-profile initiatives have included help in drafting strong laws on money laundering and asset seizure, arming counternarcotics forces, establishing special courts to prosecute narcotics trafficking or consumption, training and equipping guards at railway stations and national borders, and promoting the effective use of drug sniffing dogs (Lubin et al., 2002). On the other hand, UNODC also supports a range of drug demand reduction efforts, including drug education materials, good drug treatment protocols, and alternative development assistance to help farmers change from cultivation of opium poppies or coca to other crops. The agency has a unit focused on HIV/AIDS, with a particular focus on HIV prevention in prisons. A year in the life of UNODC may thus find its director speaking out in favor of strategies that reduce the number of drug users put unnecessarily into prison in Russia, pledging to remove references to harm reduction from UNODC materials in Geneva, and remaining silent as countries from China to Thailand commemorate the United Nations's International Day against Drug Abuse and Illicit Trafficking with mass arrests, bonfires of seized drugs, and public executions (Agence France Press, 1997; AP, 2001, 2002).

The U.N. Conventions and Reduction of Drug-Related Harm

Another commonplace of the HIV epidemic is that the pandemic requires responses other than business as usual. AIDS advocates have increasingly questioned the wisdom of treaties regulating international response to drugs that reflect no awareness whatsoever of HIV (Malinowska-Sempruch et al., 2003), or have noted that the conventions' emphasis on alleviation of human suffering and reduction of the adverse consequences of drug abuse should provide ample justification for such measures as syringe exchange (Bewley-Taylor, 2002; INCB, 2002; Fazey, 2003; Malinowska-Sempruch et al., 2003; Rossi, 2003). In March 2002, the CND itself issued a resolution that expressed "alarm" about HIV, encouraged member states to consider HIV and hepatitis C and to remember the need both for access to HIV treatment and sterile injection equipment when developing programs to reduce drug demand (CND, 2002). A year later, just before the April 2003 CND session held to mark the halfway point between the 1998 U.N. General Assembly Special Session (UNGASS) on Drugs and the 2008 goal of significant and measurable drug reduction, Greece used its presidency of the European Union to convene a high-level meeting on international drug policy. Including representatives of the European and Greek Parliament, nongovernmental organization (NGO) representatives, the European Commission, as well as researchers, scientists, and U.N. staff members, the conference affirmed the usefulness of the U.N. drug conventions, but noted that they could be improved by explicitly including support for harm reduction provisions and affirmation that drug users are not criminals but people in need of help and treatment (Hellenic Presidency of the European Union, 2003).

None of these resolutions or expressions of concern, however, has the force of law. Nor apparently, have they carried sufficient force of persuasion. When the final resolutions at the meetings of the CND were adopted in 2003, 2004, and 2005, all mentions of syringe exchange and substitution treatment had been deleted.

Whether cause or convenient excuse, the U.N. Drug Conventions have been used by national governments to justify highly punitive legal measures and failure to implement services for IDUs. Russia, which sharply stiffened penalties for all drug possession and incarcerated tens of thousands of drug users between 1998 and 2004, has pointed to the U.N. conventions for explanation of its "total prohibition" (Malinowska-Sempruch et al., 2003). Pharmacologist Edouard Babayan, Russian representative to the CND for nearly 30 years and long-time member of the INCB (INCB, 2003), is the author of the drug table used by Russian law enforcement that until 2004 recognized possession of any amount of heroin as "large" or "extra-large" and attached a prison sentence of up to seven years for possession less than a hundredth of a single dose (.005 gram) (Levinson, 2003). Babayan, Russian chief of prison health General Alexander Kononetz and others repeatedly reference the INCB and the CND to support the Russian government's decision to keep methadone illegal in Russia (Levinson, 2003; Krasnov, 2005). Similarly, a U.N. survey of government officials in seven Asian countries with IDU epidemics noted that among the reasons given for lack of substitution treatment for heroin addiction was the belief that methadone was prohibited by the spirit or letter of the conventions (UNAIDS/UNODCCP, 2000).

Although some U.N. member governments have forged ahead with nationally supported needle exchange, heroin prescription, or safer injection rooms, virtually all of these—including Australia, Germany, Great Britain, Switzerland, the Netherlands, and Canada—are members of the Western European and Other Governments (WEO) group that contributes the bulk of U.N. financing, and so may feel entitled to creative interpretation of the conventions. Recipient nations, by contrast, have shown less flexibility. Vietnam, with the support of the U.S. President's Emergency Program for AIDS Relief (PEPFAR), had approved plans for a pilot methadone maintenance treatment as of June 2005, and China has already established 49 needle-exchange sites and 34 methadone maintenance programs (IHRD, 2006). With the exception of these relatively new efforts, methadone maintenance treatment is not available except through pilot programs in any country with an established injection-driven epidemic. In Russia, despite sharp increases in HIV funding in the form of grants from the Global Fund, the World Bank, and the U.S. government, funding for needle exchange fell by nearly 30 percent between 2004 and 2005 (Sarang, 2005). Even in countries such as Vietnam and China, where governments have adopted harm reduction into their national plans and begun to provide some services, these efforts must be judged against stringent and stigmatizing law enforcement efforts to control drug users (Harring, 1991; Vietnam Committee on Human Rights [VCHR], 2000; CEEHRN, 2002; Drug Law and Health Policy Research Network [DLHPRN], 2002; Human

Rights Watch, 2003; Xinhua General News Service, 2003; Voice of Vietnam, 2003; Vietnam News Agency [VNA], 2005).

Those looking for examples of national leadership in addressing injection-driven HIV epidemics are increasingly pointing to China. The June 2005 five-year plan released by the Chinese central government identified the HIV epidemic as a priority public health concern, further energizing the "four frees and one care" campaign (free antiretroviral drugs for poor people in urban areas and everyone in rural areas; free voluntary counseling and testing; free counseling and treatment for pregnant women; free schooling for children orphaned by HIV/AIDS; and economic assistance to families affected by HIV/AIDS) launched by the government in December 2003 (Zhe, 2005; WHO, 2005c). Following receipt of a $24 million Global Fund grant to prevent the spread of HIV among drug users and commercial sex workers, the Ministry of Health proposed national guidelines that urge the promotion of needle exchange and substitution therapy as primary HIV prevention strategies for IDUs. Reports of AIDS clinics sitting empty (Human Rights Watch, 2003) are now less common than accounts of treatment initiatives. As of December 2004, WHO reported that 12,219 patients were receiving antiretroviral (ARV) therapy (WHO, 2005c), though local activists have raised questions both about the quantity and the quality of treatment provided.

The Chinese turnaround clearly demonstrates the rapid expansion of harm reduction possible when there is political will. Forty-nine needle exchange projects were established throughout rural and urban China as of March 2005, and the head of the National Center for AIDS/STD Prevention and Control (NCAIDS) Dr. Wu Zunyou has set a target of expansion to several hundred in the next two years (Dyckman, 2005). Methadone, approved by the Chinese FDA for mainland use less than 2 years ago, was being locally manufactured and provided to 34 programs across the country by the end of June 2005 (Dyckman, 2005; Thompson, 2005). The Chinese government plans for expansion to 100 programs and provision of treatment to 20,000 patients by year's end (Thompson, 2005). While even these numbers will be insufficient to address an epidemic the size of China's, the scale-up stands in marked contrast to other countries, where substitution treatment programs exist in perpetual pilot status, and where needle exchange is supported nominally or not at all by central governments.

At the same time, promising steps taken by Chinese government health professionals must be balanced against an equally aggressive, and far more punitive, campaign against drugs and drug users by the Public Security Bureau (PSB). The only drug users eligible for methadone treatment, for example, are those who have already endured two failed courses of "rehabilitation" in the highly punitive facilities run by the PSB, where residents are interned for up to six months and forced to labor with no compensation (Human Rights Watch, 2003). Sweeps in which alleged drug users are sentenced without trial to these prisonlike facilities have been a routine part of the PSB's reenergized "People's War on Drugs." In June 2005, the PSB also issued regulations urging the creation of lists of drug users at the community level, requiring that drug users present themselves for mandatory detoxification, and levying penalties on drug users who fail to submit (Japan Economic Newswire, 2005). Yunnan province also proposed penalizing public officials who fail to report drug users. Recent plans call for expansion of capacity of forced rehabilitation centers, and incarceration of as many as 68,000 addicts for up to two years (Ma, 2005). Drug users who fail to go voluntarily, or who relapse into drug use, face up to two years detention, "reeducation through labor" camps where conditions are even harsher (Xinhua News Service, 2005).

Recent reports emerging from northwest China have documented clashes occurring between AIDS activists identified as former drug users and law enforcement authorities (Human Rights Watch, 2005). Needle exchange sites have also been the targets of law enforcement, with outreach workers followed and arrested, and police waiting near syringe distribution points to capture drug users. Possession of a syringe even in the absence of drugs may soon be sufficient for arrest: the Chinese Narcotics Control Commission proposed in June 2005 that the government change the law so that drug consumption, as well as drug possession, would be considered a crime (Global News Wire, 2005a). HIV and drug control programs in China thus echo a pattern seen at the global level, where the efforts of HIV specialists seeking to contain infections are contravened by the punitive approach of those who believe that stigma and punishment are healthy.

National policies in countries with established injection-driven epidemics more generally—whether in China or Ukraine, Russia, Malaysia, or Vietnam—reveal remarkable consistency with the law-and-order approach to the problem of illicit drugs. These countries have routinely blurred lines between public health and law enforcement, leaving decisions about drug treatment in the hands of the police, requiring or encouraging physicians to collaborate with law enforcement, rounding up drug users and suspected drug users in mass arrests, and labeling drug use (and by extension, drug users) a social evil to be rooted out of society. All countries with injection-driven epidemics have mandated imprisonment or forced institutionalization for purchase of even small amounts of drugs (e.g., quantities for personal use). In Russia, rates of HIV among those in prison increased by 2,000 percent after the imposition of harsh criminal penalties. In Vietnam the government marked the turn of the century by intensifying a decade-long "social evils" campaign against drug use, forcing 25,000 drug users in Ho Chi Minh City into treatment between 2001 and 2004, and extending to five years the period of forced labor termed "rehabilitation." In Malaysia, police have the ability to detain suspects for two weeks on suspicion of being a drug user, forcibly test them, and remand anyone showing past evidence of illicit drug use to compulsory treatment centers. In early 2005, authorities announced that possession of syringes would also be punishable by imprisonment.

In all these countries, these policies of mass incarceration serve as an engine of HIV infection, uniting infected and uninfected individuals in contexts where drug use and sex are common but tools to protect against HIV transmission—whether condoms, sterile injection equipment, or opioid substitution treatment—are not.

An Alternative Approach: Drug Policy in the Context of U.N. Public Health Initiatives

Even as U.N. drug control entities urge governments to take firm, punitive actions to deal with illicit drugs, other U.N. actors have assessed the problem through the lens of public health. Principal among these are the U.N. entities most concerned with HIV/AIDS prevention among IDUs—the World Health Organization (WHO) and UNAIDS. Emphasizing the risks associated with drug use, rather than its legal status per se, WHO and UNAIDS have focused less on use of recreational drugs, and more on drug injection and exchange of sex for drugs implicated in transmission of HIV, hepatitis C, and other infectious diseases. Drawing on social science literature, they have recommended a range of interventions, including harm-reduction interventions, for reducing the spread of disease. Emphasizing vulnerability rather than criminality, they urge governments to recognize the importance of including those at risk—including active drug users—in the formation and implementation of humane policy. "Experience tells us that cooperation with drug users gets better results than persecuting them," noted UNAIDS director Peter Piot in his April 2003 address to the CND (Peter Piot, Speech to the Commission on Narcotic Drugs, Vienna, 2003). While recent controversy has forced UNAIDS, which also relies on the United States for most of its budget, to tread carefully, program representatives—armed with documentation from studies relevant to the region at hand—have often put it simply: "harm reduction works" (Cravero, 2002; Hankins, 2002).

A superficial harmony has been forged at the rhetorical level throughout the U.N. system—all U.N. actors, for example, support "comprehensive" interventions for those using illicit substances, and urge "greater political commitment" to the problem. A 2001 U.N. "systemwide" position paper stated clearly that syringe exchange programs and opioid substitution treatment were acceptable parts of a wider package of interventions including drug prevention education and drug free treatment (United Nations, 2001). At the practical level, however, the difference in emphasis between U.N. drug control entities (e.g., INCB, CND, and UNODC) and health promotion entities (e.g., WHO and UNAIDS) results in sharp contradictions in policy recommendations. These are all the more remarkable because UNODC has been a cosponsor of UNAIDS since 1999 and was the chair of the UNAIDS coordinating board in 2005.

The following are among the most striking areas of inconsistency.

• *Opioid substitution treatment.* Since 1961 the CND has classed methadone, the most affordable and best studied of available substitution treatments, as a schedule 1 substance ("especially serious risk to public health and limited, if any, therapeutic benefit"). Though UNODC joined UNAIDS and WHO in issuing a position paper in support of substitution treatment in 2004 (WHO/UNODC/UNAIDS, 2004) advocacy or financial support for the approach has been limited. Antonio Maria Costa chaired a high-level ministerial meeting for Commonwealth of Independent States (CIS) countries in April 2005 at which the Russian government insisted on the sudden removal of references to substitution treatment from the recommendations. When NGO participants objected, Costa overruled them.

U.N. health promotion agencies, by contrast, regularly advocate for substitution treatment under appropriate medical supervision as part of an effective response to HIV. Jim Kim, the director of HIV/AIDS programs at the

World Health Organization, pledged in November 2003 to investigate addition of methadone to WHO's list of essential medicines. In June 2005, WHO announced that after extensive review of the evidence, methadone and a newer substitution treatment, buprenorphine, had both been included in the list (IHRD, 2006).

• *Harm reduction.* The INCB speaks of harm reduction as linked to drug legalization efforts, and routinely reminds governments that harm reduction is no substitute for drug demand reduction. The CND has yet to adopt a single resolution acknowledging the human rights of drug users or containing the phrase harm reduction. UNODC director Costa has taken a different approach, seeking to defuse debate by diluting the meaning of the term: at the 2005 CND, for example, he suggested that arrests of drug traffickers or eradication of opium poppies were also "harm reduction."

Health promotion representatives emphasize that harm-reduction measures—specifically access to sterile syringes and substitution treatment—are scientifically tested approaches meriting support from national governments. The prevention strategy adopted by UNAIDS in 2005 prioritizes harm-reduction measures based on promoting, protecting, and respecting the human rights of drug users (UNAIDS, 2005). UNODC's own HIV unit, while avoiding the term harm reduction, has emphasized the value of a comprehensive approach, including access to sterile syringes and substitution treatment, in containing HIV in penal institutions.

• *Syringe exchange.* While acknowledging the importance of increased access to sterile injection equipment in 2002, the CND has shied away from further support even as injection-driven epidemics have grown worldwide. U.S. opposition has restricted UNODC funding for syringe exchange and forced the agency to retreat from explicit support. UNAIDS and WHO, by contrast, express consistent support for needle exchange programs as a means of reducing HIV infections.

• *International mandate.* Drug control entities refer regularly to the UN-GASS on Drugs, where participants agreed to significantly reduce or eliminate drug use by 2008, for proof of international consensus and direction on drug control. Health promotion entities reference the 2001 UNGASS on HIV/AIDS, where all member governments of the United Nations endorsed specific efforts to reduce HIV transmission that included provision of sterile injection equipment and other harm-reduction efforts. (See Table 14.1.)

Table 14.1. Seeing double at the United Nations: drug control versus public health

Drug control	Public health
A drug-free world—We can do it! (Pino Arlacchi, Director, U.N. Office on Drug Control and Crime Prevention, 1998)	The total and immediate elimination of drug injecting is . . . unlikely to be an achievable goal. (WHO, Principles for Preventing HIV Infection among Drug Users, 1997)
The discussion on drug injection rooms and some other harm-reduction measures has diverted the attention (and, in some cases, funds) of governments from important demand reduction activities. (INCB Annual Report, 2000)	The translation of well-accepted harm-reduction theory into harm-reduction reality is held back by lack of social and political will. (Catherine Hankins, Associate Director, UNAIDS, 2002)
The term use or consumption should be applied only when it refers to the use or consumption of drugs for medical or scientific purposes. . . . Drug abusers are therefore, by definition, neither consumers nor users. (INCB Annual Report, 2001)	Without the involvement of drug users themselves there can be no ongoing behavioral change and effective HIV prevention among that group. It is crucial to implement HIV preventive activities on the basis of the peer support principle, involving people from the drug-using community. (UNODC, Lessons Learned, 2001)
To promote drug use illicitly through the giving out of needles . . . would to me amount to inciting people to abuse drugs, which would be contrary to the provisions of the convention. (INCB President Philip O. Emafo, 2002)	When working with people who inject drugs, it is important to focus on harm reduction as well as rehabilitation . . . [and to] adopt a multipronged approach including needle and syringe exchange. (Innovative Approaches to HIV Prevention, UNAIDS Best Practice Collection, 2000)
Based on the belief that the deliberate use of drugs for nonmedical purposes leads to the destruction of the mind and the body, the Swedish drug control policy has as its objective a society that should be free of the evils of drug abuse . . . to achieve this ultimate goal, a drug-free society, a variety of measures are applied . . . prevention, treatment, and repressive measures. (Ambassador HS Okun, Rapporteur of the INCB, 2003)	Laws and policies that prevent drug users from accessing services must be changed. Practices that instill fear and inflict punishment on people vulnerable to HIV infection must be transformed. Stigma and discrimination that drive drug users underground and undermine prevention efforts must be eliminated. (Cathleen Cravero, Deputy Director, UNAIDS, 1998)
UNDCP [part of UNODC] has yet to adopt an official position on harm reduction. (UNDCP Legal Affairs Section, 2002)	The United Nations fully endorses the fundamental principles of harm reduction: reaching out to injecting drug users, providing sterile injecting equipment and disinfectant materials, and providing substitution treatment. (Catherine Hankins, Associate Director, UNAIDS, 2002)

Seeing Double in Thailand: Contradictions in Action

Tensions between the law enforcement and public health frameworks for responding to drug use are manifest even in countries saluted by the United Nations for their HIV prevention efforts. Thailand, for example, regularly cited as one of the few countries in the world to mount a successful effort for its response to the AIDS epidemic (UNAIDS, 2001; Ainsworth et al., 2003; UNICEF, 2003), also demonstrates how easily prevention "success" can exclude those with a history of drug use. (See Chapter 10 by Sherman, Aramrattana, and Celentano.) The Thai government has been widely praised for its 100 percent Condom Programme, which in the early 1990s helped stem rising rates of infection by requiring quality control in the manufacture of condoms, distributing approximately 60 million condoms annually free of charge to sex establishments, and working with provincial governors, chiefs of police, and chief medical officers to ensure national commitment to the program. Supplemented by such measures as alternative career development for young women in sex work, the program helped to sharply increase the use of condoms, sharply reduce sexual transmission of HIV and other sexually transmitted infections (STIs), and lower the prevalence of HIV by as much as fivefold (Nelson et al., 2002). Thailand is also the first developing nation to have implemented an effective perinatal prevention initiative, delivering short-course zidovudine to more than two-thirds of HIV-infected pregnant women in prenatal care and to nearly nine in ten of their infants, to stop the transmission of HIV (Amornwichet et al., 2002).

Instead of strong HIV prevention programs for drug users, however, the Thai government has offered them an iron fist. (See also Chapter 10.) In February 2003, the governing Thai Rak Thai (Thais Love Thais) party launched a "war" on the growing problem of methamphetamine use that has included arrest quotas for provincial police, and mass roundups of alleged drug dealers and addicts. By April, Thai newspapers were reporting that police—armed with government blacklists and offered a percentage of assets seized—had taken more than 80,000 drug traffickers into custody. Some 290,000 Thais were reportedly forced into treatment in less than three months, with police conducting forced urine tests on nightclubs and bars, and the government holding those who could not fit into established treatment centers in decommissioned army bases (Macan-Markar, 2003). Television broadcasts were soon filled not only with pictures of drugs and money seized, but with images of the large numbers of Thais—more than 2,600—shot to death during the crackdown. Officials accepted responsibility for fewer than sixty of these deaths, claiming that most resulted from drug dealers killing each other to prevent incriminating testimony. Thai and international human rights observers noted that the murders—accomplished in the style of professional gunmen, sometimes as victims were returning from police interrogation—seemed more like systematic, extrajudicial executions (Human Rights Watch, 2004).

Although Thai authorities have declared the war on drugs a "beautiful success" (Agence France Presse, 2003), its effect on programs serving drug users—including HIV prevention and research efforts—has been immediate and ugly. A study led by researchers at Chiang Mai University found that 37 percent of drug users visiting rehabilitation clinics disappeared following the start of the government crackdown and were likely to have returned to injection and risk of HIV infection (Razak et al., 2003). Programs providing risk-reduction information to drug users in the south report that many clients have stopped attending for fear of being identified by police (Paisan Suwannawong and Karyn Kaplan, Thai AIDS Treatment Action Group, personal communication, 2003). Fear of blacklisting and indiscriminate arrests have also swelled the ranks of rehabilitation centers with non-drug users, including parents who have incarcerated themselves to clear their family name, and those swept up without cause. An evaluation commissioned by the Thai government found that more than one in ten of those in compulsory treatment in the northeast had never used drugs, and that only 20 percent of those in "treatment" overall had used drugs in the previous three months (Vichai and Aramrattana, 2003).

In the context of HIV prevention for IDUs in Thailand, the war on drugs may be the latest in a long series of missteps. A pilot needle exchange program in the north has been discontinued. Long-term methadone treatment, despite a trial demonstrating efficacy more than a decade ago (Vanichseni et al., 1991), is still against the law and unavailable. The 100 percent condom program has not been implemented in prisons, whose population grew sharply due to a fivefold increase in drug-related incarcerations between 1992 and 1999, and where studies show both high rates of HIV infection and significant numbers of seroconversions behind bars (Beyrer et al., 2003). The amount of methamphetamine required for criminal charges of possession was revised downward three times between 1999 and 2001. Until mid-2003, the Thai policy on implementation of antiretroviral therapy explicitly forbade injection drug users from receiving therapy. Although the government has agreed to change the policy, IDUs continue to face severe discrimination in health care settings, or to avoid them for fear of being reported to the police (Karyn Kaplan, AIDS Treatment Action Group, personal communication, 2003).

Rates of HIV infection among drug users, meanwhile, show no sign of decline. While HIV incidence among soldiers, pregnant women, and STD clinic patients has fallen sharply since 1995, no decrease has been noted among Thai IDUs. In 1995, 32 percent of IDUs were believed to be HIV infected. By 2001, this had risen to 50 percent (Reid and Costigan, 2002). A study of military recruits in the north found that the percent of HIV-infected individuals with a history of IDU rose from 1 percent in 1991 to more than 25 percent in 1998 (Nelson et al., 2002).

Prime Minister Thaksin declared the majority of the country drug-free in honor of the king's birthday in early December 2003. After declaring to the world that he would treat drug users as patients, rather than criminals at the 2004 International AIDS Conference, however, Thaksin proceeded to renew the drug war rhetoric and arrests, as politically expedient (Global News Wire, 2005b). Whether through execution or HIV infection while incarcerated, the price paid by drug users may include their lives.

HIV Treatment, Drug Treatment, and the United Nations

WHO's declaration of a "treatment state of emergency" in a special session of the U.N. General Assembly in September 2003, and the announcement of a plan to provide HIV treatment to 3 million people worldwide by 2005, sealed the increasingly irrelevant debate about whether international HIV efforts should prioritize HIV prevention or HIV treatment. While global HIV treatment goals are moving targets—a million people were on antiretroviral therapy by mid-2005, and U.N. officials have begun to speak informally of "8 by 10"—questions about whether triple-combination antiretroviral therapy could ever be implemented in resource-poor settings have been replaced by questions on how best to "scale up." Global Fund support for new treatment efforts, negotiations of price reductions for brand-name combination therapy, and the manufacture of generics have decreased costs to prices unimaginable a decade ago. Transformation of the mechanisms to address the question of how to allocate HIV treatment to those in need, however, is also urgently needed.

Specific policy guidance on the question of how best to treat HIV-positive IDUs is particularly important for countries with injection-driven epidemics, whose ambivalence about drug use appears to influence national commitment to HIV treatment more generally. While HIV treatment to date has been too limited to draw clear conclusions—of the more than 3.5 million people estimated to be HIV infected in the five countries with large, injection-driven epidemics, fewer than 17,500 are on triple-combination therapy—preliminary evidence suggests that a history of injection is used explicitly or in practice to exclude IDUs from antiretroviral therapy (WHO, 2005a). In Russia, where IDUs accounted for close to 90 percent of cumulative cases of HIV in 2002, AIDS service programs in St. Petersburg and Moscow reported that none of those on triple-combination therapy were IDUs (CEEHRN, 2002). In the leading HIV clinic in Kuala Lumpur, former IDUs—75 percent of all cases of HIV in the country—are only 20 percent of those receiving antiretroviral therapy, and none are current drug users (Kamarulzaman, Malaysian AIDS Council, personal communication, 2003). In Ukraine, where IDUs were 69 percent of registered HIV cases in 2002, they were only 20 percent of those receiving triple-combination antiretroviral therapy, with AIDS centers reportedly placing drug users after all others in line for medication (CEEHRN, 2002). New advocacy and new funding had improved the situation in many countries in 2005, though access for IDUs continued to pose a serious challenge. Although China has declared a commitment to provision of antiretroviral therapy for drug users under the "four frees and one care" program, data on how many of those treated are IDUs remain difficult to obtain.

U.N. drug control entities have remained silent on these apparent disparities in treatment, as well as on the question of whether HIV treatment is part of the treatment or aftercare envisioned for drug users by the U.N. drug conventions. Despite the emphasis by large donors to U.N. drug control on drug treatment as the first bulwark against HIV infection, and a general emphasis on abstinence from illicit drugs as a key component of HIV prevention, there have been few critical assessments of treatment for substance dependence in resource-constrained settings. The anecdotes from countries with injection-driven epidemics, including repeated flogging as a means of detoxification in

Russia, and forced labor camps, brainwashing techniques, and experimental brain surgery in multiple countries, do not inspire confidence.

U.N. health entities have been far stronger about the efficacy of HIV treatment for IDUs and their right to receive it, if vague about efforts to ascertain whether this is being done. WHO's draft guidelines for antiretroviral treatment, for example, state unequivocally that treatment should be available for all, including users of injection drugs (WHO, 2002). At the same time, U.N. surveys of treatment availability have yet to make a systematic effort to identify how the route of HIV transmission has affected access to antiretroviral therapy. Ethical and economic analysis of the provision of antiretroviral therapy has frequently focused on questions of socioeconomic status as a determinant of access to treatment, but has rarely addressed specific questions raised by attitudes toward IDUs or assumptions about their relative worth (UNAIDS/ World Bank, 1998; WHO, 2005b). Given the large and rising share of infections attributed to IDU, this omission is serious.

Looking Ahead

Policy making, not unlike drug use, is a complex, chronic, and relapsing condition, with yesterday's advances turning into today's defeats. In keeping with harm reduction's emphasis on incremental positive change rather than adherence to absolutes, it is important to note that 2005 brought several promising developments, in particular, in Asia, for reducing harm and preventing HIV. China and Iran have both supported syringe exchange and methadone maintenance, not only in their own countries, but also in international fora. After years of "zero-tolerance" approaches to drug use, Malaysia announced in June 2005 that it would consider syringe exchange programs and would move forward on plans for a methadone pilot before the end of the year (Atan, 2005; *New Straits Times*, 2005). Indonesia has recently demonstrated a similar openness to harm-reduction approaches, establishing pilot methadone maintenance and needle exchange programs (Casey, 2005). A UNAIDS position paper adopted in July 2005 and meant to serve as the blueprint for the global strategy for HIV prevention calls explicitly for increased access to sterile syringes and respect for the human rights of drug users. That the United States relegated its objections to a footnote in the meeting minutes and endorsed the document also represents a welcome and important step.

The advocacy that led to adoption of that UNAIDS document points to the direction that future efforts might take in consolidating support for harm reduction within the U.N. system. Having witnessed the successful U.S. campaign to remove all mention of sterile injection equipment from resolutions at the Commission on Narcotics Drugs in March, advocates girded themselves for another battle at the adoption of the United Nations' global HIV prevention strategy in June. The group responsible for adopting the HIV prevention strategy, known as the UNAIDS Programme Coordinating Board, split after U.S. officials insisted in preliminary meetings that all references to needle exchange be removed from the document. This time, though, a global coalition mobilized to resist U.S. strong-arm tactics, successfully rallying NGOs and seeking support from those member states where harm reduction had demonstrated efficacy in reducing HIV transmission.

In the United States, HIV prevention, drug policy, and human rights groups —led by a coalition including the Harm Reduction Coalition, the International Harm Reduction Development Program of the Open Society Institute, Human Rights Watch, and Gay Men's Health Crisis—issued a sign-on letter urging U.S. Global AIDS Coordinator Randall Tobias not to allow ideology to trump the extensive scientific evidence in favor of clean needles. Advocates also rallied attention from sympathetic lawmakers and leading U.S. media: California congressman Henry Waxman sent a letter to U.S. Secretary of State Condoleezza Rice to emphasize the dangers of replacing science with ideology at UNAIDS, and a June 27 *New York Times* editorial referred to U.S. efforts to force a retreat from needle exchange as "a breathtakingly dangerous step." In Europe, HIV prevention experts briefed delegations to strengthen member states' commitment to standing up for science and to underscore the dangers of allowing a frankly ideological approach to shape the global response to HIV. At the meeting itself, NGO advocates and U.N. representatives worked the hallways, emphasizing that access to sterile injection equipment was a fundamental public health measure, and that significant evidence from the United States and elsewhere in the world supported the approach (IHRD, 2006).

In the final discussions at UNAIDS, the United States confronted almost unanimous opposition. The Dutch proposed language about a comprehensive approach to HIV prevention that included sterile injection equipment, and Canada added the importance of "respect for human rights of drug users." Delegates from Europe and Australia, where needle exchange has contained the HIV epidemic to a much greater extent than in the United States, were particularly forceful in arguing against U.S. objections. Norway noted that it would be "irresponsible" not to base HIV prevention on the evidence, and Finland suggested that to remove mention of sterile injection equipment would be "unethical." A compromise proposed by the United Kingdom, that would have included language about the right for donor nations to support only those interventions they chose, was rejected by other participants as unnecessary. Even Senegal, a country with few documented cases of HIV via injection, urged the United Nations to stick to the language in favor of harm reduction contained in the declaration of commitment adopted by all nations, including the United States, at the 2001 U.N. General Assembly Special Session on HIV/AIDS. Confronted by a unified front in Geneva and growing criticism at home, U.S. officials limited their objections to the footnote recorded in the meeting minutes. The language of the strategy itself, adopted on June 29, affirmed the importance of access to sterile injection equipment and the human rights of drug users.

It is unclear whether this new language will translate into new commitment to equity by the United States or other donor nations. In countries with injection-driven epidemics, donor nations and NGOs alike have tended to replace discussion of the particular needs of IDUs with warnings about spread to the "general population." These arguments, while good for rallying concern, often obscure the dynamics particular to sexual transmission between injection drug users and their sexual partners. The specter of a generalized epidemic, and corresponding assertions that AIDS is "everyone's problem," similarly distract attention from those means of prevention—again including harm reduction and specific campaigns that acknowledge the social dynamics of drug use—most likely to be helpful.

With large numbers of IDUs under the age of 30, countries or agencies reluctant to address the issue of injection directly have also increasingly appealed to the need to protect "young people" from HIV. This kind of mainstreaming, too, is counterproductive, because general HIV prevention campaigns targeted to "youth" are as unlikely to meet the needs of young injection drug users as campaigns seeking to reach gay men in the 1980s would have been if they had been designed simply for "men." When it comes to communicating honestly about HIV infections concentrated among injection drug users, lack of political courage is epidemic.

Finally, in the treatment arena, international analysis also has tended to obscure IDU-specific treatment issues behind more general calls for access to antiretroviral therapy (Human Rights Watch, 2003; US-Russia Working Group, 2003; Center for Strategic and International Studies [CSIS], 2005; WHO, 2005b). Wealthy countries—long used to classifying drug users as the noncompliant minority of HIV patients—may be better suited to offer funds than to offer guidance. Answers may come from countries like Brazil, which has overcome initial resistance to needle exchange to offer federal support in counties across the country, and which has included IDUs among those provided free access to treatment.

The sheer numbers of IDUs infected in Asia and the former Soviet Union will soon force questions of HIV prevention and the provision of antiretroviral therapy for drug users. An amendment to the U.N. drug conventions asserting that harm reduction is compatible with international treaties would be an important, if time-consuming and difficult, advance toward effective HIV prevention and treatment. In the current political climate, however, reform of the U.N. conventions seems highly unlikely. In the interim, greater resolve by like-minded nations to form a united front in support of harm reduction at the CND would be a positive step. A recommendation to reschedule methadone to a less restricted category by WHO, adoption of that recommendation by the CND, and expansion of INCB monitoring to include analysis of drug treatment as well as illicit drug diversion, are also important. The 2005 addition of substitution therapies to WHO's essential drugs list does nothing to change their legal status in countries that classify them as dangerous. Until these steps are taken, the United Nations' harmonized approach will exist on paper alone.

More generally, donor nations should not seek to make HIV programs for IDUs in developing countries in their own distorted image. Perhaps the most enduring lesson of HIV prevention says that international, national, and local entities must work together to address the explosion of HIV in resource-poor settings. Millions of people in Asia and the former Soviet Union can only hope that the collaboration brings less dissonance in the approach to drug use, and more commitment to give IDUs access to prevention and treatment measures known to be effective. If the United Nations, donor nations, and national governments fail to focus on drug users' needs, the result will be a contradiction of terrible fiscal and moral cost: an AIDS service structure that in many countries denies care or means of protection to those most in need.

References

Aceijas C., Oppenheimer, E., et al. In press. Antiretroviral treatment for injecting drug users in developing and transitional countries one year before the end of 'Treating 3 Million by 2005' making it happen: The WHO strategy. *Addiction.*

Agence France Presse. 1997. Thai and Burmese officials mark International Day against Drugs. Bangkok, June 26.

Agence France Presse. 2003. Majority of drug producers, traffickers arrested: Thai government. Bangkok. May 20.

Ainsworth, M., Beyrer, C., et al. 2003. AIDS and public policy: the lessons and challenges of "success" in Thailand. *Health Policy* 64 (1):13–37.

Amornwichet, P., Teeraratkul, A., et al. 2002. Preventing mother-to-child HIV transmission: the first year of Thailand's national program. *Journal of the American Medical Association* 288 (2):245–48.

Associated Press. 2001. China marks U.N. anti-drug day with executions, public rallies. Beijing. June 26.

Associated Press. 2002. China executes 64 to mark U.N. anti-drug day. Shanghai. June 26.

Atan, H. 2005. Addicts to be given methadone. *New Straits Times* (Malaysia). May 19.

Bewley-Taylor, D. R. 2002. Challenging the UN drug control conventions: Problems and possibilities. *International Journal of Drug Policy* 14:171–79.

Beyrer, C., J. Jittiwutikarn, et al. 2003. Drug use, increasing incarceration rates, and prison associated HIV risks in Thailand. *AIDS and Behavior* 7 (2):153–61.

Casey, M. 2005. Indonesia aims to stem rise in HIV cases. *Associated Press.* July 1.

Castells, M. 1991. *The informational city: a new framework for social change.* Toronto: Centre for Urban and Community Studies, University of Toronto.

Center for Strategic and International Studies (CSIS). 2004. *Diffusing China's time bomb: Sustaining the momentum of China's HIV/AIDS response.* A Report of the CSIS HIV/AIDS Delegation to China, April 13–18, 2004. Washington DC: CSIS.

Central and Eastern European Harm Reduction Network (CEEHRN). 2002. *Injecting drug users, HIV/AIDS treatment and primary care in central and eastern Europe and the former Soviet Union: Results of a region-wide survey.* Vilnius, Lithuania: CEEHRN.

Commission on Narcotic Drugs (CND). 2002. *Res.45/1 Human immunodeficiency virus/acquired immunodeficiency syndrome in the context of drug abuse.* Vienna: CND.

Cravero, K. 2002. *Address to the Commission on Narcotic Drugs.* Vienna: Commission on Narcotic Drugs.

Drug Law and Health Policy Research Network. 2002. *Drug policy and health in Ukraine.* New York: Open Society Institute.

Dyckman, W. 2005. *A preliminary report on the status of methadone maintenance therapy in China.* New York, International Harm Reduction Development Program.

Fazey, C. 2003. The Commission on Narcotic Drugs and the United Nations International Drug Control Programme: politics, policies and prospect for change. *International Journal of Drug Policy* 14:155–69.

Global Fund to Fight AIDS, Tuberculosis, and Malaria (GFATM). 2003a. *Program Grant Agreement between the Global Fund to Fight AIDS, Tuberculosis, and Malaria* and the Republic Center for Prophylactics and Control of AIDS of the Government of the Republic of Kazakhstan, December 1, 2003. Grant no. KAZ-202-G01-H. Geneva: GFATM.

Global Fund to Fight AIDS, Tuberculosis, and Malaria (GFATM). 2003b. *Program Grant Agreement between the Global Fund to Fight AIDS, Tuberculosis, and Malaria and the Ministry of Health and Family of the Government of Romania, July 1, 2003.* Grant no. ROM-202-G01-H-00. Geneva: GFATM.

Global Fund to Fight AIDS, Tuberculosis, and Malaria (GFATM). 2004a. *Program Grant Agreement between the Global Fund to Fight AIDS, Tuberculosis, and Malaria and the Georgia Health and Social Projects Implementation Center, March 1, 2004.* Grant no. GEO-202-G01-H-00. Geneva: GFATM.

Global Fund to Fight AIDS, Tuberculosis, and Malaria (GFATM). 2004b. *Program Grant Agreement between the Global Fund to Fight AIDS, Tuberculosis, and Malaria and the International HIV/AIDS Alliance, March 15, 2004.* Grant no. UKR-202-G01-H-00. Geneva: GFATM.

Global Fund to Fight AIDS, Tuberculosis, and Malaria (GFATM). 2004c. *Program Grant Agreement between the Global Fund to Fight AIDS, Tuberculosis, and Malaria and the National AIDS Center of the Government of the Republic of Kyrgyzstan, March 1, 2004.* Grant no. KGZ-202-G01-H-00. Geneva: GFATM.

Global Fund to Fight AIDS, Tuberculosis, and Malaria (GFATM). 2004d. *Program Grant Agreement between the Global Fund to Fight AIDS, Tuberculosis, and Malaria and the Open Health Institute, August 15, 2004.* Grant no. RUS-304-G01-H. Geneva: GFATM.

Global Fund to Fight AIDS, Tuberculosis, and Malaria (GFATM). 2004e. *Program Grant Agreement between the Global Fund to Fight AIDS, Tuberculosis, and Malaria and the Russian Health Care Foundation, September 1, 2005.* Grant no. RUS-405-G03-H. Geneva: GFATM.

Global Fund to Fight AIDS, Tuberculosis, and Malaria (GFATM). 2005. *Program Grant Agreement between the Global Fund to Fight AIDS, Tuberculosis, and Malaria and the Ministry of Health of the Government of the Republic of Azerbaijan, June 1, 2005.* Grant no. AZE-405-G01-H. Geneva: GFATM.

Global News Wire. 2005a. Law to make drug taking criminal. *China Daily.* June 23, 2005.

Global News Wire. 2005b. Thai government launches third round of all-out war on drugs. *Thai Press Reports.* April 20, 2005.

Hankins, C. 2002. *Opening Ceremony Address.* Presented at the 13th International Conference on Drug Related Harm, Ljubljana, Slovenia.

Harring, S. 1991. Death, drugs and development: Malaysia's mandatory death penalty for traffickers and the international war on drugs. *Columbia Journal of Transnational Law* 29 (2):368–405.

Hellenic Presidency of the European Union. 2003. Report on the High Level Conference on Drugs. Athens: Hellenic Presidency of the European Union.

Human Rights Watch. 2003. *Locked doors: The human rights of people with HIV/AIDS in China.* New York: Human Rights Watch.

Human Rights Watch. 2004. *Not enough graves: The war on drugs, HIV/AIDS, and violations of human rights.* New York: Human Rights Watch.

Human Rights Watch. 2005. *Restrictions on AIDS activists in China.* New York: Human Rights Watch.

International Harm Reduction Development Program (IHRD). 2006. *Harm reduction developments 2005: Countries with injection-driven epidemics.* New York: International Harm Reduction Development Program of the Open Society Institute.

International Narcotics Control Board (INCB). 1997. *Preventing drug abuse in an environment of illicit drug promotion: Report of the International Narcotics Control Board for 1997.* Vienna: International Narcotics Control Board.

International Narcotics Control Board (INCB). 2000. *Report of the International Narcotics Control Board for 2000.* Vienna: INCB.

International Narcotics Control Board (INCB). 2002a. *Report of the International Narcotics Control Board for 2002.* Vienna: INCB.

International Narcotics Control Board (INCB). 2002b. *Flexibility of treaty provisions as regards harm reduction approaches.* Vienna: INCB.

International Narcotics Control Board (INCB). 2003a. *Report of the International Narcotics Control Board for 2003.* Vienna: INCB.

International Narcotics Control Board (INCB). 2003b. *Role of the International Narcotics Control Board.* www.incb.org.

International Narcotics Control Board (INCB). 2004. *Report of the International Narcotics Control Board for 2004.* Vienna: INCB.

Jakarta Post. 2005. Reported AIDS cases soar, shared needles lead transmission. *Jakarta Post.* Jakarta. June 25, 2005.

Japan Economic Newswire. 2005. Beijing demands all drug users register with police. Beijing. May 12, 2005.

Joint United Nations Programme on HIV/AIDS (UNAIDS). 2001. *AIDS epidemic update—December 2001.* Geneva: UNAIDS.

Joint United Nations Programme on HIV/AIDS (UNAIDS). 2002. *Report on the global HIV/AIDS epidemic.* Geneva: UNAIDS.

Joint United Nations Programme on HIV/AIDS (UNAIDS). 2003. *Report on the Global HIV/AIDS Epidemic.* Geneva: UNAIDS.

Joint United Nations Programme on HIV/AIDS (UNAIDS). 2004. *Report on the global HIV/AIDS epidemic.* Geneva: UNAIDS.

Joint United Nations Programme on HIV/AIDS (UNAIDS). 2005. *UNAIDS/PCB(17)/05.329. Intensifying HIV prevention.* UNAIDS Position Policy Paper. Geneva: UNAIDS.

Joint United Nations Programme on HIV/AIDS (UNAIDS). / United Nations Office for Drug Control and Crime Prevention (UNODCCP). 2000. *Drug use and HIV vulnerability.* Geneva/Vienna: UNAIDS and UNODCCP.

Joint United Nations Programme on HIV/AIDS (UNAIDS) / World Bank. 1998. *Background materials and outputs from an on-line conference.* Antiretroviral Treatment in Developing Countries: Questions of Economics, Equity and Ethics. www.worldbank.org/aids-econ/arv/index.htm (accessed December 2, 2005).

Krajewski, K. 1999. "How flexible are the United Nations drug conventions?" *International Journal of Drug Policy* 10:329–38.

Krasnov, V. N., Ivanets, N. et al. 2005. Memorandum: Say no to methadone programs in Russian Federation. Meditsinskaya Gazeta. March 30.

Levinson, L. 2003. *Russian Drug Policy: Need for a Change. Stating the Problem and Revealing the Actual Picture.* Mobilizing Allies in Fight for Human Rights and Harm Reduction (Conference proceedings), Budapest, Hungary. June 1.

Lubin, N., Klaits, A., et al. 2002. *Narcotics interdiction in Afghanistan and Central Asia: Challenges for international assistance.* New York: Open Society Institute.

Ma, J. 2005. All Yunnan addicts bound for rehab; New offensive against narcotics will see drug treatment centres expanded to house 68,000 people. *South China Morning Post.* Kunming. June 22.

Macan-Markar, M. 2003. Thailand: 'Victory' in anti-drug war comes with high cost. *Inter Press Service.* Bangkok. May 2.

Malinowska-Sempruch, K., Hoover, J., et al. 2003. *Unintended consequences: Drug policies fuel the HIV epidemic in Russia and Ukraine.* New York: Open Society Institute.

Nelson, K. E., S. Eiumtrakul, et al. 2002. HIV infection in young men in northern Thailand, 1991–1998: increasing role of injection drug use. *Journal of Acquired Immune Deficiency Syndrome* 29 (1):62–68.

New Straits Times. 2005. Success dependent on scale. Kuala Lumpur. June 7, p. 14.

Parker, R. 2002. The global HIV/AIDS pandemic, structural inequalities, and the politics of international health. *American Journal of Public Health* 92:343–47.

Razak, M., J. Jittiwutikarn, et al. 2003. HIV prevalence and risks among injection and noninjection drug users in northern Thailand: Need for comprehensive HIV prevention programs. *Journal of Acquired Immune Deficiency Syndrome* 33: 259–66.

Reid, G., and Costigan, G. 2002. Revisiting 'The Hidden Epidemic": A situation assessment of drug use in Asia in the context of HIV/AIDS. Fairfield, Australia: Centre for Harm Reduction at the Burnet Institute.

Reuters. 2005. China gets grant to stop AIDS among drug users. June 2.

Room, R. 2003. Impact and implications of the international drug control treaties on IDU and HIV/AIDS prevention and policy. In *Reducing the risk, harms and costs of HIV/AIDS and injection drug use (IDU): A synthesis of the evidence base for development of policies and programs,* ed. J. Rehm, B. Fischer, and H. Emma. Toronto: Health Canada.

Rossi, C. 2003. A critical reading of the reports of the International Narcotics Control Board and of the US Bureau for International Narcotics and Law Enforcement Affairs. *World Drugs Report.* New York: International Antiprohibitionist League.

Sarang, A. 2005. Statement to the Prevention Roundtable, U.N. General Assembly Session on HIV/AIDS. New York. June 2.

Schaepe, H. 1999. INCB position on shooting galleries. Letter to Father J. M. George. New South Wales, 2003.

Strathdee, S., and Poundstone, K. 2003. The international epidemiology and burden of disease of injection drug use and HIV/AIDS. In *Reducing the risks, harms and costs of HIV/AIDS and injection drug use (IDU): A synthesis of the evidence base for* development of policies and programs, ed. J. Rehm, B. Fischer, and H. Emma. Toronto: Health Canada.

Thompson, D. 2005. In search of harm reduction. *The Standard.* Hong Kong. June 23.

United Nations. 1971. *Convention on psychotropic substances.* Geneva: United Nations.

United Nations. 1988. *United Nations convention against illicit traffic in narcotic drugs and psychotropic substances, 1988,* International Narcotics Control Board.

United Nations. 2001. Preventing the transmission of HIV among drug abusers: A position paper of the United Nations System, United Nations High-Level Committee on Programme. www.cicad.oas.org/en/Resources/UNHIVAIDS.pdf.

United Nations Children's Fund (UNICEF). 2003. *Former prime minister of Thailand leads the fight against HIV/AIDS* (Press Release). New York: UNICEF.

U.S.-Russia Working Group. 2003. *On the frontline of an epidemic.* New York/Moscow: TransAtlantic Partners against AIDS/East-West Institute.

Vanichseni, S., Wongsuwan, B., et al. 1991. A controlled trial of methadone maintenance in a population of intravenous drug users in Bangkok: implications for prevention of HIV. *International Journal of Addiction* 26 (12):1313–20.

Vichai, P., and Aramrattana, A. 2003. *Results of rapid assessment of drug users entering Thai treatment facilities.* Bangkok: ONCB Thailand.

Vietnam Committee on Human Rights. 2000. Notes on criminal penalties for drug users in Vietnam. Boissy Saint Leger: Vietnam Committee on Human Rights.

VNA. 2005. Vietnam accepts methadone as heroin substitute to control HIV infection. Hanoi. June 16.

Voice of Vietnam. 2003. HCM City maximizes drug control effort. www.vov.org. July 20, 2003.

Watts, J. 2004. China's shift in HIV/AIDS policy marks turnaround on health. *The Lancet* 363 (9418):1370–71.

World Health Organization (WHO). 2002. Scaling up retroviral therapy in resource-limited settings: Guidelines for a public health approach. Geneva: WHO, 1–58.

World Health Organization (WHO). 2005a. *"3 by 5" progress report.* December 2004. Geneva: WHO.

World Health Organization (WHO). 2005b. *Progress on global access to HIV antiretroviral therapy: An update on "3 by 5."* June 2005. Geneva: WHO.

World Health Organization (WHO). 2005c. Summary country profile for HIV/AIDS treatment scale-up: China. June 2005. Geneva: WHO.

World Health Organization (WHO)/United Nations Office on Drugs and Crime (UNODC)/Joint United Nations Programme on HIV/AIDS (UNAIDS). 2004. *Substitution maintenance therapy in the management of opioid dependence and HIV/AIDS prevention.* Position paper. France, WHO/UNODC/UNAIDS.

Wolfe, D. 2004. Condemned to death. *The Nation.* April 26: 14–22.

Xinhua General News Service. 2003. 2003 declared year of war against drugs in Malaysia. January 22.

Xinhua News Service. 2005. China plans to expand drug-relief reformatories. *China View.* June 26.

Zhe, Z. 2005. Cabinet sets up nine steps to fight AIDS. *China Daily.* June 16, p. 2.

15

Human Rights and Public Health Ethics

Responding to the Global HIV/AIDS Pandemic

Jonathan Cohen, J.D., Nancy Kass, Sc.D., and
Chris Beyrer, M.D., M.P.H.

The global pandemic of HIV/AIDS remains the most important infectious disease threat to human health of our time. At this writing (mid-2005) perhaps 40 million men, women, and children are living with HIV infection and more than 25 million people have already died. In 2004, the world saw 5 million people become newly infected, underscoring the undone work of prevention, and 3 million deaths, stark evidence of our ongoing failure to provide treatment and care to the many millions who need it. Over the past decade, the global investment in HIV education, prevention, and treatment has been unprecedented. Major recent efforts have included the establishment of the Global Fund to Fight AIDS, Tuberculosis, and Malaria, the World Health Organization's "Three by Five" Program, which proposed to provide 3 million persons with antiretroviral treatment by the end of 2005, and the President's Emergency Plan for AIDS Relief (PEPFAR), a commitment from U.S. President George W. Bush to provide $15 billion over 5 years to international AIDS relief. All of these initiatives share common goals of expanding AIDS treatment access and preventing further HIV infections; yet their implementation and methods have raised an array of ethical and human rights questions.

Since its inception, this pandemic has been different from those of influenza, smallpox, or polio. All were greatly feared viral epidemics with a global reach, yet none generated the kinds of social opprobrium against the infected that the AIDS pandemic has so regularly done. The global AIDS pandemic consistently has been fraught with moral, political, and human rights challenges. Indeed, it is perhaps not overstating the case to say that the human challenges raised by HIV/AIDS—its social stigma, its disproportionate burdens on the poor, its gender and sexual minority dimensions, its associations with drug use, sex work, and morality—have driven a range of advances in thought and work around public health, human rights, and public health ethics. Such work, it is argued, reveals significant overlap between human rights and ethics but also reveals some important differences. Indeed, while the human rights and ethics mandates in the context of any given public health challenge, such as HIV, may be the same, the target of their mandates may not be identical. Greater clarity in understanding similarities and differences in these domains may be of benefit to public health practitioners, ethicists, and human rights professionals.

In this chapter, we will explore three examples of public health interventions designed to reduce the spread of HIV infection, and/or mitigate its impact: (1) the use of condoms and safer sex messages for HIV prevention; (2) the routinization of HIV testing as a means of streamlining HIV surveillance, prevention, and access to treatment and care; and (3) the effort to provide antiretroviral treatment in an equitable and nondiscriminatory manner. Through these examples, we hope to illustrate that the tools of both human rights and public health ethics should be used to examine the appropriateness of any public health proposal, program, or investigation, and used as a means of improving such undertakings before implementation. It is our thesis that human rights and public health ethics are distinct yet complementary tools for evaluating and analyzing public health interventions; although they overlap in important and meaningful ways, each should be applied independently to ensure that public health research and practice are implemented with rigor and with moral and professional integrity. Use (or nonuse) of these tools in the context of HIV has been particularly critical. HIV has an unfortunate history of public and private responses that have demonstrated dramatic violations of both human rights and ethics, and, the history of AIDS likewise is fraught with examples of flawed approaches that have violated rights *and* worsened epidemic spread. And although we believe it is illustrative to describe through case examples related to HIV the role that human rights and ethics analyses perform in furthering public health, how human rights and public health ethics affect public health emerges elsewhere as well. Indeed, Chapter 3 by Wan Yanhai and Li Xiaorong suggests that this has been the case for severe acute respiratory syndrome (SARS) in China, and Chapter 2 by Lee et al. identifies similar interactions of relevance to malaria in Burma's conflict zones.

A second theme is that the expansion of HIV/AIDS prevention, treatment, and care programs into developing and transitional countries, as well as the operational research accompanying these programs, should account for the human rights contexts in which programs are implemented (Beyrer and Kass, 2002). In some cases, this context may be so repressive as to make the prospect of ethically sound and rights-respecting HIV/AIDS programs seem remote—witness, for example, the difficulty of ensuring confidentiality in HIV testing in countries like Burma and Belarus. In others, war, civil conflict, and other active humanitarian crises impede the delivery of HIV/AIDS programs and contribute to HIV risk among targeted populations. Even in stable democracies, systematic human rights abuses against people living with AIDS and populations at highest risk of infection (often those most in need of services) can undermine the potential for prevention, treatment, and care programs to be implemented in a manner consistent with human rights and ethical principles. The expansion of HIV/AIDS programs into any environment requires an analysis of its human rights culture, or the extent to which people living with or affected by HIV are vulnerable to violations of their human rights. Both human rights and public health ethics require a balancing of interests that is sensitive to context rather than "one size fits all" approaches. Both also recognize that there may be multiple moral requirements, as well as epidemiological ones, not all of which necessarily can be maximized within any single program. Both recognize that public health practice has legitimate demands of its own, such as the safety of the blood supply, which both rights and ethics frameworks must accommodate to remain relevant to practitioners and to the wider public.

This chapter is not the first effort to apply human rights and ethical frameworks to various challenges in public health, or to compare the methods and targets of human rights and ethics work. Previous studies, including a monumental work by Cook, Dickens, and Fathalla in 2003, have examined the interplay among law, ethics, and medicine in the context of reproductive health (Cook, Dickens, and Fathalla, 2003). Legal and/or ethical analysis of specific program interventions, such as HIV testing and treatment, can be found in selected academic studies (Bayer, 1994; Gostin, 2004). We attempt to build on this work by focusing on three unique ethical and human rights challenges posed by the global AIDS epidemic, and by addressing challenges that exist at the level of policy rather than clinical practice. It is hoped that by engaging with our three case studies, policy makers will grasp the importance of applying human rights and ethical principles to difficult policy decisions related to HIV prevention and control, in particular, in environments where the human rights of those most affected by HIV are being threatened. Finally, after exploring the three case studies mentioned above, we address the differing intended targets of ethical debate and human rights investigations, because it is in this arena that these frameworks may most sharply diverge in "real world" HIV/AIDS epidemic settings.

Frameworks

Human rights have been referred to as the legal expression of individuals' "ethical rights as human beings" (Cook, Dickens, and Fathalla, 2003). The modern human rights movement, expressed in the Universal Declaration of Human Rights (1948) and subsequent treaties, was largely a response to the flagrantly unethical laws, policies, and practices of Nazi Germany. These treaties now form the basis for more specific guarantees in national laws and constitutions, as well as for a range of legal procedures at the national and international level for protesting human rights violations. Human rights practitioners tend to be lawyers and advocates who do the work of documenting human rights abuses, drafting legal documents, filing complaints before national human rights commissions, and suing governments. The concept of "human rights" remains a rallying cry for anyone aggrieved by their government or other power holder, but it is as much a professionalized legal enterprise as a normative framework. The legal integrity of human rights analysis, as much as its moral appeal, is what gives the human rights movement its authority and force.

For the purposes of this chapter, the application of human rights principles to public health challenges such as HIV/AIDS means at least three things. First, it means ensuring that HIV education, prevention, and treatment programs do not infringe on the human rights of those they are intended to benefit. A classic example is forced HIV testing: while intended to diagnose HIV cases and thus advance public health goals, it represents an unnecessary and disproportionate restriction on individual autonomy and on informed consent, and thus infringes on human rights. Second, human rights analysis means ensuring that all individuals, including the most marginalized, enjoy equal access to HIV/AIDS programs. In the context of HIV/AIDS, these groups usually include injection drug users, sex workers, gay men, prisoners, and others whose history of marginalization and abuse has placed them at the highest risk of both HIV infection and inequality in access. Third, human rights analysis means identifying human rights abuses that fuel HIV risk (such as violence against women and police harassment of needle and syringe exchange sites), and taking steps at the policy level to curb these abuses. This should be seen not only as a moral imperative in itself, but also as essential to effective and sustainable health policy.

At least two misconceptions about human rights tend to complicate their application to public health crises such as HIV/AIDS. The first is that HIV/AIDS occupies the realm of "economic, social, and cultural rights" (such as the right to health care) as opposed to "civil and political rights," such as the right to free expression, association, and due process of law. In fact, many of the human rights abuses that most increase HIV risk—imprisonment without due process, censorship of health information, violence and discrimination against women—are precisely civil and political rights abuses as defined by the International Covenant on Civil and Political Rights (ICCPR, 1966) and most national constitutions. The fact that these abuses worsen health outcomes underscores what has been called the "indivisibility" of human rights norms—the notion that civil and political rights and economic, social, and cultural rights are mutually reinforcing and derive from a single principle—the concept of fundamental human dignity.

A second, related misconception is that human rights impose an undue limit on state sovereignty and restrict the legislative branch of government in its effort either to give effect to the "will of the people" (usually the majority) and/or enact effective public health policy. In fact, human rights guarantees are almost always embodied in constitutions or international treaties that have been ratified by national legislatures, and are enforced by judges that are either elected or appointed by elected officials. Moreover, human rights guarantees admit of certain limitations, as long as these limitations can be shown to be necessary and proportionate to a legitimate policy objective. Human rights analysis precisely involves identifying the rights infringement in question (usually by reference to a specific legal guarantee), and then balancing that infringement against competing policy objectives. Most important, perhaps, human rights aim to give voice to minorities who may be marginalized or disenfranchised by the democratic process. Thus, there is nothing undemocratic or threatening to public policy about enforcing robust human rights norms (including in the context of HIV/AIDS), and in fact it would be problematic not to do so.

This is not to say that human rights practitioners do not regularly criticize the conduct of governments, nor call on them to rethink their policy choices. Human rights investigations aim precisely to target state actors when governments or their agents have either failed to protect vulnerable individuals or groups, or when they have actively participated in rights violations, as the two chapters in this volume on the Thai drug war demonstrate. Such human rights investigations may lead to concrete legal actions and other specific advocacy campaigns targeting governments, actions that move well beyond the opprobrium of ethical bodies deciding that research projects or programs are ethically flawed.

Public Health Ethics Frameworks

Although many frameworks for medical ethics analysis have been put forward, frameworks for the ethics of *public health* work are a more recent contribution. Even though the foundations of both public health and medical ethics are similar, they also differ in some critical ways. Most notably, while both require the provision of benefit and the minimizing of harm, public health targets this requirement to communities as a whole, and measures benefit across society. Medical ethics, by contrast, is more likely to focus exclusively on the well-being of individuals. Public health, further, is afforded legal authority to ensure that the *public's* health is improved and/or not threatened and, at times, can use rather invasive measures, from medical isolation and quarantine to mandatory hospitalization, as seen with SARS, to secure that.

Public health ethics, then, provides a framework for balancing the important and core value of public or societal benefit with restraint to ensure that individual rights and values are not ignored or compromised whenever possible. Public health ethics also puts emphasis on justice, again, as a societal goal and a societal good.

Public health ethics shares many core values with human rights but, again, it is different in some critical ways. Public health ethics, at its core, is concerned with ensuring that public health interventions provide benefit and minimize harms, respect individuals' dignity and rights to the greatest extent possible, and are implemented fairly. These values are completely consistent with those of human rights covenants and paradigms. Unlike human rights, however, ethics is not founded in law. Although ethics may be the basis for many laws, ethics itself has no legal standing, and "moral rightness" is not legally enforceable. Appealing to ethics in crafting and implementing public health interventions nonetheless is critical for three reasons. First, engaging in morally right action is important in and of itself. That interactions, including interactions related to public health, ought to be implemented consistent with the highest ethical standards is itself an important end. Civil societies, by definition, are bounded by shared moral rules and practices as well as by more formal laws and regulations.

Second, professional ethics requires a commitment to engaging *in one's work* in ways consistent with high ethical standards. Most of the established health professions, including medicine and nursing, have long-standing codes of professional ethics; public health, more recently, also adopted a code of ethics for public health professionals. Such professional codes help to self-regulate a profession and also serve to instill trust in the profession on the part of the public (American Public Health Association, 2000).

Third, as a means to an end, good ethics makes good public health sense. Ethics asks public health to ensure that programs will be beneficial before imposing them on the public. Ethics requires that individuals and communities be treated with dignity, and it requires that all communities receive appropriate public health intervention, not just those with more privilege. Such approaches are not relevant simply to morality; they make obvious sense for public health. Such principles help to ensure that more people get health benefit and that the "targets" of public health programs will better trust that such programs are initiated to further their own interests rather than to further some arbitrary goal on behalf of the leaders. And where public health actions *do* need to infringe on civil liberties, such as in enforcing immunization requirements for public schools, it is critically important that targeted populations perceive that these programs are fair, that they are based in sound science, and that the privileged (by resources or power) are not exempted (Beyrer, 2004).

Several approaches to considering ethics in public health proposals have been put forward (Kass, 2001; Callahan and Jennings, 2002; Childress et al., 2002; Roberts and Reich, 2002). A six-step approach is offered here (Kass, 2001).

Step 1 asks what the public health goals are of any proposed intervention, policy, or program. These goals, in general, should be expressed in terms of public health improvement, namely, in the degree to which the program will reduce morbidity or mortality. For example, an HIV screening program should have as its ultimate goal fewer incident cases of HIV, not that a certain proportion of individuals will agree to be tested.

Also relevant when considering public health goals and benefits is to whom the benefit will accrue. Public health interventions often are targeted to one set of individuals to protect *other* citizens' health. Partner notification programs or directly observed therapy for tuberculosis are designed, primarily, to protect citizens from the health threats posed by others. Restricting someone's liberty to protect him or herself poses different ethical burdens than restricting liberty to protect the interests of others.

Step 2 asks how effective the intervention or proposed program is at achieving its stated goals. Proposed interventions or programs are based on certain assumptions that lead us to believe the programs will achieve their stated goals. Step 2 asks us whether *data* exist to support these assumptions. In general, the greater the burdens posed by a program—for example, in terms of cost, constraints on liberty, or targeting particular, already vulnerable segments of the population—the stronger the evidence must be to demonstrate program effectiveness. Indeed, because many public health programs are imposed on people by governments and not sought out by those targeted, the burden of proof lies with governments or public health practitioners to prove that the program will achieve its goals. If there are no good data to demonstrate program effectiveness, the analysis can stop right there, and, ethically, the program should not be implemented. Conversely, the presence of good data alone does not justify the program; it allows us to move to the next stage of the analysis.

Step 3 asks what are the known or potential burdens of the program? If data suggest that a program is reasonably likely to achieve its stated goals, the potential burdens or harms that could result from our public health work must be identified. The majority of such harms will fall into three broad types: risks to privacy and confidentiality, especially in data-collection activities; risks to liberty and self-determination, given the power accorded public health to enact almost any measure necessary to contain disease; and risks to justice, if public health practitioners propose targeting public health interventions only to certain groups. Data collection may be viewed not simply as a violation of individuals' personal privacy; breach of confidentiality of such data—deliberate or incidental—can lead to significant and tangible harms. Personal health information, such as HIV status, can be dangerous in certain settings, if obtained by authorities and/or social acquaintances; even seemingly benign data such as vital statistics can reveal patterns about ethnic groups or neighborhoods that could lead to stigma, discrimination, violence, and/or forced relocation of identifiable groups.

Health education, in general, is thought of as the ideal public health intervention because it is completely voluntary and seeks to empower individuals to make their own decisions regarding their health. Unfortunately, however, education may not be effective in all settings, and, as such, policy makers may feel the need to resort to more restrictive measures.

Regulations and legislation, strictly speaking, are coercive, because they impose penalties for noncompliance. As such, they pose risks to liberty and self-governance. While many such measures, like mandatory child safety seats or immunizations, have demonstrated efficacy, they nonetheless are the most intrusive approach to public health. Further, the law can impose threats to justice if regulations pose undue burden on particular segments of society.

Step 4 asks how can burdens be minimized? Is the least burdensome approach being implemented? Once burdens have been identified, ethics requires programs to be modified in ways that minimize burdens without greatly reducing efficacy. If disease surveillance is equally effective with unique identifiers as with names, the former design is ethically required. If voluntary programs yield almost identical cooperation and effectiveness as mandatory ones, then voluntary programs are required. In cases where identifiable information is deemed to be necessary, it remains more respectful to inform individuals that identifiable data are being collected and for what purposes.

Step 5 asks is the program implemented fairly? Consistent with the principle of distributive justice, there must be a fair distribution of benefits and burdens in public health programs. Public health benefits, such as clean water, cannot be limited to one community alone, nor can a single population be subject to disproportionate burdens. Equity remains at least as important when restrictive measures are proposed. Injustice is wrong for its own sake, and also for the material harms that can follow. This does not mean that programs or resources must be allocated equally to all communities—rather, allocations must be *fair.* That is, differences cannot be proposed arbitrarily or based on historical assumptions about who might be at risk. Rather, targeting of programs to one community and not another must be justified with strong attention to data. Moreover, the social consequences must be considered when targeting of programs occurs, and these must be balanced against the benefits to that community or others. Discussed less frequently is the degree to which public health has any explicit role in righting existing injustices, especially given the strong link between social inequities and poor health outcomes (Starfield, 2005). Several conceptions of justice allow and even require unequal allocation of benefits to right existing inequities (Rawls, 1971; Daniels, 1985).

Step 6 asks how can the public health benefits and the accompanying burdens be balanced? Even to the extent that public health professionals can try to follow these requirements, disagreements invariably will emerge over interpretation—what types of burdens are excessive, and which types of targeting are unjustified. Procedural justice, then, requires democratic procedures to determine which public health interventions, in the end, should go forward. This process will require societies to discuss what is gained from good public health, and why such benefits often must be organized collectively. In such a process, although dissent is inevitable, dissent deserves special attention if raised by an identified subgroup, such as an ethnic minority, particular age group, or residents of a particular region. In general, the greater the burden imposed by a program, the greater must be the expected public health benefit, and the more uneven the benefit and burdens—that is, when one group is burdened to protect the health of others—the firmer must be both the scientific justification and the expected benefit.

Case Studies

Case Study 1: Condoms and Safer Sex Messages

For as long as condoms have been a staple of HIV prevention programs, they have also been a subject of intense controversy. Condoms (and specifically the male latex condom, by far the most widely used and best studied product) remain the only device with known efficacy to protect against sexual transmission of HIV; they have been associated with tenfold reductions in HIV acquisition and transmission risks, enormous reductions by any standard (Nelson et al., 1996). There is also no evidence that making condoms available for HIV prevention promotes "promiscuity" or encourages people to have sex. Yet condoms continue to attract many moral and religious objections, in particular, from those who associate them with birth control or premarital sex, or who think they are ineffective. Within Roman Catholicism, condoms have pitted purists of one type of duty-based ethics—those who believe that HIV should be prevented only by "virtuous" means such as abstinence and "self-restraint"—against those who view the lifesaving potential of condoms as a pragmatic or utilitarian imperative. A middle ground has been advocated by some Catholic theologians suggesting that condoms are consistent with the ethical principle of toleration (the idea that condoms should be tolerated as long as there is no viable alternative) or the principle of cooperation (that one can view birth control as morally wrong while still making an accommodation for a public health crisis) (Fuller and Keenan, 21–29).

The use of condoms against HIV has recently come under the spotlight in the context of U.S. government-funded "abstinence-only-until-marriage" programs, which promote sexual abstinence until marriage as the exclusive means of preventing sexual transmission of HIV. Abstinence-only programs stand in stark contrast to comprehensive sex education, in that they cannot, as a condition of funding, promote or endorse the use of condoms as an effective HIV-prevention strategy. These programs have been funded domestically by the U.S. government since the 1980s and are increasingly being exported to the developing world under President George W. Bush's Emergency Plan for AIDS Relief (U.S. Leadership against HIV/AIDS, Tuberculosis, and Malaria Act, 2003; Sexuality Information and Education Council of the United States [SIECUS], 2004). Abstinence-only programs enjoy strong support among religious conservatives in the United States and have been embraced by religious leaders in many developing countries as well.

How might the debate over condoms and abstinence-only programs be analyzed through the lens of human rights and public health ethics? From a human rights point of view, an appropriate point of departure is the prohibition on censorship, which is expressed by the right "to seek and impart information of all kinds" in the International Covenant on Civil and Political Rights. To the extent that abstinence-only programs censor, withhold, or distort information about condoms as a method of HIV prevention, they represent a flagrant violation of the right to information. But these programs do more than censor information—they censor information that has the potential to save people's lives. In this way, abstinence-only approaches should be viewed as implicating the right to the highest attainable standard of health (guaranteed in the Covenant on Economic, Social and Cultural Rights), and ultimately the right to life. As one Catholic nun in the Philippines has put it, "The church may take a stand against condoms as contraception, but when used to prevent a deadly illness, the right to life is higher" (Human Rights Watch, 2004c).

Additionally, to the extent that abstinence-only-until-marriage approaches promote *marriage* as a safeguard against HIV infection, they potentially endanger the lives of individuals who face a high risk of HIV infection from their spouses. The message that marriage is a zone of safety against HIV is misleading in many settings, in particular, in societies where male risk taking is likely to be substantial before marriage or in those where domestic violence, marital rape, and customary practices such as polygyny, bride price, and wife inheritance can increase risks (Go et al., 2003; Clark, 2004; Esen, 2004). Here is where, as emphasized above, an attention to *context* is an essential part of evaluating the human rights and ethical dimensions of a public health intervention. Although it is hard to imagine a context in which it is appropriate to present marriage as broadly protective against HIV, the message is false and misleading in sub-Saharan Africa and in South and Southeast Asia, in particular, where several studies have shown that marriage is a primary risk factor for incident and prevalent HIV infection in women (Go et al., 2003; Clark, 2004).

As noted above, human rights analysis requires balancing any alleged infringement of human rights (in this case, censorship of health information) against competing policy objectives (in this case, the promotion of marriage or of a particular kind of sexual morality). Assuming the promotion of a particular brand of sexual morality is a legitimate policy objective (which is open to dispute); the lifesaving potential of condoms clearly overrides any such objective. As argued by Human Rights Watch in a 2003 report on access to condoms in the Philippines, narrow visions of sexual morality are not an adequate justification for consigning people to premature and preventable death from HIV, absent some equally effective alternative to condoms for preventing HIV infection. Abstinence-only programs do not constitute such an alternative in the face of overwhelming evidence of their lack of effectiveness and, therefore, their potential harms.

Not only does human rights support evidence-based decisions, but also public health ethics similarly support implementing public health programs only when they are consistent with sound scientific data. Although other societal values surely are relevant for public policy, public health cannot endorse programs that are likely to put individuals at risk, or that deny them information that could protect their lives. Further, the rejection of scientific evidence, or the creation of doubt about existing evidence where doubt does not exist in the scientific community, is an unsound basis for public health policy and surely contradicts tenets of both public health ethics and human rights. Such obfuscations can serve to undermine the element of trust in public bodies that is essential if governments are to be effective in epidemic contexts. The South African government's "uncertainty" about HIV being the cause of AIDS has led, in the view of many, to a paralyzing inability to promote evidence-based approaches (Kapp, 2005).

Case Study 2: Approaches to HIV Testing

Despite extraordinary advances in HIV treatment, HIV remains an incurable disease. For that reason, public health professionals have devoted the bulk of their attention in HIV to disease prevention. A core piece of many of these prevention efforts has been HIV testing. An assumption is that HIV testing, when conducted well, both informs individuals about risks for HIV (whether or not they are infected), allows people who are found to be infected to take special precautions to prevent the further spread of the disease, and serves as a gateway to diagnosis and treatment. The way HIV-testing programs are organized, however, has implications both for human rights and for ethics.

Specifically, HIV-testing programs can vary by design, in the degree of voluntariness afforded by the program, in whether the provider or the client is expected to initiate the discussion about testing, and in how much information related to HIV is provided to clients, and to the extent that testing is linked to access to care, including antiretroviral therapy.

We expand here on previous work and describe five ways in which HIV-testing programs could be organized for the general population or for subpopulations of import (Faden et al., 1991). We then focus on the implications of these models for human rights and for ethics.

The first type of program design is called "strictly mandatory." Exactly as it sounds, a strictly mandatory program requires clients to be tested for HIV, and clients have no right to refuse. The second type of program is called "conditionally mandatory." A *conditionally* mandatory program, by contrast, is one in which testing is required of clients if they want to join or have access to a particular program, but there is no requirement that they join such programs. Conditionally mandatory HIV testing is the policy, for example, for new recruits to the U.S. Army, candidates for the Peace Corps, potential immigrants to the United States, and for applicants for certain levels of life insurance. There is no requirement in the United States for anyone to join the military or obtain life insurance. If someone wants access to those opportunities, however, it is required, with no right of refusal, that they be tested for HIV. The remaining three program designs all are voluntary, but vary in how explicitly that is communicated, and on who initiates the testing. The third type of program design is the "routine provision" of HIV tests. In a program of "routine provision," providers conduct HIV tests, in particular settings, as a matter of routine. In the same way that syphilis tests are conducted routinely during prenatal care and pap smears are conducted routinely during gynecologic examinations, HIV tests can be conducted routinely in a variety of health care settings. Technically, patients in all of these situations can refuse the test and sign a statement to that effect. In reality, however, organizing a program to have providers administer it routinely assures that the vast majority of patients entering that program will have an HIV test conducted. Option four, the "routine offering" of HIV tests, is somewhat different. A program organized in this way requires health care providers to offer an HIV test to every client entering the program, but more explicitly leaves the decision up to the client about whether to be tested. The provider initiates the discussion to ensure that every patient is given the opportunity to be tested, but the patient must decide explicitly to have the test conducted. "Patient-initiated" testing is what we will call the fifth model. Under this arrangement, a client must know about, and request, an HIV test for the test to be conducted. That is, providers neither inform nor initiate discussions about HIV, but HIV tests are available to anyone who knows to request one.

In all five of these models, clients might be either provided or not provided with HIV counseling, in which basic education about HIV, transmission, and the test itself, would be conveyed. Mandatory programs might provide excellent information—even in the context of requiring that the test be performed—and routine-offer programs might provide little to no information about HIV, even in making sure to ask everyone whether they want to be tested. Thus, whereas one consideration critical to both human rights and to ethics is the degree of choice offered clients about the test, another is how much information clients are given about HIV when HIV tests are performed.

Voluntary counseling and testing is currently the international norm, delineating that programs ultimately must be voluntary, and information about HIV disease and HIV testing must be provided in any testing program. Voluntary counseling and testing programs can be, and have been, organized through routine-conduct programs, routine-offering programs, and client-initiated programs. The availability of unprecedented resources for highly active antiretroviral therapy (HAART) has led some commentators to call for massively increased mandatory or "routine-conduct" testing programs (Holbrooke and Furman, 2004; Ross, 2004; Bozette, 2005). The logic behind these calls is that few individuals will take the initiative to have HIV tests without being promoted by a health care provider, and that without knowing their HIV status they will not benefit from treatment programs that could prolong their lives and protect their partners or the unborn. The estimate that 95 percent of people living with AIDS worldwide in 2004 did not know they were HIV-positive has further galvanized support for provider-initiated testing. Although this shift in thinking has concerned some human rights advocates as an increased opportunity for involuntary testing, many public health ethicists have argued that routine offering can provide a sound balance of public health goals and rights, and can be destigmatizing by making HIV testing routine (Bayer, 1994; Kass, 2000).

Although five models for testing exist, these approaches are neither neutral nor equivalent, from human rights and ethics perspectives. Some distinctions about the program are morally relevant notwithstanding the context, for example, that voluntary programs are, prima facie, more respectful of individual choice than are mandatory programs. Other distinctions, however, arise when one examines the context in which a program would be set: for example, it may be more important to zealously safeguard informed consent in contexts where the consequences of an HIV test may be devastating to the individual involved. Such contextual considerations ultimately must drive the choice of program design. Some considerations derive from the public health context: if there is evidence that individuals will opt out of a voluntary program, and that there are severe public health consequences of less than universal testing, public health has the legal and, often, moral authority, to intervene with a mandatory initiative. The bar for this is extraordinarily high, however, and the burden of proof will be on public health to demonstrate both that a voluntary program would not be effective and that the public health burdens of less than universal participation outweigh the ethical burden of trampling on individuals' free choice about HIV testing. Such a moral mandate is more likely to occur in contexts such as tuberculosis (TB) or avian flu, where communicability of disease is greater.

The ethically acceptable approach will depend, as above, on the potential harms and benefits from each. We will focus here on how the human rights context often predicts the range and severity of harms that can result from each of these approaches and, in turn, which approach would be ethically preferable for a given context. If there are concrete legal protections against AIDS-related discrimination in employment, insurance, immigration, and education, as well as against abuses against HIV-positive individuals, such as domestic violence, involuntary disclosure of test results, and deportation, then HIV testing may be less fraught with human rights concerns. The presence or absence of protections around these issues helps to determine which type of design will be ethically acceptable, as the risk/benefit ratio does not flow from a given testing approach but rather from the interaction between approach and context. In considering any of these testing approaches, a human rights framework would thus call for a review of the rights context in a given setting and, in particular, of the existence of legal and policy protections against AIDS-related human rights violations. And here the fundamental assumption of state beneficence, of trust that the actions of the state are taken for the benefit of citizens, is of primary importance for whether programs will be acceptable to populations or face widespread refusal.

The debate among various approaches to HIV testing has, not surprisingly, been called "perhaps the most challenging question in HIV/AIDS policy today" (De Cock, Marum, and Mbori-Ngacha, 2003). In an article in *The Lancet*, Kevin De Cock of the U.S. Centers for Disease Control and Prevention (CDC) and colleagues argued that current approaches favoring client-initiated voluntary testing and counseling were "an obstacle to scale-up of services and attainment of targets." They suggested that "universal voluntary knowledge of HIV serostatus should be a prevention goal" and, to that end, recommended the adoption of three specific practices: HIV testing for all women attending antenatal clinics "unless women actively refuse"; routine HIV testing in sexually transmitted infection clinics; and "universal" HIV testing among patients with tuberculosis or attending hospitals with symptoms potentially attributable to HIV. De Cock and colleagues suggested that HIV prevention messages emphasizing "ABC" (Abstain, Be faithful, use Condoms) ignored the possibility that monogamous couples might not know each other's HIV status, and recommended that "ABC" be replaced with prevention messages emphasizing the importance of HIV testing. They concluded that "the provision of information with ability of patients to decline HIV testing, *informed right of refusal* or the opt-out approach, balances autonomy with usual medical practice and meets ethical standards of informed consent." From a public health ethics perspective this approach is certainly justifiable, all else being equal. How does opt-out fare with the context-specific analyses of human rights?

In practice settings of compromised rights, those offered HIV tests by their health providers (as opposed to those who initiate a test) may not be fully informed of their right of refusal and, even if they are, may feel subjectively as though they have no option to refuse. Recent research by Human Rights Watch in the Philippines and the Dominican Republic has validated this concern (Human Rights Watch, 2004a, 2004b). The fact that many patients may genuinely feel they have no choice to opt out of a test offered by their physician, or be apprehensive about asserting that choice even if they know they have it, suggests at the very least that specific safeguards should be implemented and enforced to ensure that the informed right of refusal is a meaningful one. From an ethics perspective, this point cannot be overemphasized. The difference in burden posed by what we might call an operationally mandatory versus a truly voluntary opt-out program is enormous, and yet the difference in benefits to individuals and communities may be small, given that reasonable rates of acceptance of testing in voluntary programs with sound informed consent procedures is possible.

Informed consent is not the only intervention required to safeguard patients' rights and well-being, however. A second human rights concern is the involuntary disclosure of confidential HIV test results. Intentionally or not, medical facilities may disclose HIV test results to other doctors, hospital administrators, epidemiologists conducting HIV surveillance, government authorities, family members, or diverse others. In some cases, confidentiality may be breached even without the patient first being informed of his or her HIV status. Often this will depend on the country involved: the sharing of confidential medical information may be less likely in a jurisdiction with a culture of respect for patients' rights than one with a history of authoritarian or even paternalistic public health practices. The repercussions of involuntary disclosure of HIV status will also be context dependent: in some countries, in particular, those that are lax in protecting the legal rights of people living with AIDS, disclosure may lead to employment discrimination, retaliatory violence from spouses or other sex partners, general stigma from the community, and discriminatory treatment by public officials (including, ironically, health officials). These repercussions are often likeliest to fall disproportionately on women, who are more likely than men to come into contact with formal health services (most obviously antenatal services) and thus more likely to receive routine HIV testing. Human rights groups have accordingly called for well-funded safeguards, ranging from emergency help lines for battered women to effective prosecution of perpetrators of sexual violence, to accompany any routine testing scheme (Csete, Schleifer, and Cohen, 2004). In addition, before HIV-screening programs are initiated, there must be discussion of to whom, if anyone, results will be disclosed, other than the patient. Ethics requires a strong justification for involuntary disclosure of any medical information, in particular, information as socially and personally sensitive as HIV. In some contexts, public policy allows HIV results to be reported to local public health departments by name—another setting in which state beneficence is so crucial. Although there clearly is public health rationale for such practices, such disclosures not only pose a violation of one's personhood, they also can risk serious harm in terms of discrimination in multiple realms. Such reporting, then, is subject not only to the requirement of balancing benefits and harms, but also to minimizing harms. This includes clear procedural require-ments for confidentiality (such as unique identifiers or, as technically possible, encrypted or password-protected information), enforced policies that limit the numbers of persons able to access personally identifiable information, and procedures for unlinking names from HIV status in the majority of contexts where data are collected.

A third human rights concern is whether routine HIV testing will have harmful consequences in societies where there is a widespread stigma associ-ated with HIV/AIDS. In places where HIV is thought of as a curse, a contagion, or a punishment for sexual promiscuity, it may not be unreasonable to leave the decision of whether to have an HIV test entirely with the individual. This may be even more important where individuals who know their HIV status expose themselves to criminal liability for "knowingly" transmitting HIV to others. To be sure, some have argued convincingly that routine testing is the best way to "demystify" HIV/AIDS and alleviate this stigma. However, for rou-tine testing to succeed in doing so, it should be combined with rigorous infor-mation and education campaigns that provide factual information about HIV transmission, which itself is an intervention designed to promote benefit and minimize harms.

Finally, from a human rights perspective, any approach to HIV testing should recognize that people have a right of access to HIV testing as part of the broader right to health care enshrined in the International Covenant on Economic, Social and Cultural Rights (ICESCR, 1967). Considerations such as informed consent, confidentiality of test results, protections against violence and discrimination, and measures to combat stigma are not intended to be barriers to HIV testing. On the contrary, they are human rights imperatives against which the underlying "right to test" must be weighed. The 1984 Sir-acusa Principles on the Limitation and Derogation of Principles in the ICCPR provide a useful guide to this weighing process, noting that public policies (in this case HIV testing) can infringe rights if they are sanctioned by law, aimed at a legitimate public health goal, necessary to achieve that goal, no more intrusive or restrictive than necessary, and nondiscriminatory in appli-cation (U.N. Economic and Social Council [UN ECOSOC], 1984). These prin-ciples should be interpreted as a strong presumption in favor of strategies that protect people's right to choose, but not as a requirement to adopt any one approach to testing. The International Guidelines on HIV/AIDS and Human Rights, issued as nonbinding policy guidance to governments by the Office of the High Commissioner for Human Rights (OHCHR) and the Joint United Nations Programme on HIV/AIDS (UNAIDS) in 1996, state that all diagnostic HIV testing of individuals "should only be performed with the specific informed consent of that individual" except where specific judicial authorization is granted to perform a mandatory test (OHCHR/UNAIDS, 1996).

It is unfortunate that in some debates over routine testing, both human rights and ethics perspectives have been misconstrued as standing in the way of effective public health practice. This misunderstanding may stem in part from early debates over HIV testing, in which both human rights advocates and ethicists successfully argued that *mandatory* testing constituted not only an infringement on bodily autonomy, but also a threat to public health by fostering mistrust for health care providers and driving HIV-positive people "underground" (Bayer et al., 1986; Childress, 1987; Hunter, 1987). The fact that human rights advocates now fear a return to mandatory testing under the guise of routine provider-initiated testing should not be viewed as obstructionist, but rather as a good faith attempt to imbue important public health interventions with equally important human rights safeguards. Moreover, critics of the human rights approach often fail to realize that the importance of HIV testing—both to the individual and to the community—is part of the human rights calculus. Human rights law recognizes not only "civil and political" rights such as bodily autonomy and freedom from coercion, but also "economic and social" rights such as the right to the highest attainable standard of health, which entitles people to the best HIV prevention strategies available. Ethics, too, has been misrepresented as caring about individual autonomy at the expense of sound public health. Ethics, by definition, is a balancing strategy where multiple moral considerations and pulls coexist. Indeed, a distinction between public health ethics and traditional medical ethics is the more explicit acknowledgment of the importance of *public* health, and the measures to protect and promote public health that often can be achieved only through collective action. At the same time, one of the important responsibilities of public health ethics is scrutinizing public health interventions—in particular, invasive ones—to ensure not only that they can deliver the public health benefits by which they are justified, but also that they explicitly consider what individual violations might simultaneously occur, and create disclosures, interventions, and safeguards, as relevant, to diffuse the impact.

In both human rights and ethics frameworks, the question of HIV testing hinges in critical ways on context. The social harms of the disclosure of sensitive information and loss of confidentiality have everything to do with the rule of law, citizens' right to redress (or the absence thereof), and prevailing climates of openness or fear. For public health programs responding to widespread epidemics (such as HIV, SARS, or influenza), "one size fits all" programmatic approaches can be applied evenly across countries and work well in some, while creating great suffering in others.

Case Study 3: Equity in Access to Antiretroviral Therapy

Even the most ambitious targets for expanding access to antiretroviral therapy—for example, the World Health Organization's aim to treat 3 million people in developing countries by the end of 2005—recognize that many people in need of treatment will not receive it. This has generated inquiry over who should receive priority in government-funded programs (assuming anyone should receive priority), and how to establish fair and transparent procedures for making this decision (McCoy, 2003; UNAIDS/WHO, 2004). Simply ignoring this issue and providing treatment on a "first come, first served" basis will almost certainly result (and has resulted) in certain sectors of society being systematically excluded from programs. These sectors are likely to be those traditionally excluded from HIV/AIDS services, such as the rural poor, migrants and ethnic minorities, and stigmatized groups (such as sex workers, injection drug users, prisoners, and lesbian, gay, bisexual, and transgender persons) who traditionally face discrimination in the health sector.

The issue of equity in treatment rollout is complicated because, in some countries, the overwhelming majority of people in need of antiretroviral therapy come from politically marginalized or unpopular groups. Perhaps the clearest example of this is injection drug users, who are consistently underrepresented in national treatment programs despite accounting for the overwhelming majority of people in need of treatment in many countries. In Ukraine, for example, injection drug users represent more than 80 percent of those currently in need of treatment, but less than 5 percent of those currently receiving it (Kim, 2004). A similar pattern can be seen across the region of Eastern Europe and the former Soviet Union, where injection drug users represent the vast majority of people living with HIV/AIDS and in need of treatment. Similar data should be collected for other marginalized groups, such as sex workers, men who have sex with men, and prisoners (United Nations Reference Group on HIV/AIDS, 2005).

The reason for such underrepresentation in treatment rollouts may be an underlying pattern of human rights abuse that renders certain populations less able to obtain basic health care. Thailand is a case in point: since the beginning of the AIDS epidemic, the Thai government has systematically excluded injection drug users from its HIV/AIDS programs and has instead pursued a policy of "zero tolerance" of drugs that has resulted in the mass incarceration of drug users, accompanied by forced treatment (Human Rights Watch, 2004a). Drug users have faced brutal discrimination by public officials, violations of due process in the criminal justice system, and a climate of fear that has forced them in many cases to escape into hiding (see Chapter 1 by Kerr, Kaplan, Suwannawong, and Wood) (Human Rights Watch, 2004a). It should come as no surprise that drug users' account for a reported 0 percent of individuals receiving HIV/AIDS treatment in Thailand, despite representing the fastest-growing group of new HIV infections in the country (U.N. Reference Group on HIV/AIDS, 2005). This disparity underscores the importance of addressing a full range of human rights violations to achieve the particular human rights guarantee of equal access to HIV/AIDS treatment.

In sub-Saharan Africa, some experts have predicted that entrenched gender discrimination will result in women and girls being less able to reap the benefits of increased access to antiretroviral therapy than their male counterparts (Center for Health and Gender Equity [CHANGE], 2004). There is reason to believe this will not always be so: in some contexts, women are the first to receive treatment because of their greater frequency of contact with the health care system (especially antenatal care), as well as the priority placed on preventing transmission of HIV from mothers to newborn children. However, as treatment programs move beyond reproductive health contexts and into the "general population," and in particular, where costs or user fees are imposed on patients, women may be more likely to be excluded than men. Women's unequal ability to control family property or to achieve economic independence from their husbands, often a result of unequal property laws as well as entrenched cultural norms with regard to gender roles, means that simple costs like transportation to the hospital or user fees for health services may be beyond their means. Anecdotal evidence suggests that married women who do succeed in obtaining antiretroviral medicines may have those medicines confiscated by their husbands, who in some cases may have sent their wives for testing and treatment as a proxy for going themselves.

Both globally and in sub-Saharan Africa, women account for more than half of people infected with HIV. The range of gender-based human rights violations that contribute to this disparity—rape, domestic violence, sexual coercion, unequal access to property and education, and traditional practices such as widow inheritance, and bride price—may likewise impede women's equal access to HIV treatment (Human Rights Watch, 2005a). If a woman declines an HIV test for fear of retaliatory violence from her husband, this could result in her not receiving the treatment for which she might otherwise be eligible. Similarly, if a woman lacks meaningful avenues of justice for rape and domestic violence, she might fail to report these crimes and obtain otherwise available HIV diagnosis and treatment. Simply adopting a nondiscrimination policy in the delivery of HIV drugs is unlikely to produce substantive gender equality unless specific steps are taken to address women's systemic barriers to health care.

Under human rights law, the guiding principle for equitable access to antiretroviral treatment is that of nondiscrimination and equality under the law. This principle accepts that governments have difficult choices to make and that not every "social good" can be made universally available. Governments are restricted, however, from intentionally or unintentionally denying social benefits to individuals on the basis of, among other things, race, sex, national or ethnic origin, religion, and political viewpoint. Sometimes such denial will be justified, as where pregnant women are given preference for treatment to prevent HIV transmission from parent to child. But such decisions should never be based on unfounded or stereotypical assumptions about marginalized groups—such as the assumption that injection drug users should not qualify for treatment programs because they are "noncompliant" or incapable of conforming to a treatment regimen. In the case of antiretroviral treatment, they should be based on clinically relevant criteria and, beyond that, on criteria that are justified in the circumstances and that do not offend human dignity.

The procedures by which these criteria for treatment access are set should likewise be subject to both human rights and ethics standards. International human rights law recognizes the "right to participate," which should include a positive obligation on governments to solicit the views of affected populations in formulating public policy (ICCPR, 1966). But more urgently, authoritarian governments that place restrictions on civil society, including crackdowns on AIDS activism and censorship of the press, risk adopting AIDS policies that do not reflect the needs of their population. These "first-generation" human rights guarantees (freedom of speech, freedom of the press, freedom of association) are essential to treatment rollouts to the extent that they foster the political participation of the widest range of stakeholders possible. Procedural justice, as mandated by ethics in creating significant public health policy, has such rights as its cornerstone. China until quite recently has been a case in point: here, the routine jailing of AIDS activists and restrictions on the press have, among other abuses, contributed to an environment in which treatment criteria are set from the "top down" and may not reflect sound public health criteria.

Finally, human rights law requires that governments be proactive in removing systemic barriers that marginalize discrete groups from social benefits, in particular, where those groups are distinguished by personal characteristics such as race, gender, and ethnic origin. It is not enough for governments to adopt sound medical and equitable social criteria for treatment eligibility; they must go the extra step of ensuring that people ultimately are able to access treatment on a nondiscriminatory basis. This is often expressed in terms of "formal" versus "substantive" equality. Under a system of formal equality, it may be sufficient to establish nondiscriminatory eligibility criteria and "let the chips fall" where they may. Substantive equality, by contrast, recognizes that many groups who would otherwise meet the existing criteria may be excluded for systemic reasons—for example, lack of access to resources, lack of knowledge that treatment programs are available, or inability to speak the local language. Human rights law requires that governments take positive steps to remove these systemic barriers and make the existing criteria for eligibility work for everyone.

Thus far we have discussed allocation schemes in what ethics would call "negative obligations"—those outcomes we must ensure do not happen. But there may be justifications from human rights, ethics, or public health perspectives about priorities for allocating antiretroviral therapy for what *ought* to occur. Some have argued that the very poor child survival outcomes for children in developing countries without a healthy mother argue that mothers should have priority access, because so many others within families depend on their survival (Zaba et al., 2005). In a different context, South African communities faced with limited resources have argued that community members willing to be publicly open about their HIV status, and committing to advocating for access for others, should be given priority and kept alive, because their survival is the most likely to benefit others. In settings where economic disparities are wide, such as in the newly industrialized states of Asia (Hong Kong, Singapore, Malaysia, and Thailand), some have argued that the poor should be prioritized in public programs, because the wealthy can and will afford private-sector care (World Bank, 1997). These are painful debates and decisions whatever the context, and they are unlikely to decline as the rollouts of antiretroviral therapy reach increasingly more countries and communities affected by AIDS.

Looking Ahead

In some sense, public health, human rights, and ethics have universal and deeply shared values. It is the mission of public health to improve health, reduce morbidity, and reduce mortality wherever it does its work. Particular public health methods, although perhaps individually better suited to one locale than to another, in general derive from a well-accepted set of tools in the public health "tool box." Human rights and ethics, too, have basic sets of principles and rules in common that are intended to guide and/or dictate behavior in a variety of situations to ensure that human rights and ethics norms are not compromised in the pursuit of good public health outcomes.

While the principles and values of human rights and public health ethics are shared, in general, a significant difference between them remains in terms of targets and redress. Ethicists generally have little legal power to challenge what may be viewed as unethical practices or programs, even where the target of such ethical critique or advocacy is government or publicly sanctioned policies. Human rights, on the other hand, not only explicitly targets governments or the policies they endorse; international tribunals, war crimes trials, and the like are among the most potent tools of human rights advocates. Thus, whereas human rights organizations explicitly try to challenge rights violations through existing legal systems, ethical frameworks try to shape shared societal norms for morally appropriate behavior, norms that, in turn, may be reflected in the law. Human rights, further, often channels its arguments through media or advocacy, whereas in ethics the media and advocacy are less likely to be the primary means of communicating. In certain contexts, the goals of public health, ethics, and human rights can be well aligned. Public health, as a branch of government, has extraordinary power to further the public's health in ways that are beneficial, careful, and fair. But it is because such significant power, wherever it is given, so easily can be abused, that both ethics and human rights have created their own sets of checks and balances. Ethics and human rights provide the moral and legal "brakes" to redirect public health to more constructive tactics, and to highlight to public health professionals, through advocacy, argumentation, and accountability, what are and are not justifiable uses of state power and intervention in the name of furthering public health.

It has been the thesis of this chapter that the human rights context in which public health work, in general, and HIV work, in particular, is conducted will have an extraordinary impact on which public health tools ultimately must be selected to have ethically sound public health responses. The relationship of citizens to their governments has a tremendous impact on public health status in different locales and, indeed, the degree to which governments believe that they have a responsibility to care for the health of their public varies strikingly from country to country. Similarly, when public health seeks to intervene, the human rights or political context into which it enters also will influence to a great degree both what the public health benefits of a given intervention might be, and the ways in which a given intervention is ethically acceptable, ethically unacceptable, or ethically required.

References

American Public Health Association (APHA). 2000. *Guide to implementing model standards.* www.apha.org (accessed December 7, 2005).

Bayer, R. 1994. AIDS: Human rights and responsibilities. *Hospital Practice* 29 (2):155–64.

Bayer, R., Levine, C., and Wolf, S. M. 1986. HIV antibody screening: An ethical framework for evaluating proposed programs. *Journal of the American Medical Association* 256:1768–74.

Beyrer, C. 2004. Public health, human rights, and the beneficence of states. *Human Rights Review* 5 (1):28–33.

Beyrer, C., and Kass, N. 2002. Human rights, politics, and reviews of research ethics. *The Lancet* 360:246–51.

Bozzette, S. A. 2005. Routine screening for HIV infection: Timely and cost-effective. *New England Journal of Medicine* 352 (6):70–85.

Callahan, D., and Jennings, B. 2002. Ethics and public health: Forging a strong relationship. *American Journal of Public Health* 92 (2):169–76.

Center for Health and Gender Equity (CHANGE). 2004. *Gender, AIDS, and ARV therapies: Ensuring that women gain equitable access to drugs within U.S. funded treatment initiatives. CHANGE: Takoma Park, MD.* www.genderhealth.org.

Childress, J. F. 1987. An ethical framework for assessing policies to screen for antibodies for HIV. *AIDS Public Policy Journal* 2:28–31.

Childress, J. F., Faden R. R., Gaare, R., Gostin, L. O., Kahn, J., Bonnie, R. J., Kass, N. E., Mastroianni, A., Moreno, J. D., and Nieburg, P. 2002. Public health ethics: Mapping the terrain. *Journal of Law, Medicine, and Ethics* 30:170–78.

Clark, S. 2004. Early marriage and HIV risks in sub-Saharan Africa. *Studies in Family Planning* 35 (3):149–60.

Cook, R. J., Dickens, B. M., and Fathalla, M. 2003. *Reproductive health and human rights: Integrating medicine, ethics, and law.* Oxford: Oxford University Press.

Csete, J., Schleifer, R., and Cohen, J. 2004. Opt-out testing for HIV in Africa: a caution. *The Lancet* 363:493–94.

Daniels, N. 1985. *Just health care.* Cambridge: Cambridge University Press.

De Cock, K. M., Marum, E., and Mbori-Ngacha, D. 2003. A serostatus-based approach to HIV/AIDS prevention and care in Africa. *The Lancet* 362:1847–49.

Esen, U. I. 2004. African women, bride price, and AIDS. *The Lancet* 363:716.

Faden, R., Kass, N., and Powers, M. 1991. *Warrants for screening programs: Public health, legal and ethical frameworks.* Vol. 3 of *AIDS, Women and the next generation: Towards a morally acceptable public policy on HIV screening of pregnant women and newborns,* ed. Ruth Faden, Gail Geller, and Madison Powers, 26. New York: Oxford University Press.

Go, V. F., Sethulakshmi, C. J., Bentley, M. E., Sivaram, S., Srikrishnan, A. K., Solomon, S., and Celentano, D. D. 2003. When HIV-prevention messages and gender norms clash: the impact of domestic violence on women's HIV risk in slums of Chennai, India. *AIDS and Behavior* 7 (3):263–72.

Gostin, L. O. 2004. Testing and screening in the HIV/AIDS epidemic: A pubic health and human rights approach. In *The AIDS pandemic: Complacency, injustice, and unfulfilled expectations,* ed. L. O. Gostin, 133–50. Chapel Hill: University of North Carolina Press.

Holbrooke, R., and Furman, R. 2004. A global battle's missing weapon. *New York Times.* February 10.

Hunter, N. D. 1987. AIDS prevention and civil liberties: The false security of mandatory testing. *AIDS Public Policy Journal* 2:1–10.

Human Rights Watch. 2004a. *Not enough graves: Thailand's war on drugs, HIV/AIDS and violations of human rights.* Vol. 16, no. 8(C). New York (July 2004).

Human Rights Watch. 2004b. *A test of inequality: Discrimination against women living with HIV in the Dominican Republic.* Vol. 16, no. 4(B) (July 2004).

Human Rights Watch. 2004c. *Unprotected: Sex, condoms, and the human right to health in the Philippines.* Vol. 16, no. 6(C) (May 2004).

Human Rights Watch. 2005a. *Dose of reality: Women's rights in the fight against HIV/AIDS.* New York (March 2005).

Human Rights Watch. 2005b. *The less they know, the better: Abstinence-only HIV/AIDS programs in Uganda.* Vol. 17, no. 4(A) (March 2005).

International Covenant on Civil and Political Rights (INCCPR). 1966. G.A. res. 2200A (XXI), 21 U.N. GAOR Supp. (No. 16) at 52, U.N. Doc. A/6316 article 19.

International Covenant on Economic, Social and Cultural Rights (ICESCR). 1966. GA Res. 2200 (XXI), 21 UN GAOR, 21st Sess., Supp. No. 16, at 49, UN Doc. A/6316 (1966), article 12.

Joint United Nations Programme on HIV/AIDS and World Health Organization (UNAIDS/WHO). 2004. *Guidance on ethics and equitable access to HIV treatment and care.* Geneva: WHO.

Kapp, C. 2005. Court case shines spotlight on South African AIDS policy. *The Lancet* 366 (9482):291.

Kass, N. 2000. A change in approach to prenatal HIV screening. *American Journal of Public Health* 90:1026–27.

Kass, N. 2001. An ethics framework for public health. *American Journal of Public Health* 91:1776–82.

Keenan, J. F., Fuller, J. D., Cahill, L. S., and Kelly, K., eds. 2000. *Catholic Ethicists on HIV/AIDS Prevention*, 21–29. London: Continuum International.

Kim, J. 2004. WHO's HIV/AIDS strategy under the spotlight. *Bulletin of the World Health Organization* 82 (6):474–76.

McCoy, D. 2003. *Health sector responses to HIV/AIDS and treatment access in southern Africa: Addressing equity.* Regional Network for Equity in Southern Africa (EQUINET) in cooperation with Oxfam Great Britain. October 2003.

Nelson, K. E., Celentano, D. D., Eiumtrakul, S., Hoover, D., Beyrer, C., Suprasert, S., Kuntolbutra, S., and Khamboonruang, C. 1996. Changes in sexual behavior and a decline in HIV infection among young men in Thailand. *New England Journal of Medicine* 335 (5):297–303.

Office of the High Commissioner for Human Rights (OHCHR) and Joint United Nations Programme on HIV/AIDS (UNAIDS). 1996. *HIV/AIDS and human rights: International guidelines.* Geneva: OHCHR and UNAIDS.

Rawls, J. 1971. *A theory of justice.* Cambridge: Belknap Press of Harvard University Press.

Roberts, M., and Reich, M. 2002. Ethical analysis in public health. *The Lancet* 359: 1055–59.

Ross, E. 2004. Agencies seek routine AIDS tests in developing world. *Associated Press.* July 11.

Sexuality Information and Education Council of the United States. 2004. Federal spending for abstinence-only-until-marriage programs (1982–2006). Available at: www.siecus.org/policy/states/2004/Federal%20Graph.pdf (accessed December 7, 2005).

Starfield, B. 2005. Equity, social determinants, and children's rights: coming to grips with the challenges. *Ambulatory Pediatrics* 5 (3):134–37.

United Nations Reference Group on HIV/AIDS. 2005. *Treatment and care for drug users living with HIV/AIDS*. Available at: www.idurefgroup.org/background_papers.php (accessed December 7, 2005).

United Nations Economic and Social Council, U.N. Sub-Commission on Prevention of Discrimination and Protection of Minorities. 1984. *Siracusa principles on the limitation and derogation of principles in the International Covenant on Civil and Political Rights*, Annex, UN Doc E/CN.4/1984/4.

U.S. Leadership against HIV/AIDS, Tuberculosis, and Malaria Act of 2003, ss. 402(b)(3), 403(a).

World Bank. 1997. *Confronting AIDS: Public Priorities in a Global Epidemic*, 206–233. London: Oxford University Press.

Zaba, B., Whitworth, J., Marston, M., Nakivingi, J., Rubertentwari, A., Urassa, M., Issingo, R., Mwaluko, G., Flyod, S., Nyondon, A., and Crampin, A. 2005. HIV and mortality of mothers and children: evidence from cohort studies in Uganda, Tanzania, and Malawi. *Epidemiology* 16 (3):275–80.

16

Gender and Sexual Health Rights

Burma

Voravit Suwanvanichkij, M.D., M.P.H., Heather Kuiper, M.P.H.,
Alice Khin, M.B.B.S., M.Med., Terrence Smith, M.D., M.P.H.,
and Cynthia Maung, M.B.B.S.

Violations of human rights have specific and disproportionately harmful effects on the physical and mental health of girls and women, especially on their reproductive and sexual health. In areas where women are socially and economically subordinate to men, these violations are particularly devastating. In the case of sexual violence, the resulting harms are often compounded by social stigma. In modern conflict settings, rape has been used as a tool of war and ethnic cleansing. Although global attention was focused on this most acutely as a result of the civil war in the Balkans in the 1990s, this has also recently been seen in West Africa, Sudan, and the Great Lakes Region of Central Africa. This violation plays on the social status of women, where the victims of this egregious rights violation are often subjected to social isolation and shame. (See Chapters 8 and 11.) We have been working in another conflict setting, eastern Burma, which continues to simmer as we write. At the Mae Tao Clinic, located on the border of Thailand and Burma, we serve the health needs of internally displaced persons (IDPs) and other Burmese migrants, including girls and women affected by sexual violence, neglect, and the downstream effects of social discrimination. In this chapter we use our experiences to explore gender and health rights in a setting of sharply limited resources. These observations apply globally and complement the case studies and research strategies presented elsewhere in this text.

Human rights law and policy recognizes that rights include basic civil and political rights as well as social, economic, and cultural rights. The interplay of health consequences and rights violations occurs over a continuum, spanning from essential civil liberties to economic rights, including access to a minimum standard of health care. We believe it is a rights violation against women when civil society fails to provide access to gender-based health services such as family planning, prevention of sexually transmitted infections (STIs), and prenatal care; and to such a degree that girls and women live at substantially increased risk of consequences such as septic abortion, maternal death, and fetal wastage. It is our view that health indicators uniquely affecting women provide an accurate picture of the rights status of women and of civil society in general.

Gender and Sexual Rights: The Burmese Experience

The Burmese military junta came to power 1962, when General Ne Win initiated a coup against the lawfully elected civil government (International Crisis Group [ICG], 2003). Since that time, the population has been ruled by a succession of military juntas. The current junta, the State Peace and Development Council (SPDC), is one of the worst dictatorships in the world, where the abrogation of political rights has led to a steady decline in both the economy and the population's health status. Particularly hard hit have been Burma's ethnic minorities in geographic parts of the nation where armed groups resist government control (Altsean, 2005; U.S. Department of State, 2005). As part of its war against insurgents, the Tatmadaw or Burmese military employs a campaign known as the Four Cuts Policy (see also Chapter 2) that denies the population access to food, funds, recruits, and information (ICG, 2003; Risser et al., 2004). Central to this strategy is the forced relocation of civilians from contested areas to "relocation centers" more firmly under control of the central administration, and with it deliberate destruction of rice fields and food storage facilities (Thailand Burma Border Consortium [TBBC], 2004; Altsean, 2005). The forced relocation of indigenous populations has been regularly accompanied by summary executions, rape, confiscation of land and property, torture, forced labor (often on public works or as army porters), and compulsory contributions to the military (Belak, 2002; EarthRights International, 2003; Risser et al., 2004; Amnesty International [AI], 2005; U.S. Department of State, 2005). Relocation sites often are fenced off and resemble concentration camps. There is insufficient food, unclean water, and a lack of basic health services (Fink, 2001). Between 1996 and 2002, about 2,500 villages in Burma's eastern frontiers were destroyed or forcibly relocated, resulting in the displacement of more than 600,000 mostly ethnic minority Burmese (Risser et al., 2004; TBBC, 2004). The brunt of this occurred in Shan State where between 1996 and 1998, 1,400 villages in a 7,000-square-mile area were forcibly relocated and the population subjected to forced labor; villagers caught outside relocation sites were often subjected to extrajudicial execution (Shan Human Rights Foundation [SHRF], 1998; Fink, 2001; Belak, 2002). Those who fled successfully have become IDPs or refugees in neighboring countries, in particular, Thailand, where an estimated 2 million Burmese reside. These individuals typically are not provided with even the most basic health and education services. Coupled with their lack of legal protections, they are highly vulnerable to exploitation, including sexual exploitation and forced labor.

Where women lack political rights and economic equality, poor health status is common. In Burma, females are disproportionately poor and are expected to be the family caretaker, often withdrawing early from school to meet this social obligation and perpetuating this cycle of poverty (Altsean, 2001; Women's League of Burma [WLB], 2002; U.S. Department of State, 2005). These political and social trends drive down the overall health status of Burmese women.

Trafficking is another rights violation, which the United Nations and member states have charged the Burmese junta (U.S. Department of State, 2004). In response to these allegations, the junta instituted a policy prohibiting women under age 25 from crossing international boundaries without a guardian (Physicians for Human Rights [PHR], 2004; U.S. Department of State, 2005). Paradoxically, this has forced women seeking work abroad to hire agents to facilitate crossing borders, putting them at further risk for being violated and exploited (National Coalition Government of the Union of

Burma [NCGUB], 2002; PHR, 2004; Kachin Women's Association Thailand [KWAT], 2005).

In addition to state-sponsored violence, women face gender-based violence at home. In Burma an estimated 3–15 percent of women report having experienced some form of physical or mental violence; and this is may be an underestimate because cultural norms demand privacy in the husband-wife relationship (Belak, 2002; NCGUB, 2002; Mae Tao Clinic, 2004). Poverty and financial dependence on a husband further contribute to subordinate status. If a woman leaves, she may not be able to support herself or her children (Belak, 2002; NCGUB, 2002; WLB, 2002). The societal value placed on virginity before marriage and monogamy within marriage further dissuades females from reporting sexual violence (Belak, 2002).

Women in conflict zones, including refugees and IDPs, face even higher risks of sexual violence and negative health effects. This vulnerability is corroborated by our experience providing health services along the Burma-Thai border. In May 2002, the Shan Women's Action Network (SWAN) and the Shan Human Rights Foundation (SHRF) released the report *License to Rape*, which documented 173 incidents of rape and other forms of sexual violence involving 625 girls and women by *Tatmadaw* soldiers in Shan State between 1996 and 2001 (SHRF and SWAN, 2002a). Most of these crimes occurred in areas of forced relocation in central Shan State, an area of increasing military activity and anti-insurgency activities by the SPDC (SHRF and SWAN, 2002a; Risser et al., 2004). As is common where such atrocities take place, the government responded by issuing denials along with statements that the findings were invented to smear the state's image (New Light of Myanmar, 2002; SHRF and SWAN, 2002b). They also warned the population not to discuss rape and violence. Since the release of this report, however, others have investigated this issue, corroborating the findings of SWAN and SHRF that rape and sexual violence are committed systematically and with impunity by SPDC soldiers, in particular, against ethnic minority women (Apple and Martin, 2003; EarthRights International (ERI), 2003; Karne Women's Organization [KWO], 2004; WLB, 2004; Woman and Child Rights Project and Human Rights Foundation of Monland [WCRP and HURFOM], 2005). Few services are available to address the needs of survivors (Ba-thike, 1997; Belak, 2002).

Women's Health Is a Human Right

The 1978 Alma-Ata Declaration of the WHO recognizes "that health, which is the state of complete physical, mental and social well-being, and not merely the absence of disease or infirmity, is a fundamental human right and that the attainment of the highest possible level of health is a most important world-wide social goal, whose realization requires the action of many other social and economic sectors, in addition to the health sector" (World Health Organization [WHO], 1978). In many countries, the health status of women is unacceptably substandard and is seen by many as an abrogation of their basic human rights. Here, the fields of public health and human rights advocacy are complementary. Public health's statistical tools can provide useful measures of rights when they assess the status of populations, especially vulnerable populations such as girls and women, who live in settings of subordination, exploitation, and violence. These measures provide powerful documentation for legal redress while also informing health planning and service delivery. Seen in this light, measures of infant and maternal mortality are particularly useful indicators of rights. And where governments (or juntas) issue inaccurate figures to minimize actual conditions, independent assessments are called for.

Humanitarian emergencies, conflict, and resource scarcity often aggravate already difficult conditions. In such settings, measures of malnutrition, trauma, maternal and infant mortality, and sentinel diseases including HIV, malaria, and tuberculosis are particularly useful indicators (Swiss and Giller, 1993; Gasseer et al., 2004). Today, 99 percent of the yearly estimated 580,000 maternal deaths worldwide occur in developing countries (Starrs, 1998; Goldman and Glei, 2003). Expressed per 100,000 live births, the highest maternal mortality rate is in Africa (1,000), followed by Asia (280), Oceania (260), Latin America and the Caribbean (190), Europe (28), and North America (11). Furthermore, for every maternal death, almost 30 women are injured or develop life-long disabilities from pregnancy and childbirth complications (Donnay, 2000). When a woman dies or is disabled, the health of her entire family, especially that of her children, also suffers (United Nations Department of International Economic and Social Affairs, 1991; Starrs 1998). Maternal mortality is a sensitive indicator of the overall health status and human rights enjoyed by girls and women and it tends to track or move with other health status indicators for the female population. It also indexes access to health care services overall and the capacity of the health care sector to respond to needs (Amowitz, Reis, and Iacopino, 2002a). Recognizing these realities, the International Safe Mother Initiative recognizes disproportionately high maternal mortality to be a human rights and social justice issue:

> For a woman to die from pregnancy and childbirth is a social injustice. Such deaths are rooted in women's powerlessness and unequal access to employment, finances, education, basic health care and other resources. These factors set the stage for poor maternal health even before a pregnancy occurs, and make it worse once pregnancy and childbearing have begun.
>
> Making motherhood safer, therefore, requires more than good quality health services. Women must be empowered, and their human rights—including their rights to good quality services and information during and after pregnancy and childbirth—must be guaranteed (Cook, 1997; Safe Mother Initiative, 1997).

Unplanned pregnancy is one consequence of rape and, like sexual violence in general, may be underreported (Swiss and Giller, 1993; Amowitz et al., 2002b). When health services are marginal, rape and resulting pregnancy can be lethal (Gasseer et al., 2004). In Burma proximate causes of maternal death are complications from unsafe abortions and postpartum hemorrhage, both treatable and preventable, and sometimes the result of rape (U.N. Population Fund [UNFPA], 2001). In areas populated predominantly by ethnic minorities, rape is committed with impunity by the *Tatmadaw* and contributes to unintended pregnancies, unsafe abortions, and other negative health repercussions (Belak, 2002).

Life expectancy is another sensitive indicator of health and rights. Here again we can point to our experience in providing medical services along the border between Burma and Thailand. About 50 years ago Thailand and Burma were at similar stages of economic and social development. Today, the average life expectancy for women in Thailand is 74.4 years but only 63.8 years in Burma (Central Intelligence Agency [CIA], 2005). Although fully accurate figures are not available, there is little doubt that a major disparity exists. One contributing factor is excess maternal mortality, which disproportionately decreases women's life expectancy in Burma's eastern conflict zones compared with elsewhere in the country. For example, anemia, often a result of prevalent malaria, malnutrition, and closely spaced pregnancies in these areas, increases the risk of maternal death due to postpartum hemorrhage (Mae Tao Clinic, 2004). Infant mortality and mortality of children under age 5 also are useful indicators. Such measures from the conflict areas of eastern Burma do not resemble national figures and are more comparable to figures from Angola, Somalia, Liberia, and Sierra Leone, which face similar underlying realities (Eh Kalu and Lee, 2005). (See Table 16.1.)

Reproductive Rights and Unsafe Abortion

Maternal mortality accounts for more than half of the deaths of women and 20 percent of hospital admissions in central Burma. Unsafe abortions are a primary cause (Ba-thike, 1997; WHO, 2000; Belak, 2002). Except when the pregnancy threatens the life of the mother, abortion is illegal in Burma. Both patient and medical practitioner involved in an abortion are subject to fines or up to three years imprisonment; ten if the procedure results in death (Sen, 2001; NCGUB, 2002; Belton and Maung, 2004). Nevertheless, abortion is commonly employed to control fertility (Beyrer and Stachowiak, 2003; WLB, 2004). The UNFPA estimates that one-in-three pregnancies in Burma ends in abortion and approximately 750,000 abortions are carried out each year, or about 2,000 per day (Ba-thike, 1997; WHO, 1997a; United Nations Development Programme and UNFDA], 2001; Belak, 2002). In one survey, 58 percent of married women in Rangoon reported having had at least one abortion; lack of formal education and low income are risk factors (Ba-thike, 1997; WHO, 1997a). These figures may be lower than the actual number because abortion is both illegal and stigmatized, being perceived as a method used by "unmarried women" to terminate unplanned pregnancies (Belak, 2002). Because of the penalties associated with abortion, they are done clandestinely and under unsanitary conditions, by the woman herself or by untrained practitioners (Chelala, 1998; Belak, 2002; NCGUB, 2002). A variety of methods are used to induce abortion, ranging from traditional herbs to insertion of foreign objects such as sticks, iron rods, porcupine quills, and slivers of bamboo into the cervix, often resulting in local infections or sepsis (Ba-thike, 1997; Belak, 2002; NCGUB, 2002). While it appears that maternal mortality ratios have slowly been declining over time in Burma, mortality rates from septic abortion complications remain high and unchanged despite its being ranked by the Ministry of Health as one of the top ten most important health problems facing the country (Ba-thike, 1997; NCGUB, 2002).

Table 16.1. Selected indicators of health status and health expenditures: Burma, eastern Burma states, and Thailand

	Burma	Thailand	United Kingdom	Rwanda	Somalia	DR Congo	Sierra Leone	Selected eastern Burma conflict zones[*]
Per capita GNI[†] (UNICEF, 2006)	220	2,540	33,940	220	130	120	200	—**
Life expectancy at birth (years) (UNICEF, 2006)	61	70	79	44	47	44	41	
MMR[‡] (UNICEF, 2006)	360	44	13	1,400	1,100	990	2,000	1,000–1,200
IMR[§] (UNICEF, 2006)	76	18	5	118	133	129	165	135
U5MR[‖] (UNICEF, 2006)	106	21	6	203	225	205	283	294
Lifetime risk of maternal death (1 in XX)[#] (UNICEF, 2006)	75	900	3,300	10	10	13	6	—**
Total health expenditures per capita, 2002 (international $)[††] (WHO, 2006)	30	321	2,160	48	N/A	14	27	
Per capita government expenditure on health, 2002 (international $)[††] (WHO, 2006)	6	223	1,801	27	N/A	4	16	
Total expenditure for health, 2002 (%GDP) (WHO, 2006)	2.2	4.4	7.7	5.3	N/A	4.0	2.9	

*Unpublished data from the Backpack Health Worker Team Program Health Information System for ethnic states in eastern Burma, 2003

†Gross national income per capita is the gross national income divided by the midyear population, expressed in U.S. dollars.

‡Maternal mortality rate (MMR) = probability of death of pregnancy-related causes per 100,000 live births

§Infant mortality rate (IMR) = probability of dying at under 1 year, per 1,000 live births

‖Under five mortality rate (U5MR) = probability of dying at under 5 years per 1,000 live births

#XX, one death in the total number of maternal women in the given column.

**Although no figures for lifetime risk of maternal death are available for IDPs in eastern Burma, given the similar MMRs among these areas, it is likely to resemble figures for Rwanda, Somalia, Sierra Leone, and the Democratic Republic of the Congo (formerly Zaire).

††Computed by WHO for comparability among member states

The fear of arrest and social stigmatization that drives women to get clandestine abortions also prevents them from seeking health services when complications develop. The consequences can be catastrophic (Belak, 2002). The incidence of women hospitalized for complications of abortion in ethnic minority Mon, Chin, Karenni, and Kachin States is even higher than in the general population (Ba-thike, 1997; Belton, 2002). At the Mae Tao Clinic, unsafe abortion accounted for approximately 16 percent of cases in the reproductive health outpatient department in 2002. In 2003, 352 patients were admitted to the reproductive health inpatient ward for complications resulting from abortions, accounting for half of nonobstetric admissions there and consuming almost one-third of the entire clinic's operating budget (Mae Tao Clinic, 2004). A contributing factor is the frequency of repeat abortions, itself a result of systemwide failures to provide postabortion contraception (Belak, 2002). At the Mae Tao Clinic, 26 percent of patients admitted for complications of abortion had a prior history of an abortion (Mae Tao Clinic, 2004).

What we observed in Mae Sot is seen elsewhere in the world where family-planning services are either unavailable or unlawful. Burma is an extreme case, as the use of modern contraceptives by reproductive-age women is estimated at 17–22 percent, among the lowest in the world. It is even lower in ethnic minority areas (Chelala, 1998; Belak, 2002; Beyrer and Stachowiak, 2003). Contraception was only legally introduced in Burma in 1991 and condoms in 1993. Under still-existing colonial-era laws against prostitution, possession of condoms by a woman is considered evidence of involvement in sex work and is grounds for arrest and imprisonment for up to three years (Belak, 2002; NCGUB, 2002; Low Htaw, 2004). According to a former WHO employee involved in HIV prevention, "the government issued a law to legalize the use of condoms but the problem is that only the police know this information. Women are still unaware of it. And prostitution itself is still illegal. That is one of the major problems" (Low Htaw, 2004). As in other countries where cultural taboos and strict government censorship limit disseminating information about sex and reproductive health, modern contraception is used far too infrequently, is misused, or is refused. This is especially so in remote villages along the frontiers (Ba-thike, 1997; Belak, 2002; NCGUB, 2002). A survey of villagers and IDPs primarily in Karen State conducted at the Mae Tao Clinic by the Backpack Health Worker Team Program[1] (see Lee et al.) found that 34.3 percent of respondents felt that discussing reproductive health issues was taboo and 31.6 percent opposed educating youth on pregnancy prevention. Less than 35 percent of survey participants used contraception and of those not wanting more children, only 59 percent were taking steps to prevent pregnancy. Most had little awareness of birth control methods except for oral contraceptives (40%) and Depo-Provera (44%). Despite this, use of these methods was still very low: 8.9 percent and 10.4 percent, respectively (Mae Tao Clinic, 2003). In another survey done among Burmese migrant factory workers in Mae Sot, only 15 percent of young women had ever seen a condom and only 1.4 percent had ever used one (Mullany et al., 2003).

The consequence of inadequate public education and access to contraceptive technologies in Burma means that women too often turn to quack practitioners or rely on street pharmacies to purchase products with dubious contraceptive efficacy (Ba-thike, 1997; Belak, 2002; Belton, 2002). This situation is worse in the conflict zone of eastern Burma where the *Tatmadaw* often forbid the sale of medications to villagers in an attempt to block supplies from reaching ethnic insurgents. Possessing medications can result in arrest and extrajudicial execution (Karen Human Rights Group [KHRG], 2001). Where counseling about birth spacing is available it typically is not provided in indigenous minority languages and the providers are ethnic Burmese unfamiliar with local languages, customs, and norms. This further limits access for ethnic minority women and fails to address local cultural attitudes and misconceptions (Belak, 2002; U.S. Department of State, 2005). Our experiences caring for Burmese migrants along the frontiers underscores the theme that, where there is repressive government and civil strife, girls and women suffer particular harms as a result of lack of knowledge about and access to reproductive health information and relevant services, especially safe and effective contraception.

Indicators of Maternal Mortality and Morbidity

Preventing morbidity and mortality that results from complications of abortion and delivery often can be accomplished with relatively simple, cost-effective measures. Failing to do so is an abrogation of women's rights, especially when it is a consequence of governmental neglect. According to the International Safe Motherhood Initiative, more than three-quarters of all maternal deaths in developing countries take place during or soon after

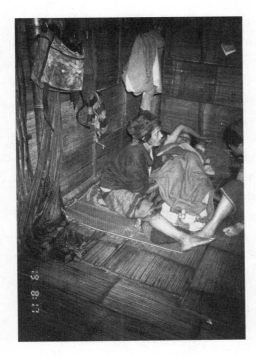

Figure 16.1. Woman delivering a baby in the Burmese rainforest attended by a traditional birth attendant. Photo courtesy of Karen Human Rights Group

childbirth, and the "single most critical intervention for safe motherhood is to ensure that a health worker with midwifery skills is present at every birth, and transportation to a health facility in case of an emergency" (AbouZahr, 1997). However, according to the World Health Organization (WHO), skilled attendants are present at only 53 percent of births in the developing world, whereas in developed countries, skilled attendance is nearly universal (WHO, 1997b). Indeed, most maternal and neonatal deaths in developing countries take place at home and thus away from health facilities and skilled health workers (Costello et al., 2004). Emerging data suggest that the use of community-based interventions, such as birth attendants, reduces complications such as perinatal mortality and postpartum hemorrhage (Sibley and Sipe, 2004; Jokhio et al., 2005; Prata et al., 2005). (See Figure 16.1.)

In this regard, again, Burma compares poorly. Roughly 80 percent of deliveries take place at home with 46 percent assisted by traditional birth attendants (TBAs) that are only minimally skilled, 38 percent by nurses or midwives, and 9 percent by physicians. Only 16 percent of births occur in hospitals (WHO, 1997a; Agence France Presse [AFP], 2005). Based on a recent reproductive health survey in ethnic states we conducted at the Mae Tao Clinic, these figures are even worse in the ethnic conflict zones. Only 16.1 percent of women said they had received antenatal care from a trained medical provider in a hospital and clinic, or from a trained medic. Seventy-seven percent gave birth at home, 74 percent of these with the assistance of a TBA; only 8 percent delivered in a clinic or hospital. Between 5 and 35 percent of women reported giving birth while hiding in the jungle during times of instability (Mae Tao Clinic, 2003). We found many factors at play, including that the cost of care often is prohibitive, physical access is difficult, information is censored or unavailable in local languages, and staff members are insufficiently trained, lack proper equipment and supplies, and are not culturally appropriate (Belak, 2002; U.S. Department of State, 2005). The outcome is a glaring absence of antenatal care, skilled delivery, and postpartum care, resulting in excess maternal morbidity and mortality (Belak, 2002; Belton, 2002; NCGUB, 2002; TBBC, 2004). These issues are further aggravated by a high prevalence in Burma of malnutrition and infectious diseases like malaria, especially in the conflict zones. Multiple closely spaced pregnancies further increase the risk for maternal anemia and low neonatal birth-weight and contribute to poor health outcomes for mothers and infants (KHRG, 2004).

AIDS, Sexually Transmitted Infections, and Malaria

HIV/AIDS and malaria are among the most important infectious diseases in the developing world. Across Asia, including in Burma, most women acquire HIV through heterosexual contact. Cultural forces often stand in the way of proven prevention modalities, in particular, in regard to prevention of sexual transmission. In response to concerns about public health measures to combat the transmission of HIV, Lt-Gen. Khin Nyunt, then secretary-1 of Burma's ruling SPDC, said, "We are a very conservative, religious society and it was rather against our culture to put condoms on show as a means of prevention" (*Myanmar Times*, 2001). Meanwhile poverty, prostitution, and a booming illegal economy that includes trade in narcotics continue to fuel the spread of HIV in one of the worst epidemics in Asia (ICG, 2002, 2004; PHR, 2004). Funding to address the problem falls far short of what is needed, with the 2004 National AIDS budget for Burma reaching only 22,000 USD, one of the lowest levels of support documented worldwide (Broadmoor, 2003; ICG,

2004). Basic surveillance data for Burma are poor. Official figures from the National AIDS Program (NAP) in December 2004 cite about 340,000 people living with HIV infection. However, estimates using 1999 sentinel surveillance place the figure closer to 687,000, or 3.46 percent of reproductive age adults, suggesting a widespread, generalized epidemic (Beyrer et al., 2003). Although found all over the country, HIV/AIDS is most prevalent in the Shan and Kachin States, along the eastern frontiers (Beyrer et al., 2003). This finding is supported by data obtained in 2001 from Shan migrant construction workers living in northern Thailand. Their HIV prevalence is double that of comparable northern Thais, who already have the highest HIV prevalence in Thailand (Srithanaviboonchai et al., 2002). A major force driving this epidemic is injecting drugs. Sentinel surveillance data obtained from injection drug users in Muse, near the Chinese border, showed that 92.3 percent were HIV positive (Beyrer et al., 2003). Assessments of pregnant women receiving antenatal care revealed that this population still remains relatively free of HIV (ranging from 1.4 to 4.9%). The concern is for the future, because girls and women in their reproductive years are now in the midst of a rapidly spreading HIV epidemic (ICG, 2002; Beyrer et al., 2003).

Throughout the developing world the factors already discussed that contribute to adverse reproductive health also place girls and women at risk for HIV/AIDS and other sexually transmitted diseases: social subordination and social stigma, outright government censorship of and more passive failing to provide public health education, failing to provide AIDS prevention and testing services, including condoms, and sexual violence (Belak, 2002; Broadmoor, 2003; Mullany et al., 2003). In the situation we have observed firsthand in Burma, sexual violence is particularly egregious because it is part of a government policy to violate and intimidate ethnic minorities. As in many parts of the developing world, poor ethnic minority Burmese girls and women are disproportionately at risk for acquiring HIV. In Burma the few national AIDS programs to provide services like condoms and voluntary counseling and testing (VCT), antiretroviral drugs for preventing mother-to-child transmission (PMTCT), and for treating active HIV infection are located in cities and towns and run by ethnic Burmese instead of ethnic minorities (Belak, 2002; Min Thwe, 2004). The dire shortage of equipment and supplies that exists throughout the country is at its worst in rural areas. Needles often are reused, and blood is not always screened before transfusion. This also disproportionately affects women of reproductive age because they are at risk for anemia as a result of frequent pregnancies, malaria infection (see below), and depo-Provera injection for contraception (Belak, 2002). An infected mother is still expected to care for her ill children and husband. Over time, she will not be able to work and will sink further into poverty (Altsean, 2001).

Poor economic conditions continue to drive women and girls into sex work, enormously increasing their risk of acquiring HIV and other STIs. In Burma, the government's antitrafficking measures actually seem to increase trafficking, sexual exploitation, and exposure to STIs (Belak, 2002; PHR, 2004; Altsean, 2005). In a 1999 sentinel surveillance study, 52 percent of sex workers in Rangoon and Mandalay were HIV positive (Belak, 2002; Beyrer et al., 2003). Reliable data are not available for Shan girls trafficked into Thailand for sex work, but the rate of HIV infection might be even higher (Beyrer, 2001; Beyrer et al., 2003).

Malaria is endemic in developing nations throughout the tropical world and can be found throughout rural Burma. About 60 percent of the population is at risk, in particular, those along the Thai-Burma border where we provide medical services. Effective national measures for prompt diagnosis, treatment, and disease control do not exist (Nosten et al., 1991b; Ejov et al., 1999; Htay-Aung et al., 1999; WHO, 2000). Insecticide-treated mosquito nets are not affordable or available in rural areas where they are needed (Ejov et al., 1999; Lin et al., 2000; Kyawt-Kyawt-Swe and Pearson, 2004). Where they are owned, people in conflict zones forced to flee into the jungle for safety will usually leave these behind, taking only the bare essentials with them (Committee for Internally Displaced Karen People, 2004). In one prospective study of primarily Karen women living in camps on the Thai-Burma border, 10 percent of women of child-bearing age were pregnant at any given time and the proportion of women developing malaria at some time during pregnancy was about 37 percent (Nosten et al., 1991b). Pregnant women face potentially dire consequences from malaria, which can be fatal: pregnancy reduces immunity and increases complications such as severe anemia, spontaneous abortion, stillbirth, and premature delivery (WHO, 2003). Because government-sponsored health services are essentially nonexistent in the malaria-endemic areas of Burma, there is the widespread misuse of counterfeit, unsafe, and adulterated drugs. In turn, this drives the problem of increasing malaria drug resistance and treatment failure, a consequence disproportionately borne by women during pregnancy (Nosten et al., 1991a; Belak, 2002; Newton et al., 2002; Dondorp et al., 2004).

Applying Human Rights to Public Health: Law and Policy

The right to health is recognized in numerous international documents and agreements including the Universal Declaration of Human Rights (Article 25.1, "Everyone has the right to a standard of living adequate for the health of himself and of his family, including food, clothing, housing and medical care and necessary social services") and the International Covenant on Economic, Social and Cultural Rights ("The right to health is closely related to and dependent upon the realization of other human rights . . . including the rights to food, housing, work, education, human dignity, life, nondiscrimination, equality, the prohibition against torture, privacy, access to information, and the freedoms of association, assembly and movement. These and other rights and freedoms address integral components of the right to health") (United Nations, 1948, 1966a). The latter document further recognizes the duty of signatory states to reduce "the stillbirth-rate and of infant mortality and for the health development of the child" (United Nations, 1966a). A state is required to "demonstrate that every effort has been made to use all resources that are at its disposition in an effort to satisfy, as a matter of priority, those minimum obligations" (United Nations, 2000). There are obligations spelled out in article 5 (e) (iv) of the International Convention on the Elimination of All Forms of Racial Discrimination of 1965, articles 11.1 (f) and 12 of the Convention on the Elimination of All Forms of Discrimination against Women of 1979, and in article 24 of the Convention on the Rights of the Child of 1989, as well as in regional documents such as the European Social Charter of 1961 as revised (art. 11), the African Charter on Human and Peoples' Rights of 1981 (art. 16), and the Additional Protocol to the American Convention on Human Rights in the Area of Economic, Social and Cultural Rights of 1988 (art. 10) (United Nations, 2000).

Because reproductive health is so essential to family and society, it receives special status in the context of rights and health. For example, General Comment 14 of the United Nations Committee on Economic, Social and Cultural Rights, 2000, stated, "Reproductive health means that women and men have the freedom to decide if and when to reproduce and the right to be informed and to have access to safe, effective, affordable and acceptable methods of fam-

ily planning of their choice as well as the right of access to appropriate health-
care services that will, for example, enable women to go safely through pregnancy and childbirth" (United Nations, 2000). However, as Rebecca Cook,
author of WHO's *Advancing Safe Motherhood through Human Rights*, points
out, human rights historically have been applied to compel governments to
prevent torture or ensure free speech, but they have not been applied aggres-
sively to require governments to address preventable causes of death, such as
deaths related to motherhood. "That has always been left to the health sector—it hasn't been viewed as a significant problem of social justice." Cook
further notes, "The recharacterization of maternal mortality from a health
disadvantage to a social injustice places governments under a legal obligation
to remedy the injustice" (Cook, 1997; Safe Motherhood Initiative, 1997; Kennedy, 2001).

The need to hold governments and policy makers accountable is especially
relevant in the age of HIV/AIDS and other sexually transmitted infections
where women are at heightened risk because of social inequities and biologic
vulnerabilities. In this context we cite the withdrawal of funding to Burma by
the Global Fund to Fight AIDS, Tuberculosis, and Malaria. Despite the high
prevalence of these diseases within the country, their decision was a bold
step to hold the military government responsible for creating "an increasingly restrictive environment for implementation . . . which effectively prevents the implementation of performance-based and time-bound programs in
the country, breaches the Government of Myanmar's commitment to provide
unencumbered access, and frustrates the ability of the Principal Recipient to
carry out its obligations" (Global Fund, 2005). Several groups[2] have analyzed
and put forward policy perspectives regarding societal obligations relevant to
gender, reproductive, and sexual health.

- The right to the highest attainable standard of health
  The "highest attainable standard of health" must include the right
  to reproductive health services, including maternal health information
  and care that enables women to survive pregnancy and childbirth. In
  particular, the International Covenant on Economic, Social and Cultural Rights explicitly holds the state responsible for reducing the "stillbirth rate and of infant mortality and for the healthy development of

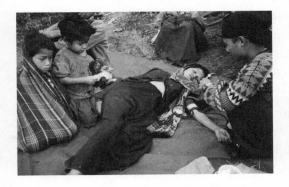

Figure 16.2. Internally displaced woman in eastern Burma with untreated fever. Photo courtesy of Karen Human Rights Group

the child" (United Nations, 1966a). Doing so requires improving maternal health through access to family planning, pregnancy-related care, emergency obstetrical services, and access to information with resources to act on the information. Article 10(2) provides that "special protection should be accorded to mothers during a reasonable period before and after childbirth" (United Nations, 2000). This covenant also holds states responsible for, "the prevention, treatment and control of epidemic, endemic, and occupational and other diseases," and obligates them to address the spread of diseases such as STIs and HIV/AIDS, which adversely affect sexual and reproductive health. Implicitly, states must take responsibility in addressing their underlying social determinants (United Nations, 2000). (See Figure 16.2.)

- The right to information

   Everyone, including children, has the right to "seek, receive and impart information of all kinds," according to article 19 of the International Covenant on Civil and Political Rights (United Nations, 1966b). Access to information is essential to secure the right to the highest attainable standard of health.

- The rights to life, liberty, and security

   These fundamental rights are pledged in article 6 of the International Covenant on Civil and Political Rights and article 3 of the Universal Declaration of Human Rights and states are bound to prevent their violation or abridgement (United Nations, 1948, 1966b). In terms of women's reproductive health, violations include the targeted assault on girls and women and children as a strategy for suppressing a population or ethnic group. States also are in violation if they are deliberately negligent in providing essential services to ensure a woman's ability to have a healthy pregnancy and childbirth and to decide if, when, and how often to bear children. Sexual violence and the threat of sexual violence are recognized as being at "the core of women's subordination in society . . . the single greatest threat to the self-determination of . . . women" (Human Rights Watch, 2004); a state not only must go beyond not sponsoring violence but it must also protect its citizens from violence and its consequences, including providing HIV prophylaxis and pregnancy prevention to the survivors of assault (Human Rights Watch, 2004).

• The right to equality and nondiscrimination on grounds such as sex, marital status, race, age, and class.

Articles 2.2 and 3 of the U.N. Covenant for Economic, Social and Cultural Rights (UNCESCR) prohibit "discrimination in access to health care and underlying determinants of health, as well as to means and entitlements for their procurement" (United Nations, 1966a). The United Nations Convention on the Elimination of All Forms of Discrimination against Women (CEDAW) prohibits policies and programs that "require women seeking health services to obtain authorization from their husbands, or that criminalize medical procedures that only women need, such as abortion" or that place women at heightened risk for trafficking and violence. CEDAW also says that lack of permission by husband, partner, parents, or health authorities should not restrict a woman's (married or unmarried) access to appropriate care. States are required to legally prohibit "child marriage, rape, sexual abuse" (United Nations, 1979; Safe Motherhood Initiative, 1997).

Nondiscrimination also encompasses a right to appropriate technology; the U.N. Committee of the UNCESCR suggests that health services should not "favour expensive curative health services which are often accessible only to a small, privileged fraction of the population." And in situations where resources are constrained, "the vulnerable members of society must be protected by the adoption of relatively low-cost targeted programmes" (United Nations, 2000). This applies to health care services like safe and effective contraception; voluntary counseling and testing and antiretroviral drugs to prevent transmission of HIV from mother to child, immunization, and malaria prevention and prophylaxis that, in the arena of health services, are relatively low-cost and easy to provide.

A political vision of gender rights and women's health requires translating scientific and legal insights into action and law. While not binding, several international consensus documents define sexual and reproductive rights in the context of actions governments should take to uphold them. In 1993, the World Conference on Human Rights held in Vienna called for a Declaration on the Elimination of Violence against Women. This was the first international human rights instrument that made specific reference to sexual rights for women. In 1994 the Programme of Action adopted by the International Conference on Population and Development (ICPD) in Cairo further advanced this directive by developing a comprehensive framework that explicitly named reproductive health and sexual health as part of human rights for all people including refugees and internally displaced persons (UNFPA, 1994). The 1995 Platform for Action of the Fourth World Conference on Women in Beijing reaffirmed this commitment and included discrimination against women as a significant factor contributing to the rate of complications and deaths in pregnancy and childbirth. By doing so, it specifically acknowledged that excess maternal mortality and morbidity reflect inequalities and inadequacies in access to health services and that they can be prevented by providing timely reproductive health services, including contraception, safe abortion, and obstetric care (United Nations, 1995). Both the ICPD and the Platform for Action recognize that unsafe abortion is a violation of a woman's rights. In its international policy agenda the September 2000 Millennium Declaration further highlighted the growing international consensus that women's reproductive health is a human right. To be pursued over the next 25 years, its Millennium Development Goals or MDGs gave health a predominant role, in particular, concerning maternal health, women's empowerment, and gender equality. It also called for reducing child mortality, including infant mortality.

Linking Public Health and Human Rights: Data, Policies, and Programs

Accurate and reliable documentation of health outcomes through population-based measurement is one way to hold rights abusers accountable for their actions. Good studies can link variables that increase health risks to rights and identify vulnerable groups. Certainly, regular health surveillance should monitor violence against women and its outcomes, and assess access to health care and the state's response to health needs for girls and women (Amowitz, Reis, and Iacopino, 2002a). The goal is to have objective data on health that correlate to specific rights violations, and to use this information to guide policy and action. Particular effort should be made during humanitarian relief operations and conflict to research women's health issues to guide services needed for survivors (Iacopino et al., 2001; Amowitz et al., 2002b; Gasseer et al., 2004). Research should also assess access to food, potable water, housing, healthy occupation, and similar determinants of health as they affect gender and rights (United Nations, 2000).

The policy imperative is that states are responsible for regularly assessing the health status of girls, women, and children and to look for disparities in access and outcomes; and to consider these as rights violations, and, where possible, to eliminate them. Even allowing for disparities in development across nations, it still is the responsibility of governments to "demonstrate that every effort has been made to use all resources that are at its disposition in an effort to satisfy, as a matter of priority, those minimum obligations" (United Nations, 2000). In this context, it is essential to consider that reproductive health includes the freedom for both women and men "to decide if and when to reproduce and the right to be informed and to have access to safe, effective, affordable and acceptable methods of family planning of their choice as well as the right of access to appropriate health-care services that will, for example, enable women to go safely through pregnancy and childbirth" (United Nations, 2000).

Programs should be driven by both data and policy, and interventions should follow rights-based principles such as not to place undue burden or further disparity and to allocate resources per a full assessment of all alternatives. We draw on our own efforts to reduce maternal mortality to illustrate some of the practical dimensions of linking public health and human rights. Data from the Backpack Health Worker Team (BPHWT) and Mae Tao Clinic (MTC) document a high maternal mortality rate of 1000 to 1200 per 100,000 live births inside of Burma's conflict zones.[3] Most deaths are due to postpartum hemorrhage and sepsis, both treatable and/or preventable with timely and appropriate interventions. Excess maternal mortality also contributes to high infant and child mortality in these areas. In collaboration with other organizations that support ethnic minority IDPs in the region, MTC and BPHWT developed a multilevel strategy to reduce maternal mortality. We increased on-the-ground access and capacity for delivering emergency obstetrical care[4] by establishing the MTC as a regional center for Comprehensive Emergency Obstetrical Care, and developed a network of mobile Centers for Capacity Building and Referral Care (CCRs) that extend far into eastern Burma to train TBAs and provide potentially lifesaving Basic Emergency Obstetrical Care for women and girls who would otherwise have no care. Significant was the decision to invest in the TBAs as part of the core strategy; if we focused solely on providing more fully trained medical professionals, many of the most needy would not be served at all. TBAs attend roughly three quarters of all deliveries and are respected, integral members of the IDP communities (Mae Tao Clinic, 2003). Furthermore, TBAs are receptive to learning new skills and putting them into practice[5] (Shaw, 2004). This program thus falls in line with the policy perspective of the U.N. Committee of UNCESCR that health services should not "favour expensive curative health services which are often accessible only to a small, privileged fraction of the population" (United Nations, 2000). This program based in Mae Sot is just one way to incorporate gender-based rights and health in a community setting. No doubt there are other models, but our approach demonstrates that this can be done even in settings where resources are constrained and the governance is inadequate.

Looking Ahead

The trend worldwide is to incorporate gender and rights considerations into health policy. In settings of civil strife and repressive military regimes, a first priority usually includes demilitarizing the country, maintaining civil order, and stopping abuses such as forced labor, population transfers, seizing property, and sexual violence and the exploitation of women and girls. In many cases this requires the assistance of international bodies, such as the United Nations Special Rapporteur on Human Rights, who take the first step to investigate abuses and thereby establish a framework for holding perpetrators accountable for their actions. Providing for the health and safety of girls and women, often ethnic-minority girls and women, must be a high priority.

A first necessary step is gathering accurate independent health data linked to rights conditions in places where governments either deliberately or negligently fail to track basic health statistics. Chapter 3 discusses an epidemic among blood donors in China where there is still no accurate assessment about who was and is infected with a variety of transmittable diseases. Until

a good epidemiological study occurs, it is probably not possible to provide adequate health services to those in need. In Burma we are all too aware of the
paucity of information available on the general health status of the population
and, specifically, data pertaining to women's health in areas such as HIV, sexual violence or rape, illicit abortions, and maternal morbidity and mortality.

One must also address transnational issues. Examples of rights violations
and health consequences transcending national boundaries are presented
elsewhere in this volume, including the civil conflicts in Sierra Leone and the
Democratic Republic of Congo and the breakup of the former Yugoslavia. As
described by Cathy Zimmerman, transnational issues also surface regularly
where girls and women are trafficked. Wherever abuses occur across borders,
international cooperation and assistance are needed. Our experience working in Mae Sot is that the long and porous 2000-kilometer border between
Burma and Thailand erects a largely artificial barrier when it comes to health
needs. Populations move across rather freely and bring with them their medical problems. In such settings, donors should eliminate funding restrictions
based on frontiers, especially so in conflict zones where international assistance often is the only source of health care (TBBC, 2004). Above all, donors
must be aware of the pitfalls of providing humanitarian supplies and funds
to corrupt, violent, and negligent regimes without also insisting on extensive
monitoring and oversight. We have learned this firsthand with the Burmese
military junta, where too often donor resources do not make it to the people
for whom they are intended (Associated Press, 2004).

Notes

1. The Backpack Health Worker Team Program, in partnership with the Mae Tao
Clinic (MTC), serves civilians affected by the upheaval in eastern Burma. It is distinct
from the MTC, however, in that its cadres of mobile medic teams provide health and
public health care to villagers and IDPs *inside* of Burma, where virtually no other
organizations are able to function.

2. This material synthesizes work by the U.N. committees overseeing the International Bill of Rights, the World Health Organization, Human Rights Watch, the Alan
Guttmacher Institute, and the Safe Motherhood Initiative. In the case of quotations,
direct reference is made to a specific document; otherwise, general referral to the
reference section of this chapter provides credit.

3. Maternal mortality also contributes to high infant and child mortality.

4. Basic Emergency Obstetrical Care (BEOC) includes: administration of antibiot-
ics, oxytocics, or anticonvulsants; manual removal of the placenta; removal of retained products following miscarriage or abortion, and assisted vaginal delivery with

forceps or vacuum extractor. Comprehensive Emergency Obstetrical Care (CEOC) includes BEOC, plus: cesarean section and safe blood transfusion (UNFPA: www.unfpa .org/mothers/obstetric.htm).

5. An evaluation of TBA training by the Backpack Health Worker Team found that TBAs undergoing training made significant positive changes in their practice; for example, the percentage of TBAs reporting hand washing increased (from 46% to 83%), as it did for using sterile practices to cut umbilical cords (11% to 61%), and for applying antiseptic to the cord (14% to 66%).

References

AbouZahr, C. 1997. Improving access to quality maternal health services. Paper presented at the Safe Motherhood Technical Consultation, Sri Lanka, 18–23 October 1997. www.safemotherhood.org/facts_and_figures/care_during_childbirth.htm (accessed November 22, 2005).

Agence France Presse. 2005. UNICEF expands Myanmar HIV/AIDS Program. May 21, 2005.

Altsean. 2001. *Women's report card on Burma, 2001.* Bangkok: Altsean.

Altsean. 2005. *Interim report card, July 2004–February 2005: A summary of political and human rights developments in Burma.* Bangkok: Altsean.

Amnesty International. 2005. *Myanmar: Leaving home.* http://web.amnesty.org/library/print/ENGASA160232005 (accessed November 22, 2005).

Amowitz, L. L., Reis, C., and Iacopino, V. 2002. *Maternal mortality in Herat Province, Afghanistan: The need to protect women's rights.* Boston: Physicians for Human Rights. www.phrusa.org/research/afghanistan/maternal_mortality.html (accessed November 22, 2005).

Amowitz, L. L., Reis, C., Lyons, K. H., Vann, B., Mansaray, B., Akinsulure-Smith, A. M, Taylor, L., and Iacopino, V. 2002. Prevalence of war-related sexual violence and other human rights abuses among internally displaced persons in Sierra Leone. *Journal of the American Medical Association* 287 (4):513–21.

Apple, B., and Martin, V. 2003. *No safe place: Burma's army and the rape of ethnic women.* Washington, DC: Refugees International. www.refugeesinternational .org/files/3023_file_no_safe_place.pdf (accessed November 22, 2005).

Associated Press. 2004. Thailand donates condoms, medicines to Myanmar. September 22.

Ba-thike, K. 1997. Abortion: A public health problem in Myanmar. *Reproductive Health Matters* 9 (May):94–100. www.hsph.harvard.edu/grhf-asia/suchana/9999/ rh141.html (accessed November 22, 2005).

Belak, B. 2002. *Gathering strength: Women from Burma on their rights.* Chiang Mai, Thailand: Images Asia.

Belton, S. 2002. *Lady's love powder.* www.ibiblio.org/obl/docs/Lady's_Love_Powder .htm (accessed November 22, 2005).

Belton, S., and Maung, C. 2004. Fertility and abortion: Burmese women's health on the Thai-Burma border. *Forced Migration Review* 19:36–37.

Beyrer, C. 2001. Shan women and girls and the sex industry in Southeast Asia: Political causes and human rights implications. *Social Science and Medicine* 53 (4):543–50.

Beyrer, C., Razak, M. H., Labrique, A., and Brookmeyer, R. 2003. Assessing the magnitude of the HIV/AIDS epidemic in Burma. *Journal of Acquired Immune Deficiency Syndromes* 32:311–17.

Beyrer, C., and Stachowiak, J. 2003. Health consequences of the trafficking of women and girls in Southeast Asia. *Brown Review of World Affairs* 10 (1):105–19.

Broadmoor, T. 2003. Edging towards disaster. *The Irrawaddy*, May. www.irrawaddy .org/database/2003/vol11.4/cover.html (accessed November 22, 2005).

Central Intelligence Agency (CIA). 2005. *The World Factbook, 2005.* www.cia.gov/ cia/publications/factbook/ (accessed November 22, 2005).

Chelala, C. 1998. What's ailing Burma: The state of women and children's health. *Burma Debate* Spring 1998 5(2). www.burmadebate.org/archives/spring98health .html (accessed November 22, 2005).

Committee for Internally Displaced Karen People. 2004. Mother finds hope in Law Thi Hta. *Internally Displaced People News* 2 (2):7.

Cook, R. J. 1997. Advancing safe motherhood through human rights. Paper presented at Safe Motherhood Technical Consultation, Sri Lanka, 18–23 October.

Costello, A., Osrin, D., and Manandhar, D. 2004. Reducing maternal and neonatal mortality in the poorest communities. *British Medical Journal* 329:1166–68.

Dondorp, A. M., Newton, P. N., Mayxay, M., Van Damme, W., Smithius, F. M., Yeung, S., Petit, A., Lynam, A. J., Johnson, A., Hien, T. T., McGready, R., Farrar, J. J., Looareesuwan, S., Day, N. P., Green, M. D., and White, N. J. 2004. Fake antimalarials in Southeast Asia are a major impediment to malaria control: Multinational cross-sectional survey on the prevalence of fake antimalarials. *Tropical Medicine and International Health* 9 (12):1241–46.

Donnay, F. 2000. Maternal survival in developing countries: What has been done, what can be achieved in the next decade. *International Journal of Gynaecology and Obstetrics* 70 (1):89–97.

EarthRights International. 2003. *Entrenched: An investigative report on the systematic use of forced labor by the Burmese Army in a rural area.* Chiang Mai, Thailand: EarthRights International.

Eh Kalu, and Lee, K. 2005. In the Black Zone: Mortality rates and conflict-related human rights abuses among internally displaced Mon, Karen and Karenni people of Eastern Burma. Paper presented at Lessons Learned from Rights-Based Approaches to Health, Atlanta, Georgia, 14–16 April.

Ejov, M. N., Tun T., Aung, S., Lwin, S., and Sein, K. 1999. Hospital-based study of severe malaria and associated deaths in Myanmar. *Bulletin of the World Health Organization* 77 (4):310–14.

Fink, C. 2001. *Living silence: Burma under military rule.* Bangkok: White Lotus Company.

Gasseer, N. A., Dresden, E., Keeney, G. B., and Warren, N. 2004. Status of women and infants in complex humanitarian emergencies. *Journal of Midwifery and Women's Health* 49 (4) (Suppl. 1):7–13.

Global Fund to Fight AIDS, Tuberculosis and Malaria (GFATM). 2005. Fact sheet: Termination of grants to Myanmar. August 18. www.theglobalfund.org/en/media _center/press/pr_050819_factsheet.pdf (accessed November 22, 2005).

Goldman, N., and Glei, D. A. 2003. Evaluation of midwifery care: Results from a survey in rural Guatemala. *Social Science and Medicine* 56:685–700.

Htay-Aung, M. S., Thaung S., Mya, M. M., Than S. M., Hlaing T., Soe-Soe, Druilhe P., and Queuche, F. 1999. Well-breeding *Anopheles dirus* and their role in malaria transmission in Myanmar. *Southeast Asian Journal of Tropical Medicine and Public Health* 30 (3):447–53.

Human Rights Watch. 2004. South Africa's Obligations under International and National Law. In *Deadly delay: South Africa's efforts to prevent HIV in survivors of sexual violence.* Chap. 7. www.hrw.org/reports/2004/southafrica0304/7.htm (accessed November 22, 2005).

Iacopino, V., Frank, M. W., Bauer, H. M., Keller, A. S., Fink, S. L., Ford, D., Pallin, D. J., and Waldman, R. 2001. A population-based assessment of human rights abuses committed against ethnic Albanian refugees from Kosovo. *American Journal of Public Health* 91 (12):2013–18.

International Crisis Group. 2002. *Myanmar: The HIV/AIDS crisis.* April 2. www.crisis group.org (accessed November 22, 2005).

International Crisis Group. 2003. *Myanmar backgrounder: Ethnic minority politics.* May 7. www.crisisgroup.org (accessed November 22, 2005).

International Crisis Group. 2004. *Myanmar: Update on HIV/AIDS policy.* December 16. www.crisisgroup.org (accessed November 22, 2005).

Jokhio, A. H., Winter, H. R., and Cheng, K. K. 2005. An intervention involving traditional birth attendants and perinatal and maternal mortality in Pakistan. *New England Journal of Medicine* 352 (20):2091–99.

Kachin Women's Association Thailand. 2005. *Driven away: Trafficking of Kachin women on the China-Burma border.* Chiang Mai, Thailand: Kachin Women's Association Thailand.

Karen Human Rights Group. 2001. *Flight, hunger, and survival: Repression and displacement in the villages of Papun and Nyaunglebin districts.* www.khrg.org (accessed November 22, 2005).

Karen Human Rights Group. 2004. *Enduring hunger and repression: food scarcity, internal displacement, and the continued use of forced labor in Toungoo District.* www .khrg.org.

Karen Women's Organization. 2004. *Shattering silences: Karen women speak out about the Burmese military regime's use of rape as a strategy of war in Karen State.* Mae Sariang, Thailand: Karen Women's Organization.

Kennedy, S. 2001. Acting globally: Public health law; Rebecca Cook puts social science and public health research in a legal context. *Edge* Spring 2 (1). www.research .utoronto.ca/edge/spring2001/leaders/rebeccaCook.htm (accessed November 22, 2005).

Kyawt-Kyawt-Swe, and Pearson, A. 2004. Knowledge, attitudes and practices with regard to malaria control in an endemic rural area of Myanmar. *Southeast Asian Journal of Tropical Medicine and Public Health* 35 (1):53–62.

Lin, K., Aung, S., Lwin, S., Min, H., Aye, N. N., and Webber, R. 2000. Promotion of insecticide-treated mosquito nets in Myanmar. *Southeast Asian Journal of Tropical Medicine and Public Health* 31 (3):444–47.

Low Htaw. 2004. Carrying condoms is a crime for Burmese women. *BurmaNet News.* July 16. http://six.pairlist.net/pipermail/burmanet/20040716/000495.html (accessed November 22, 2005).

Mae Tao Clinic. 2003. *Reproductive health survey* (unpublished data). Mae Sot, Thailand: Mae Tao Clinic.

Mae Tao Clinic. 2004. *Annual report, 2003.* Mae Sot, Thailand: Mae Tao Clinic.

Min Thwe. 2004. HIV/AIDS education and prevention in Myanmar. *AIDS Education and Prevention* 16 (Suppl. A):170–77.

Mullany, L. C., Maung, C., and Beyrer, C. 2003. HIV knowledge, attitudes, and practices among Burmese migrant factory workers in Tak Province, Thailand. *AIDS Care* 15 (1):63–70.

Myanmar Times. 2001. Special feature. January 15–21. www.myanmar-information.net/infosheet/2001/010122.htm (accessed November 22, 2005).

National Coalition Government of the Union of Burma. 2002. *Burma human rights yearbook, 2001–2002.* Nonthaburi, Thailand: National Coalition Government of the Union of Burma.

The New Light of Myanmar. Briefing on false allegations on sexual violence against women held. August 24, 2002. www.myanmar.gov.mm/NLM-2002/enlm/august 24.htm#(3) (accessed November 22, 2005).

Newton, P. N., White, N. J., Rozendaal, J. A., and Green, M. D. 2002. Murder by fake drugs. *British Medical Journal* 324 (7341):800–801.

Nosten, F., ter Kuile, F., Chongsuphajaisiddhi, T., Luxemburger, C., Webster, H. K., Edstein, M., Phaipun, L., Thew, K. L., and White, N. J. 1991a. Mefloquine-resistance falciparum malaria on the Thai-Burmese border. *The Lancet* 337 (8750):1140–43.

Nosten, F., ter Kuile, F., Maelankirri, L., Decludt, B., and White, N. J. 1991b. Malaria during pregnancy in an area of unstable endemicity. *Transactions of the Royal Society of Tropical Medicine and Hygiene* 85 (4):424–29.

Physicians for Human Rights (PHR). 2004. No status: Migration, trafficking and exploitation of women in Thailand: Health and HIV/AIDS risks for Burmese and hill tribe women and girls. www.phrusa.org/campaigns/aids/pdf/nostatus.pdf (accessed November 22, 2005).

Prata, N., Mbaruku, G., Campbell, M., Potts, M., and Vahidnia, F. 2005. Controlling postpartum hemorrhage after home births in Tanzania. *International Journal of Gynaecology and Obstetrics* 90 (1):51–55.

Risser, G., Oum Kher, and Sein Htun. 2004. *Running the gauntlet: The impact of internal displacement in Southern Shan state.* Bangkok: Institute of Asian Studies, Chulalongkorn University

Safe Motherhood Initiative. 1997. Advance safe motherhood through human rights. In *The safe motherhood action agenda: Priorities for the next decade.* www.safemotherhood.org/resources/pdf/aa-04_advance.pdf (accessed November 22, 2005).

Sen, B. K. 2001. Women and the law in Burma. *Legal Issues on Burma Journal* 9: 28–43.

Shan Human Rights Foundation. 1998. *Dispossessed: A report on forced relocation and extrajudicial killings in Shan State, Burma.* Chiang Mai, Thailand: Shan Human Rights Foundation.

Shan Human Rights Foundation and Shan Women's Action Network. 2002a. *License to rape: The Burmese military regime's use of sexual violence in the ongoing war in Shan State.* Chiang Mai, Thailand: Shan Human Rights Foundation and Shan Women's Action Network.

Shan Human Rights Foundation and Shan Women's Action Network. 2002b. *A mockery of justice.* Chiang Mai, Thailand: Shan Human Rights Foundation and Shan Women's Action Network. www.shanwomen.org/pdf/mockery_of_justice.pdf (accessed November 22, 2005).

Shaw, M. 2004. *Rethinking the training of birth attendants: A model for the Karen of Burma.* Master's thesis, University of California, Berkeley, School of Public Health.

Sibley, L., and Sipe, T. A. 2004. What can a meta-analysis tell us about traditional birth attendant training and pregnancy outcomes? *Midwifery* 20 (1):51–60.

Srithanaviboonchai, K., Choi, K. H., van Griensven, F., Hudes, E. S., Visutratana, S., and Mandel, J. S. 2002. HIV-1 in ethnic Shan migrant workers in northern Thailand. *AIDS* 16 (6):929–31.

Starrs, A. 1998. *The safe motherhood action agenda: Priorities for the next decade.* Report of the Safe Motherhood Technical Consultation, Sri Lanka, 18–23 October 1997. New York: Family Care International.

Swiss, S., and Giller, J. E. 1993. Rape as a crime of war: A medical perspective. *Journal of the American Medical Association* 270 (5):612–15.

Thailand Burma Border Consortium. 2004. *Internal displacement and vulnerability in Eastern Burma.* Bangkok: Thailand Burma Border Consortium.

United Nations. 1948. *Universal Declaration of Human Rights.* www.un.org/Overview/rights.html (accessed November 22, 2005).

United Nations. 1966a. *International Covenant for Economic, Social and Cultural Rights.* www.unhchr.ch/html/menu3/b/a_cescr.htm (accessed November 22, 2005).

United Nations. 1966b. *International Covenant on Civil and Political Rights, Article 19.* www.unhchr.ch/html/menu3/b/a_ccpr.htm (accessed November 22, 2005).

United Nations. 1979. *Convention on the elimination of all forms of discrimination against women.* Drafted by the Commission on the Status of Women (CSW) www.un.org/womenwatch/daw/csw/index.html (accessed November 22, 2005).

United Nations. 1995. *Beijing platform for action.* Fourth World Conference on Women. www.un.org/womenwatch/daw/beijing/platform/ (accessed November 22, 2005).

United Nations. 2000. *General Comment no. 14 (2000): Substantive issues arising in the implementation of the International Covenant on Economic, Social and Cultural Rights.* Economic and Social Council: Committee on Economic, Social, and Cultural Rights. www.unhchr.ch/tbs/doc.nsf/(symbol)/E.C.12.2000.4.En?OpenDocument (accessed November 22, 2005).

United Nations Children's Fund (UNICEF). 2005. *Information by country.* www.unicef.org/infobycountry/index.html (accessed November 22, 2005).

United Nations Children's Fund (UNICEF). 2006. *Information by country.* www.unicef.org/infobycountry/index.html (accessed November 22, 2005).

United Nations Department of International Economic and Social Affairs. 1991. *The world's women: Trends and statistics.* New York: United Nations.

United Nations Development Programme and United Nations Population Fund (UN-FPA). 2001. *United Nations Population Fund Proposed Projects and Programmes: Recommendation by the Executive Director, Proposed Special Assistance to Myanmar.* July 13, 2001.

United Nations Population Fund (UNFPA). 1994. Programme of Action of the International Conference on Population and Development. www.unfpa.org/icpd/icpd _poa.htm (accessed November 22, 2005).

United Nations Population Fund (UNFPA). 2001. Population and reproductive health situation in Myanmar. Available at: UNFPA Myanmar website. http://myanmar. unfpa.org/about.htm (accessed November 22, 2005).

U.S. Department of State. 2004. *Trafficking in persons report, June 2004.* www.state .gov/g/tip/rls/tiprpt/2004/ (accessed November 22, 2005).

U.S. Department of State. 2005. *Burma: Country reports on human rights practices 2004,* February 28, 2005. www.state.gov/g/drl/rls/hrrpt/2004/41637.htm (accessed November 22, 2005).

Woman and Child Rights Project (WCRP) and Human Rights Foundation of Monland (HURFROM). 2005. *Catwalk to the barracks: Conscription of women for sexual slavery and other practices of sexual violence by troops of the Burmese military regime in Mon areas.* Bangkok: WCRP and HURFOM.

Women's League of Burma (WLB). 2002. *Breaking the silence.* www.ibiblio.org/obl/ docs/breaking_the_silence.htm (accessed November 22, 2005).

Women's League of Burma (WLB). 2004. *System of impunity: Nationwide patterns of sexual violence by the military regime's army and authorities in Burma.* Chiangmai, Thailand: WLB.

World Health Organization (WHO). 1978. *Declaration of Alma-Ata,* September 6–12, 1978. www.who.int/hpr/NPH/docs/declaration_almaata.pdf (accessed November 22, 2005).

World Health Organization (WHO). 1997a. *An assessment of the contraceptive method mix in Myanmar.* Geneva: WHO. www.who.int/reproductive-health/publications/ HRP_ITT_97_1/assessment_contraceptive_method_mix_Myanmar.pdf (accessed November 22, 2005).

World Health Organization (WHO). 1997b. *Coverage of maternity care: A listing of available information.* 4th ed. Geneva: WHO. www.safemotherhood.org/facts_and _figures/care_during_childbirth.htm (accessed November 22, 2005).

World Health Organization (WHO). 2000. *WHO Country Cooperation Strategy (CCS), Myanmar.* Geneva: WHO. www.who.int/countries/en/cooperation_strategy _mmr_en.pdf (accessed November 22, 2005).

World Health Organization (WHO). 2003. *Lives at risk: Malaria in pregnancy.* www .who.int/features/2003/04b/en/ (accessed November 22, 2005).

World Health Organization (WHO). 2004. Country health profile—Myanmar: Trends in health status. http://w3.whosea.org/EN/Section313/Section1522_6853.htm (accessed November 22, 2005).

World Health Organization (WHO). 2006. *Countries.* www.who.int/countries/en/ #M (accessed November 22, 2005).

17

Advocacy Strategies for Affording the
Right to Health

Holly Burkhalter

For most of the past thirty years, U.S.-based international human rights organizations have focused on civil and political rights. But the other half of the
international "Bill of Rights" which animates so many human rights activists in
the developing world—economic, social, and cultural rights—has been largely
absent from the agenda of organizations like Amnesty International, Human
Rights Watch, and my own organization, Physicians for Human Rights (PHR).
Some in the conventional human rights movement do not consider economic
rights to be human rights as such, and several of the establishment groups are
carrying on lively debates over which—if any—of our methodology and tactics
can be successfully brought to bear on economic rights issues at all.

Since its founding in 1986, Physicians for Human Rights has engaged in
monitoring and advocacy on civil and political rights violations. Three years
ago, the organization undertook an effort to apply international law and PHR
capacities to the right to health. We began this work by supporting the right
of poor people with HIV/AIDS in sub-Saharan Africa to obtain antiretroviral
drugs. We have broadened our campaign to include research and advocacy
on health systems and health workers. Our Washington, D.C.–based staff has
waded deep into the "weeds" of foreign assistance policies on HIV/AIDS. It is a

far cry from the human rights advocacy I was accustomed to during my previous two decades at Human Rights Watch and Physicians for Human Rights, where such issues as war crimes, torture, political repression, and unjust imprisonment were our priorities. I've found that some of the tools of the civil and political rights agenda serve us well when we promote the right to health, but it is also clear that advocating for international health requires new strategies, skills, and partnerships.

In this chapter I discuss the work of health and human rights advocates and describe some of the approaches we have used to secure an unprecedented amount of additional U.S. foreign assistance to confront the global pandemic as well as the difficulties we've faced in the context of U.S. policy toward the global AIDS pandemic.

The first and perhaps most important task of the international HIV/AIDS advocacy movement was the creation of a moral and political imperative to provide the antiretroviral treatment required for individuals with full-blown AIDS. Access to treatment for the majority of people living with AIDS in the poorest countries of the world—Africa and the Caribbean—has been a possibility only in the past several years, thanks to new resources from the Global Fund to Fight AIDS, Tuberculosis, and Malaria (GFATM), the U.S. government, and other donors. As recently as 2001, a mere 30,000 Africans who needed highly active antiretroviral therapy (HAART) were receiving these medications. Most of them purchased the expensive treatment themselves. Offering the same medications, which had been in routine use since 1997 in the United States and Europe, to nearly 4 million Africans with AIDS who needed them immediately to survive was not even a matter of serious discussion among most health professionals and policy makers in the United States and internationally until 2001.

Since then, a sea change has occurred in public opinion and national and donor policy with regard to AIDS treatment. Even while supplies, infrastructure and access to HAART lag far behind need in poor countries, in particular, in sub-Saharan Africa and the Caribbean, the concept of consigning people with AIDS to certain death is neither politically nor morally tenable in 2006.

The Tactics of Shame and Blame

Ken Roth, executive director of Human Rights Watch, suggests in a public dialogue about economic, social, and cultural rights that the advocacy tools of the international civil and political rights movement are for the most part ill-suited to promoting government compliance with economic rights standards. As he puts it, "our ability to investigate, expose and shame" is "the core of our methodology . . . The principal power of groups like Human Rights Watch is our ability to hold official conduct up to scrutiny and to generate public outrage." Roth has stated that the methodology of Human Rights Watch and groups like it is best directed toward abuses that have specific victims, perpetrators, and remedies, but ill suited to promoting compliance with economic rights norms.

There is a vital role for shaming and generating moral outrage as tools for advancing the cause of economic rights. Generating moral outrage over the world's brutal double standard with regard to who should live with and who should die of HIV/AIDS was crucial to moving forward to secure the right to HAART for people with AIDS in poor countries.

The first and perhaps most important targets of shaming and blaming in this context were pharmaceutical companies and the U.S. government, which promoted regimens and regulations to safeguard their profits. This role was taken up with particular alacrity by HealthGAP [Global Access Project]. The small activist nongovernmental organization was formed in 1999 in association with ACT-UP, the front-line U.S. treatment access group, which agitated successfully in the United States for the development of drugs to treat the disease.

HealthGAP's first campaign was to highlight the role of the Clinton Administration in protecting U.S. pharmaceutical companies from actions by foreign governments to obtain access to low-cost generic alternatives for treating HIV/AIDS. The group learned from a whistle-blower inside the executive branch that the administration was pressuring the Government of South Africa to rescind its Medicines Act. The statute addressed such issues as compulsory licensing of generic drugs. HealthGAP activists launched the issue—and themselves—at Vice President Al Gore, the target they thought they could best influence through shame. Activists disrupted the vice president's campaign launch by leaping before the news cameras and chanting "Gore's Greed Kills, AIDS Drugs for Africa!" Paul Davis of HealthGAP put it this way: "The first issue of the 2000 presidential campaign was Al Gore versus Nelson Mandela."

HealthGappers trailed Vice President Gore at other campaign events around the United States, flinging blood-drenched pills, waving signs, and chanting. Their goal, recalls Davis, was to get the Clinton Administration to cry "Uncle," and in January 2000 they got their wish. President Clinton issued an executive order that reneged on access to low-cost generics in the context of the African Growth and Opportunity Act. Within months the Indian generic manufacturers announced the production of copies of U.S.-made antiretrovirals for $350 per year. The U.S. price was at the time in the range of $10,000.

The Importance of Expertise

In addition to civil disobedience and the in-your-face activism that has been a signature of the right-to-treatment movement in the United States, HealthGAP developed extensive expertise on the technical aspects of drug development and trade. Along with trade, patent, and pharmacologic experts at the Consumer Project on Technology and Médecins sans Frontières, Health-GAP activists went head to head with lobbyists and experts from some of the most prosperous and politically connected pharmaceutical companies in the world. They did so by becoming as technically expert as their adversaries on every aspect of international trade in medicine, observing trade meetings, and publicizing and denouncing every action taken by the companies and governments that set back the cause of access to low-cost, high-quality medicine for the treatment of HIV/AIDS and tuberculosis.

The treatment access campaign is not the first human rights initiative to require technical expertise. The International Campaign to Ban Landmines (ICBL), for example, required immense technical expertise on the weapon itself and all aspects of production, export, stockpiling, and use. Antimine activists Steve Goose of Human Rights Watch and Jodi Williams of the ICBL are among the world's leading experts on the weapon. They became alternative sources of credible information for governments, who had in the past depended for technical information on military personnel who did not want to give up the weapon.

Similarly, the treatment access movement became an alternative source of information about pharmaceutical development and trade. Several Health-GAP and Médecins sans Frontières experts advise developing country governments, and they are the brain trust for the nongovernmental organization (NGO) movement in the United States and worldwide. Although much remains to be done, generic triple-combination therapy to treat full-blown HIV/

AIDS can now be obtained for approximately $200–300 per year. Armed with up-to-the-minute reconnaissance and fueled with moral outrage, HealthGAP and its allies around the world became an extraordinary force that played a role in the quest for available generic medicines for the poor that was and is wholly disproportionate to their small size and modest assets.

Breaking through the Zero-Sum Barrier

At the same time as AIDS activists were waging all-out war on the price of treatment, they had to confront conventional wisdom about widespread scale-up of antiretroviral therapy for the poor in Africa. In countries that spent only a few pennies per capita per day on health, the notion of offering sophisticated and still prohibitively expensive pharmaceuticals to millions of people was, for most policy makers and many in the public health community, simply unthinkable.

South African Justice Edwin Cameron's speech at the XIII International AIDS Conference in Durban, South Africa, in 2000 was, for many researchers and activists, a political and moral watershed. Justice Cameron, an HIV-positive gay man, condemned the fact that he thrived because he could afford to buy the medicines he needed while millions of others died. He spoke directly to the issue of the right of the individual to live: "All these efforts [by governments and international agencies] are indisputably commendable. But whether taken individually or together, they fail to command the urgency and sense of purpose appropriate to an emergency room where a patient is dying. The analogy is understated—for the patients who are dying number in their tens of millions. For each of them, and for all their families and loved ones, the emergency is dire and immediate. What is more, the treatment that can save them exists. What is needed is only that it be made accessible to them."

It would be nearly three years before national governments, the United States, and most other donors began to heed that call. The Bush Administration's director of the U.S. Agency for International Development, Andrew Natsios, stated bluntly before a Congressional panel in June 2001 that antiretroviral treatment for Africans would be impossible because they wouldn't be able to take their medication at specific times. "People do not know what watches and clocks are. They do not use Western means for telling time. They use the sun." Natsios went on to make the case that, given available resources, prevention, not treatment, had to be paramount.

In his view that prevention and palliative care should be provided, not treatment of the disease with antiretroviral medications, Andrew Natsios had good company. The U.N. Declaration of Commitment on HIV/AIDS, adopted by the General Assembly in June 2001, paid lip service to treatment but stated that "prevention of HIV must be the mainstay of the national, regional and international response to the epidemic." The document set specific two-year, four-year, and ten-year prevention targets, including ambitious reductions of prevalence among specific age groups, as well as specific benchmarks for prevention of mother-to-child transmission. In contrast, there were no specific targets or strategies for antiretroviral treatment, other than cautious language calling on states to "make every effort to provide progressively and in a sustainable manner, the highest attainable standard of treatment for HIV/AIDS, including . . . effective use of quality-controlled anti-retroviral therapy in a careful and monitored manner."

The medical profession itself was divided on the question of providing expensive and sophisticated drugs to people in countries whose annual per capita health spending was inadequate for easily preventable and treatable diseases. In May 2002 the *Lancet* published a study comparing the cost effectiveness of treatment versus prevention. The authors concluded that prevention was 28 times more cost effective than AIDS-drug cocktails (Marseille, 2002). In the spirited exchange with treatment proponents that followed, the authors noted the following: "In general, we believe that after 6–8 years in a country unable to finance both adequate prevention and treatment, a strong-treatment approach would mean not only more people being treated but also more symptomatic individuals remaining untreated than would a strong-prevention approach. This is because with inadequate prevention, the need for treatment further outpaces the financial and infrastructural capacity to deliver it. This conclusion, and indeed most of our arguments, depends crucially on the premise that on the time scale that matters, the prevention/HAART-funding trade-off is real—i.e. more for one really does mean less for the other."

The numbers of new HIV exposures every year clearly dwarfed the tiny numbers receiving HAART in sub-Saharan Africa, suggesting that even expanded treatment wouldn't begin to keep pace with incidence. But at the same time, the data stood as an indictment of "prevention-only" interventions by national governments, international agencies, and wealthy donor countries, which had demonstrably failed to check the progress of the pandemic. At the end of 1997, the year when antiretroviral medicine became widespread in the West, contemporary estimates put the number of people living with HIV/AIDS worldwide at 31.6 million. The number continued to climb, reaching 40 million in 2001. Every year, 5 million or more people were becoming infected, and the number of annual AIDS-related deaths globally rose from 2.3 million in 1997 to 3 million in 2001 (U.S. National Institutes of Health, National Institute for Allergy and Infectious Disease, 1998; UNAIDS, 2004).

So long as the amount of money for all AIDS initiatives remained grossly inadequate, treatment and prevention would be in competition for resources. Although trade-offs are nothing new in poor countries, the stark difference between life and death that a handful of drugs represented for millions of poor people with AIDS in Africa added moral authority and impetus to the discussion. Activists—especially in the medical and health professions—refused to trade off prevention for treatment or treatment for prevention, and demanded that resources be made available for both.

South African activist Zackie Achmat, head of the Treatment Action Campaign, explicitly condemned the zero-sum conundrum when he spoke to thousands of researchers, policy makers, and activists at the 2002 International AIDS Conference in Barcelona, Spain. Achmat, who refused for many months to take antiretroviral drugs until they would become available generally in South Africa, addressed the conference by video, as his precarious health prevented him from attending: "it is unconscionable because what we are speaking of are current statistics and not our lives. Our lives matter. The five million people with HIV in South Africa matter. And the millions of people throughout the world with HIV, their lives matter. And so it is not simply a question of the cold statistics that we're putting to you, but a question of valuing each person's life equally."

In the United States, Achmat's cause—the right to treatment—was taken up not only by AIDS organizations, progressive doctors, and human rights activists but also by activists at the other end of the political spectrum. Health missionaries affiliated with Evangelical and Catholic missions abroad knew the reality of the AIDS pandemic in ways that U.S. policy makers did not. For missionaries in Uganda, South Africa, Kenya, and Zambia witnessing mass death and living among orphans, the need for treatment immediately to save lives was obvious. Religious conservatives made their views known spectacularly at the first-ever Christian Conference on HIV/AIDS in Washington, DC, in February 2002. Organized by Samaritan's Purse (a charity founded by Rev. Billy Graham's son, Franklin Graham), the conference drew nearly 1,000 Christians—many of them from Africa. One after another, missionaries took the stage to describe their helplessness in the face of medication they couldn't afford. One memorable moment at the conference came when an Evangelical medical doctor thundered from the lectern that no country that spent as little as the United States did on foreign assistance deserved to call itself a Christian nation.

One of the most important moments in the treatment access campaign came when guest speaker Senator Jesse Helms stood before the group beside Ugandan First Lady Janet Museveni and confessed his shame over having done so little for African victims of AIDS. Days later Helms—arguably the Senate's most conservative member—announced his intention to sponsor legislation designating $500 million to prevent mother-to-child transmission of the virus. His effort, which quickly grew to include treatment for mothers as well as newborns, was the first successful effort to provide foreign assistance funds for treatment of HIV/AIDS. It was a significant forerunner to President Bush's announcement of his own treatment initiative a year later.

The Politics of the Possible

Outrage and shame alone were not sufficient to make HAART in poor countries a political priority in the United States. The necessary addition to the moral case for the scale-up of HAART in Africa was making a persuasive case that providing expensive treatment in very poor settings was possible, and therefore morally imperative. Africa's grossly substandard health infrastructure, the cost of medicines, and the immense numbers of people in sub-Saharan Africa meeting medical criteria for receiving antiretroviral therapy daunted the prospect, as did the fact that foreign aid for health lagged far behind need. Activists had to take on each of these limiting factors and make the case to donors and national governments that treatment was possible even in the direst circumstances.

The success of Médecins sans Frontières in South Africa and Partners in Health in Haiti in providing antiretroviral drugs to AIDS patients inspired activists to demand scale-up and replication of their work. While Partners in Health and Médecins sans Frontières provided HAART to only a small number of individuals, they nonetheless demonstrated not only that sophisticated medical regimens were possible in the poorest countries of the world, but also that poor patients thrived. Partners in Health also demonstrated the role that community health workers and volunteers could play.

Scaling up HAART in poor countries was boosted enormously by two important developments. The first was U.N. Secretary General Kofi Annan's endorsement of treatment and call for $7–10 billion from national governments, international institutions, and donors in 2001 and the subsequent creation of the Global Fund to Fight AIDS, Tuberculosis, and Malaria. The second was the World Health Organization's announcement in April 2002 of a campaign to provide antiretroviral (ARV) treatment to 3 million people by the year 2005. Jim Kim, formerly of Partners in Health, joined Lee at the WHO, bringing with him a sense of urgency and commitment to the poorest, as well as practical experience in treating multi-drug-resistant TB and HIV/AIDS in very poor countries.

Partners in Health was not just a moral beacon for AIDS activists and policy makers. The "Lazarus effect" of antiretroviral therapy when applied to the poorest and sickest of their patients was persuasive and inspiring. Some years ago, Jim made the point by saying that when President Kennedy announced a goal to land an astronaut on the moon, it was not possible to do so. The goal drove the scientific exploration, technical developments, and financial means necessary to achieve it. But stopping the AIDS pandemic, in his view, did not require scientific or technological breakthroughs: preventing and treating the disease in the West was routine by 1997. Kim and fellow activists set about persuading policy makers that money was the largest impediment to scale-up of an otherwise doable proposition.

One of those who were persuaded that providing HAART to millions was possible and thus necessary was the President of the United States. President Bush's State of the Union address in January 2003 included the surprising commitment to launch an emergency HIV/AIDS initiative that would provide treatment to 2 million people in Africa by 2008. There were many factors that contributed to the Bush commitment, not the least of which was the eloquent personal appeal by Irish rock star Bono with his extensive expertise and charismatic ability to connect at a personal level with virtually anyone—including powerful, conservative senators. But it was doctors who made the case to President Bush that AIDS treatment was possible in the poorest countries of the world. Paul Farmer and Jim Kim of Partners in Health were at a secret White House meeting in 2002, as was Nils Daillaire of the Global Health Council, Eric Goosby of Pangaea Global AIDS Foundation, Tony Fauci of the National Institutes of Health, and several other medical professionals. In describing the success of small-scale treatment efforts in Haiti and South Africa, the group persuaded President Bush that scale-up to afford treatment to millions *could* be achieved and therefore *must* be achieved.

Putting the Cart before the Horse

New resources from the United States, the GFATM, and other donors made possible a significant increase in the number of individuals in Africa receiving HAART. But just as skeptics predicted, African countries' undernourished, understaffed, and poorly administered health systems sharply limited scale-up. The impoverished state of African health systems that African activists know so well only became a visible issue for their U.S. counterparts when scale-up of HAART hit a brick wall because of the shortage of doctors and nurses. Moreover, the dearth of health workers and the influx of foreign assistance for HAART created distortions in public health as poorly paid nurses and doctors migrated to better-paying jobs in foreign-funded AIDS initiatives. In short, the health infrastructure issue that AIDS activists avoided, for fear that it would derail the treatment imperative, was and is an immense impediment to achieving most public health goals, including universal treatment. It was as if we finally had an excellent cart—affordable antiretroviral drugs and money to purchase them—but lacked a horse—health workers and competent systems—to draw it.

The publication in November 2004 by the Joint Learning Initiative of a two-year investigation of human resources for health in Africa generated much-needed attention to the scope of the health worker shortage. The project projected that, to reach the U.N. Millennium Development Goals in health by 2015 (including reversing the AIDS pandemic), sub-Saharan African countries would need at least an additional 1 million trained health workers. The Joint Learning Initiative noted that death from HIV/AIDS among health workers and brain drain of African medical professionals to the United States and Europe were leaving some countries worse off with every passing year.

Over the past two years, HIV/AIDS activists have broadened their treatment and prevention agenda to now include health systems. Physicians for Human Rights, for example, challenged the executive branch's long-time refusal to provide funds for salaries of health personnel and agitated for large foreign aid increases to increase recruitment and retention of desperately needed health professionals in AIDS-burdened countries. Other donors took up the health worker challenge with alacrity. Department for International Development (DFID), the development assistance arm of the British government, broke with past precedent and in December 2004 announced it would provide approximately 55 million British pounds ($100 million) to Malawi to enable it to expand its health workforce, including increasing health workers' poverty-level salaries by 50 percent.

The International Monetary Fund's stabilization agreements and caps on public spending and hiring, which are in part responsible for the shortage of health workers and malnourished health systems in Africa's poorest countries, are at last receiving scrutiny from Western donors and international health proponents because they are impeding the United States' pledge to provide HAART to 2 million people and the WHO's road map for providing HAART to 3 million by 2005. The International Monetary Fund now faces an unprecedented chorus of demands from activists, donor governments, and international health officials to relax its public sector budget ceilings that limit health spending in AIDS-burdened countries.

PHR took up the issue of brain drain of health professionals, identifying both "pull" and "push" factors contributing to outmigration. Here again, it has been absolutely essential that health rights proponents persuade policy makers who have long been skeptical of major investments in poorly run, corrupt, or hopelessly overwhelmed health systems in Africa. Although abundant scholarship has been done on health systems and human resources within them, we activists have had to become expert in our own right. PHR's Eric Friedman researched brain drain for a year and in 2004 published a report that took on the various factors contributing to outmigration of health professionals and provided policy recommendations for addressing each of them. When health systems campaigners were asked by Bush Administration officials what such inputs would cost, PHR's Friedman and Joint Learning Initiative experts scoured available estimates of everything from training to salary increases to safe workplace supplies and equipment, and proposed cost estimates for every major investment required to stem the brain drain of health professionals. Friedman estimated that the total cost from all spigots (including both national governments and international donors) to develop and retain the health workers needed for the minimum desirable density was approximately \$2–7 billion over five years. Developing and publicizing the funding needed to achieve a tangible goal helped drive advocacy. It allowed activists to make a specific request for increased funding and to measure governments' and donors' progress toward that goal.

Harm Reduction versus Risk Avoidance

At the heart of the health and human rights movement is the vision of a better life for the poor, the abused, and the marginalized. As we have seen, the right to treatment movement, which included the secular Left, the religious Right, and the medical and health community, made a moral issue out of access for the poor to antiretroviral therapy. The growing consensus among the American public was reflected in nearly unanimous majorities in the House and Senate in support of the president's emergency AIDS program. That "big tent" consensus has made possible significant contributions to the GFATM and sustained unprecedented levels of bilateral assistance for health in Africa.

Although treatment for HIV/AIDS appears to be warmly supported across the political spectrum in Congress, tensions over what the United States should fund in the way of HIV prevention continually fray the political consensus needed to sustain high levels of foreign aid in the future. The most serious disputes have been clustered in three areas: AIDS prevention among intravenous drug users; the relative importance of abstinence, faithfulness, and condoms in generalized epidemics; and AIDS prevention among sex workers.

A thread that runs through all three is the issue of risk avoidance versus risk reduction and disagreement over what constitutes appropriate services for individuals in high-risk situations. The competing camps largely are secular AIDS activists and public health professionals on the one hand, and religious conservatives in Congress, the executive branch, and the public, on the other.

One can see the differences in perspective in the way that policy makers view certain HIV prevention measures for injection drug users. The medical literature and experience of health practitioners working with intravenous drug users is virtually unanimous as to the benefits of needle exchange as a means of preventing AIDS transmission between drug users and their partners. But U.S. law prohibits federal funds from being used for needle exchange programs domestically or abroad. Accordingly, states, cities, and philanthropies fund clean needle exchange programs, along with other services for addicts, and no fewer than seventeen federally funded studies have found the programs to be successful in reducing the risk of HIV transmission in the United States.

Many religious conservatives in Congress and the White House are fiercely opposed to harm-reduction initiatives and have brought enormous pressure to bear on the Office of the Global AIDS Coordinator on the issue. A subcommittee in Congress has commenced an investigation of the U.S. Agency for International Development (USAID). Subcommittee Chairman Mark Souder is opposed to funding programs that include needle exchange that is funded by others. He has demanded tens of thousands of USAID emails and documents for inspection. And his counterparts in the Senate favor limiting U.S. contributions to the Global Fund to Fight AIDS, Tuberculosis and Malaria because it funds needle exchange.

The reasons for far-right opposition include a fear (not borne out in the medical literature) that reducing risk will encourage individuals to inject drugs, and a conviction that harm reduction is just a short step toward drug legalization. Other religious conservatives are opposed to needle exchange because they believe it may make drug use less dangerous in terms of HIV but it in no way meets the needs of drug users, who require drug treatment, counseling, health care, and shelter. They view needle exchange as simply writing off sick people and leaving them to kill themselves, if not others.

Virtually all health professionals, human rights activists, and family members who support injection drug users would agree with the view that needle exchange is not the only service drug addicts require. But HIV infection is so prevalent among needle-sharing users that without access to clean needles the issue of drug treatment and counseling is largely irrelevant. As one activist who funds harm-reduction programs in Eastern Europe put it to me, "We're trying to keep them alive long enough to get into treatment—though there's none available here."

Congressional hostility to needle exchange is not yet a front-burner issue for most U.S.-based treatment access campaigners because their work has largely been focused on Africa, where injection drug use plays a minimal role in AIDS transmission. But in the "next wave" countries of Eastern Europe and Asia, injection drug use is overwhelmingly the cause of transmission, and the numbers of users and their sexual partners are enormous (Aciejas et al., 2004). If the United States is to play a useful role in confronting the pandemic outside of Africa, the question of needle exchange will be squarely on rights activists' agendas.

No One's Rights May Be Traded Off for Another's

Most public health proponents and secular activists strongly support interventions for individuals in high-risk situations that limit their risk but do not reject the circumstances that produce that risk or advocate life changes to eliminate risk. For example, campaigns to provide condoms to sex workers and their clients are vital HIV prevention strategies. Sex worker empowerment makes it more likely that they will be able to use condoms and enhance the effectiveness of prevention activities within the sex industry. Left-leaning and public health-oriented activists strongly favor such approaches on human rights and public health grounds. The Bush Administration and many religious conservatives in Congress and in the faith community, in contrast, oppose sex work/prostitution per se on moral grounds, and view condom dissemination as risk reduction at best and complicity in gross abuse at worst. Although they do not oppose services to women in the sex industry, they are suspicious of groups that they believe are helping organize or legalize the sex industry.

The 2003 legislation that implemented the president's emergency AIDS plan contains a provision that requires all those receiving funding under the act to affirmatively oppose prostitution and sex trafficking. Groups that work directly with sex workers are particularly upset about the requirement because they view it as stigmatization of women and men who are already marginalized, exploited, and at risk of HIV exposure. Activists working with sex workers feel that distancing themselves from these women's "work" will make it impossible for them to help organize ways to make their lives more bearable within the sex industry. Physicians for Human Rights supports that view and has joined a lawsuit with other health and humanitarian groups to protest the statutory requirement.

Note that conservative members of Congress who wrote the provision are not unsympathetic with the plight of sex workers. Indeed, it is precisely because they view prostitution as inherently exploitive, degrading, and dangerous and they oppose certain measures to reduce harm within it. It is the commercial sex industry that they abhor and the violence and abuse that usually lands women and girls there—a view shared by many feminists around the world, including me.

An important element in the tension between health activists seeking to provide services to sex workers and conservative nongovernmental organizations and policy makers is the issue of sex trafficking. The heart of the Left-Right controversy on HIV prevention in the sex industry is the fact that sexually exploited children and women and girls trafficked into the commercial sex industry through violence, fraud, and debt bondage are in prostitution and often in the same facilities that NGOs are serving. Health promoters and sex worker unionists in brothels and hotels are likely fully aware of children and trafficking victims among them but feel unable to respond to their plight without losing all access to the facilities. Moreover, on the few occasions in which law enforcement officials have intervened to remove children and trafficking victims from brothels in southeast Asia, sex worker organizations and their supporters in the secular AIDS movement in the United States have denounced the interventions because they have created difficulties for willing adults within the same brothels, who lose their employment when brothels are closed or are rounded up and even deported if they are in the country illegally.

Child protection and legal reform organizations, on the other hand, are outraged at the trade-off of children and women in sexual bondage for others in the trade. Given that people of good will tolerate the rape of children and women in no other circumstance, they are frustrated by the ubiquitous hostility from the secular Left toward police rescue of victims and angered at public protest of such interventions.

There appears to be no common ground between sex worker rights and AIDS prevention activists on the one side and antitrafficking, child rescue proponents on the other. Suspicion on the Left of religious activists who are most closely associated with child protection and law enforcement approaches, and suspicions on the Right of health providers who consider prostitution "work" and tolerate the victimization of women and children, has made even rational discourse virtually impossible.

Tensions over the issue of AIDS services in the sex industry are growing, and it is vitally important to resolve them in ways that advance the human rights and health of both groups within the commercial sex industry. Women, girls, and children in the commercial sex industry need rights protection, law enforcement, health care, AIDS prevention, and liberty, and they need it now. Barriers to leaving the sex industry are high, and for many women there are few if any alternatives to selling sex. At the same time, child prostitution and trafficking are not inevitable and can be vastly reduced if competent law enforcement is extended and protection of their rights made a priority.

The health and AIDS activist community, which has heroically championed prevention and empowerment for sex workers, has been largely missing in action when it comes to the appalling issue of children and trafficking victims in prostitution. While the restrictive legislation makes it less likely that they will take up their cause, which is largely the purview of the religious Right, it is vital that they do so. It is also vital that antitrafficking and child protection proponents squarely address the trade-offs implicit in rescue, and with national governments and donors, develop and promote protocols for rescue and rehabilitation that do not bring harm to others.

Conclusion

The worst health disaster in history, the HIV/AIDS pandemic, requires all of us to go back to school and find new tools and strategies and alliances. At the same time, we can use tactics such as documentation, shaming, and accountability that have served the civil and political rights movement so well.

Religious and secular American activists from both ends of the political spectrum have, without cooperation or intentionality, played an inestimable role in the U.S. leadership role on the international AIDS pandemic. That victory was precious, but the political consensus that produced it is fragile. It is incumbent on health and human rights activists to continue to find and expand the consensus needed to confront the pandemic until it has been stopped.

References

Aceijas, C., Stimson, G. V., Hickman, M., and Rhodes, T. United Nations Reference Group on HIV/AIDS Prevention and Care among IDU in Developing and Transitional Countries. 2004. Global overview of injecting drug use and HIV infection among injecting drug users. *AIDS* 18 (17):2295–303.

Joint United Nations Programme on HIV/AIDS (UNAIDS). AIDS Epidemic Update, December 2001. Available at: www.unaids.org/wac/2001/wad01/Epiupdate2001_en.pdf (accessed January 4, 2006). UNAIDS has since revised several earlier estimates of infections downward, including estimating the number of overall infections in 2001 to be 34.9 million.

Joint United Nations Programme on HIV/AIDS (UNAIDS). *2004 Report on the Global AIDS Epidemic* 2004. Available at: www.unaids.org/bangkok2004/GAR2004 _html/GAR2004_00_en.htm (accessed January 4, 2006).

Marseille, E., Hoffman, P. B., and Kahn, J. G. 2002. HIV prevention before HAART in sub-Saharan Africa. *The Lancet* 359:1851–56.

U.S. National Institutes of Health, National Institute for Allergy and Infectious Disease, NIAID Fact Sheet: HIV/AIDS Statistics (July 1998). Available at: www.aegis .com/factshts/niaid/1998/niaid98_fact_sheet_aidsstat.htm (accessed January 4, 2006).

Index